Challenging Cases in Allergic and Immunologic Diseases of the Skin

Massoud Mahmoudi
Editor

Challenging Cases in Allergic and Immunologic Diseases of the Skin

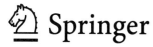

Editor
Massoud Mahmoudi
Chair, Continuing Medical Education,
El Camino Hospital,
Los Gatos, Los Gatos,
CA, USA

Assistant Clinical Professor,
Department of Medicine,
University of California,
San Francisco, San Francisco
CA, USA

Adjunct Associate Professor
Department of Medicine,
School of Osteopathic Medicine,
University of Medicine and
Dentistry of New Jersey, Stratford,
NJ, USA

Adjunct Associate Professor
Department of Medicine,
San Francisco College of Osteopathic Medicine,
Touro University, Vallejo, CA, USA
allergycure@sbc.global.net

ISBN 978-1-60761-295-7   e-ISBN 978-1-60761-296-4
DOI 10.1007/978-1-60761-296-4
Springer New York Dordrecht Heidelberg London

Library of Congress Control Number: 2010936295

© Springer Science+Business Media, LLC 2010
All rights reserved. This work may not be translated or copied in whole or in part without the written permission of the publisher (Springer Science+Business Media, LLC, 233 Spring Street, New York, NY 10013, USA), except for brief excerpts in connection with reviews or scholarly analysis. Use in connection with any form of information storage and retrieval, electronic adaptation, computer software, or by similar or dissimilar methodology now known or hereafter developed is forbidden.
The use in this publication of trade names, trademarks, service marks, and similar terms, even if they are not identified as such, is not to be taken as an expression of opinion as to whether or not they are subject to proprietary rights.
While the advice and information in this book are believed to be true and accurate at the date of going to press, neither the authors nor the editors nor the publisher can accept any legal responsibility for any errors or omissions that may be made. The publisher makes no warranty, express or implied, with respect to the material contained herein.

Printed on acid-free paper

Springer is part of Springer Science+Business Media (www.springer.com)

To the memory of my father, Mohammad H. Mahmoudi, and to my mother, Zohreh, my wife, Lily, and my son, Sam, for their continuous support and encouragement.

Preface

I am happy to present to you the Challenging Cases in Allergic and Immunologic Diseases of the skin. This book like our preceding title, Challenging cases in Allergy and Immunology, is a collection of interesting and challenging cases affecting thousands of people who suffer from allergic and immunologic skin diseases. A wide range of subjects from simple skin allergy to complex autoimmune diseases of the skin are discussed and presented in an easy-to-follow format.

This book consists of five parts and 20 chapters, and each chapter presents two cases. What makes this book unique is the style of its presentation. Each case starts with a short abstract, followed by case presentation, working diagnosis, data, final diagnosis, and discussion. For the purpose of clarification, most chapters have included several colorful photos for better illustration of the case and discussion. To further stimulate the readers' thought process, we have prepared five multiple choice questions per case with answer keys. Although most questions are short, a few are in case presentation format.

This book is intended to target clinicians, educators, fellows, residents, medical students, nurses, and allied health providers who are involved in learning or educating in the areas of allergy, immunology, or dermatology.

This collection is an effort of a distinguished group of clinicians, researchers, and educators. A combined work and contribution of allergists, dermatologists, and rheumatologists have made this title a multispecialty reference book.

I would like to extend my gratitude to all contributors, especially Professor Howard Maibach and his team who contributed four chapters on allergic contact dermatitis and one on contact urticaria syndrome, and my mentor professor Lloyd Cleaver and his team who contributed three chapters on urticaria, atopic dermatitis, and psoriasis.

Finally, I am indebted to Humana and Springer for leading the role in allergy and immunology education evidenced by hundreds of titles in this area, and Richard Lansing, the executive editor, who initially accepted my proposal and guided me during the preparation of the previous and the present title. I also would like to thank Amanda Quinn for editorial assistance and the entire editorial and production team at Humana/Springer.

I hope you find this collection and the previous title *"Challenging Case in Allergy and Immunology"* useful resources and use them to guide your trainee. I am looking forward to hear your comments, and I will be happy to address them in the future edition of this book. I can be reached at allergycure@sbcglobal.net.

Los Gatos CA   Massoud Mahmoudi

Contents

Part I Urticaria and Angioedema 1

1. **Urticaria** 3
   Lloyd J. Cleaver and Jonathan L. Cleaver

2. **Cold Urticaria** 25
   Grace Peace Yu, Alan A. Wanderer, and Massoud Mahmoudi

3. **Contact Urticaria Syndrome** 45
   Zack Thompson and Howard I. Maibach

4. **Idiopathic Angioedema** 59
   Cristina J. Ramos-Romey and Timothy J. Craig

5. **Hereditary Angioedema** 73
   Michael J. Prematta and Timothy Craig

Part II Skin Manifestation of Drug Allergy 89

6. **Stevens–Johnson Syndrome/Toxic Epidermal Necrolysis** 91
   Satoshi Yoshida

7. **Serum Sickness and Serum Sickness-Like Reaction** 111
   Neha Reshamwala and Massoud Mahmoudi

Part III Allergic Contact Dermatitis 125

8. **Preservatives** 127
   Sara Flores and Howard Maibach

9. **Allergic Contact Dermatitis: Rubber Allergies** 141
   Peter Burke and Howard I. Maibach

10	**Jewelry: Nickel and Metal-Based Allergic Contact Dermatitis**............	153
	Peter Burke and Howard I. Maibach	
11	**Allergic Contact Dermatitis to Fragrances**..	169
	Sarah J. Gilpin and Howard I. Maibach	

Part IV Other Allergies Affecting Skin and Mucous Membranes 181

12	**Atopic Dermatitis**..	183
	Albert E. Rivera and Lloyd J. Cleaver	
13	**Allergic Reactions Affecting Mucosal Surfaces**	201
	J. Wesley Sublett and Jonathan A. Bernstein	

Part V Immunologic Diseases of the Skin... 215

14	**Vasculitis**	217
	Satoshi Yoshida	
15	**Cutaneous Mastocytosis**	237
	Jason R. Catanzaro and Haig Tcheurekdjian	
16	**Cutaneous Lupus**	251
	Lisa G. Criscione-Schreiber	
17	**Psoriasis**	267
	Lloyd Cleaver, Nathan Cleaver, and Katherine Johnson	
18	**Scleroderma**...	287
	Elena Schiopu and James R. Seibold	
19	**Autoimmune Blistering Diseases of the Skin and Mucous Membranes**	303
	Timothy Patton and Neil J. Korman	
20	**Alopecia Areata**..	323
	Luciano J. Iorizzo III and Mary Gail Mercurio	

Index 339

Contributors

Jonathan A. Bernstein, M.D. FAAAAI, FACAAI
Division of Immunology/Allergy Section, Department
of Internal Medicine, University of Cincinnati College of Medicine,
231 Albert Sabin Way, ML#563, Cincinnati, OH 45267-0563, USA

Peter Burke, D.O.
Philadelphia College of Osteopathic Medicine, Philadelphia, PA 19131, USA and
University of California San Francisco, San Francisco, CA 94143-0989, USA

Jason R. Catanzaro, M.D.
Departments of Medicine and Pediatrics, University Hospitals Case Medical
Center/Rainbow Babies and Children's Hospital, Case Western Reserve
University, Cleveland, OH, USA

Jonathan L. Cleaver
Kirksville College of Osteopathic Medicine, A.T. Still University, Kirksville,
MO, USA

Lloyd J. Cleaver, D.O., FACOD
Department of Dermatology, A.T. Still University/Northeast Regional Medical
Center, 700 W. Jefferson Street, Kirksville, MO 63501, USA

Nathan Cleaver
Kirksville College of Osteopathic Medicine, A.T. Still University, Kirksville,
MO, USA

Timothy J. Craig, D.O.
Section of Allergy and Immunology, Penn State Milton
S. Hershey College of Medicine, Penn State University, Hershey, PA, USA

Lisa G. Criscione-Schreiber, M.D.
Division of Rheumatology and Immunology, Duke University, Box 3490 DUMC,
Room 4021 Duke South, Purple Zone, Durham, NC 27710, USA

Sara Flores
Department of Dermatology, School of Medicine, University of California, San Francisco, San Francisco, CA, USA

Sarah J. Gilpin, M.P.H.
University of Minnesota, 4000 Pheasant Ridge Dr, Blaine, MN 55449, USA

Luciano J. Iorizzo III, M.D.
Department of Dermatology, University of Rochester, Rochester, NY, USA

Katherine Johnson
Kirksville College of Osteopathic Medicine, A.T. Still University, Kirksville, MO, USA

Neil J. Korman, M.D., Ph.D.
Professor, Department of Dermatology, University Hospitals Case Medical Center, Cleveland, OH, USA

Massoud Mahmoudi, D.O., Ph.D., M.S., RM (NRM), FASCMS, FACOI, FAOCAI, FACP, FCCP, FAAAAI
Chair, Continuing Medical Education, E1 Camino Hospital, Los Gatos, Los Gatos, CA, USA;
Assistant Clinical Professor, Department of Medicine, University of California, San Francisco, San Francisco, CA, USA;
Adjunct Associate Professor, Department of Medicine, School of Osteopathic Medicine, University of Medicine and Dentistry of New Jersey, Stratford, NJ, USA;
Adjunct Associate Professor, Department of Medicine, San Francisco College of Osteopathic Medicine, Touro University, Vallejo, CA, USA

Howard I. Maibach, M.D.
Professor, Department of Dermatology, School of Medicine, University of California, San Francisco, San Francisco, CA, USA

Mary Gail Mercurio, M.D.
Associate Professor, Department of Dermatology, University of Rochester, Rochester, NY, USA

Timothy Patton D.O.
Assistant Professor, Department of Dermatology, University of Pittsburg, Pittsburg, PA, USA

Michael J.Prematta
Penn State Milton S. Hershey College of Medicine, Section of Allergy and Immunology, Penn State University, Hershey, PA, USA

Contributors

Cristina J. Ramos-Romey, M.D.
Section of Allergy and Immunology Penn State Milton S. Hershey College of Medicine, Penn State University, Hershey, PA, USA

Neha Reshamwala, M.D.
Division of Allergy and Immunology, Department of Pediatrics, School of Medicine, Stanford University, Stanford, CA, USA

Albert E. Rivera, D.O.
Northeast Regional Medical Center, 700 West Jefferson Street, Kirksville 63501, MO, USA

Elena Schiopu, M.D.
Division of Rheumatology, University of Michigan, 24 Frank Lloyd Wright Drive, Lobby M, Suite 2500, PO Box 481, Ann Arbor, MI 48106, USA

James R. Seibold, M.D.
Professor and Chief Division of Rheumatology, University of Connecticut Health Center, Farmington, CT, USA

J. Wesley Sublett, M.D., MPH
Division of Immunology/Allergy Section, Department of Internal Medicine, University of Cincinnati College of Medicine, Cincinnati, OH, USA

Haig Tcheurekdjian, M.D.
Assistant Clinical Professor, Allergy/Immunology Associates, Inc, Cleveland, OH, USA and Departments of Medicine and Pediatrics, Case Western Reserve University, Cleveland, OH, USA

Zack Thompson
University of California San Francisco, 2901 Cityplace West Blvd., Apt. 442, Dallas, TX 75204-0360, USA

Grace Peace Yu, M.D., M.Sc.
Stanford University School of Medicine, Department of Pediatrics, Division of Allergy and Immunology, Stanford, CA, USA

Satoshi Yoshida, M.D., Ph.D., FAAAAI, FACAAI
Department of Allergy and Immunology, Johns Hopkins Medicine International, Tokyo Midtown Medical Center, Tokyo, Japan

Alan A. Wanderer, M.D.
Clinical Professor of Pediatrics, Allergy, and Clinical Immunology, University of Colorado, Denver, CO, USA

Part I
Urticaria and Angioedema

Chapter 1
Urticaria

Lloyd J. Cleaver and Jonathan L. Cleaver

Abstract Urticaria is a common problem that can be a challenge not only for the patient, but also for a physician. Urticaria is classified based on clinical presentation and stimulus. The correct identification of the urticaria subtype is crucial for the management and treatment of the patient. A thorough history and physical examination are imperative in working up this diagnostic conundrum.

Keywords Acute urticaria • Chronic urticaria • Physical urticaria • Cholinergic urticaria • Angioedema • Urticaria and angioedema diagnosis and treatment

Case 1

The patient is a 68-year-old white female who was referred for a new evolving rash for 1 week. The patient initially developed red, dime to nickel sized "itchy bumps" on her back. This rash continued to progress over the next week and eventually involved her bilateral arms, legs, back, abdomen, and face. She complained of an intense itch as well as some associated pain at the lesions that was keeping her awake at night. She had received intramuscular injections of triamcinolone. She stated that this has slowed the formation of new lesions, relieved the tightness in her throat and chest, but there was still an intense itch present. The patient denied any other systemic symptoms present since the start of her "rash." The patient was on multiple medicines, including pramipexole, medroxyprogesterone, propranolol, atorvastatin, gabapentin, fenofibrate, aspirin, amlodipine, vitamin B1, vitamin B12, and a multivitamin. The patient had recently been switched from omeprazole to ranitidine approximately 3–4 days before the first lesion appeared. She has a significant past

L.J. Cleaver (✉)
Department of Dermatology, A.T. Still University/Northeast Regional Medical Center,
700 W. Jefferson Street, Kirksville, MO 63501, USA
e-mail: LCleaver@atsu.edu

M. Mahmoudi (ed.), *Challenging Cases in Allergic and Immunologic Diseases of the Skin*,
DOI 10.1007/978-1-60761-296-4_1, © Springer Science+Business Media, LLC 2010

medical history of squamous cell carcinoma with metastasis to the neck with the treatment of chemotherapy and radiation, chronic bronchitis, hypertension, myocardial infarction, chronic kidney disease, and frequent bladder infections.

Upon physical examination, the patient demonstrated multiple erythematous, wheal-based, annular to serpiginous, targetoid lesions. The lesions were present on the bilateral legs, arms, back, abdomen, and minimal involvement of the face (Figs. 1.1– 1.3). No involvement was noted of the mucosal membranes and the patient had no adenopathy present of the cervical, axillary, inguinal, or supraclavicular nodes.

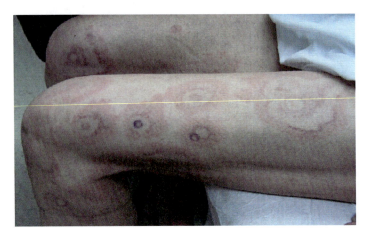

Fig. 1.1 Targetoid, erythematous to violaceous, edematous lesions with central clearing and whealing on the periphery

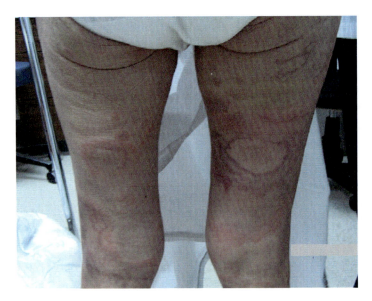

Fig. 1.2 Targetoid, erythematous to violaceous, edematous lesions with central clearing and whealing on the periphery

1 Urticaria

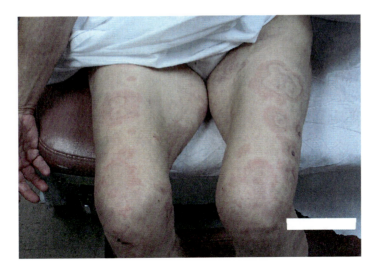

Fig. 1.3 Targetoid, erythematous to violaceous, edematous lesions with central clearing and whealing on the periphery

With the Presented Data What Is Your Working Diagnosis?

The clinical presentation of extremely pruritic targetoid urticaria-like lesions that respond to previously given IM steroids most likely suggests some type of urticaria. The tenderness of some of the lesions, the systemic involvement, and the tightness in the throat and chest suggest possibly a vasculitic component. Urticarial vasculitis was favored.

Differential Diagnosis

Acute urticaria, erythema multiforme, urticaria vasculitis, drug eruption, Sweet's syndrome, neutrophilic vasculitis.

Workup

1. A detailed history is imperative in gathering more information once any type of urticaria is suspected. The authors have an urticaria sheet that all patients fill out. This patient had started ranitidine approximately 5–7 days prior to the development of the first lesion.
2. A punch biopsy was performed at the center of an active lesion and another at the periphery. The punch biopsy demonstrated a small vessel vasculitis with endothelial swelling and purpura. There was mild focal fibrin deposition, angiocentric inflammatory infiltrate consisting predominantly of neutrophils, and leukocytoclasis.

3. Serum complement levels (CH50, C3, C4, and anti-C1q) were all within normal levels. Antinuclear antibody (ANA) was negative, and urinary analysis demonstrated moderate amounts of protein. Complete blood count (CBC) and complete metabolic panel (CMP) were unremarkable.

What Is Your Diagnosis and Why?

The diagnosis is urticarial vasculitis secondary to the use of ranitidine. The acute onset of her urticarial breakout after the new use of ranitidine is a large clue to the diagnosis. The punch biopsy is fairly specific for a leukocytoclastic vasculitis consistent with urticarial vasculitis. Urticarial vasculitis has a propensity for eosinophils over other types of vasculitis. Sweet'ssyndrome demonstrates a more intense dermal infiltrate with marked upper dermal edema. The syndrome typically possesses karyorrhexis and lacks vessel wall necrosis, fibrin, and vasocentric neutrophils, which are features of urticarial vasculitis. The punch biopsy along with clinical features is the standard for diagnosing urticarial vasculitis, but it does not help determine the etiology. Acute urticaria does not demonstrate vasculitic changes.

Management and Follow-Up

The patient was instructed to stop the ranitidine immediately. She was prescribed fexofenadine 180 mg to take daily, hydroxyzine 25 mg at night, and fluocinonide 0.05% cream to apply to the red itchy areas twice a day. The patient was also given pramoxine hydrochloride 1% to apply throughout the day. The lesions completely cleared within 1 week and the proteinuria cleared within 4 weeks. The patient was later rechallenged with the ranitidine and had an acute urticarial dermatitis. Since avoiding ranitidine, the patient has been symptom free.

Questions

1. The proper management of urticarial vasculitis includes which of the following?
    (a) Topical corticosteroids are usually not necessary as adjunctive therapy for symptomatic relief.
    (b) Undergo immediate radioallergosorbent testing (RAST).
    (c) Potent antihistamines.
    (d) Long-term oral steroids.

2. How can urticarial vasculitis be differentiated from chronic urticaria?

    (a) Lesions that persist greater than 24 h.
    (b) Location of lesions – truncal distribution.
    (c) The severity of pruritus.
    (d) Triggering stimulus.

3. Which of the following statements is true?

    (a) Urticarial vasculitis may present with both chronic urticaria and angioedema.
    (b) The diagnosis of urticarial vasculitis can be made without histological confirmation.
    (c) Urticarial vasculitis typically occurs in elderly males.
    (d) Urticarial vaculitis lesions are typically asymptomatic.

4. Which of the following is not a known association with urticarial vasculitis?

    (a) Hepatitis.
    (b) Medications.
    (c) Systemic Lupus erythematosus.
    (d) Congestive heart failure.

5. Which of these treatments would be the most appropriate long-term treatment?

    (a) Use of an immunosuppressant.
    (b) Daily topical steroid use.
    (c) First generation antihistamines.
    (d) Avoidance of trigger.

Answers: 1(c), 2(a), 3(a), 4(d), 5(d)

Case 2

A 28-year-old female presented to the dermatology clinic for a second opinion regarding recurrent "hives." These hives have been troubling the patient on a routine basis for the last 4 years. She has been diagnosed by her doctor as having pressure and heat urticaria. She has had two episodes of hospitalizations for swelling of the lips and difficulty in breathing. She now carries an epinephrine pen with her. She has been treated for these "hives" with hydroxyzine on an as-need basis and fexofenadine 180 mg a day. She stated that this only helps, but does not control her symptoms. Her last big flare occurred postpartum of her third child. She had extensive angioedema and systemic urticaria while she was hospitalized and treated.

The patient's medical history was significant for Wolf–Parkinson–White arrhythmia; three vaginally delivered healthy children, and tubal ligation. RAST was done previously and was only reactive to dust mites. Her biological father had systemic lupus erythematosus. The patient denied use of any alcohol or drugs, but does smoke one pack of cigarettes per day. The review of systems was otherwise unremarkable.

On physical examination, there were few erythematous and blanchable wheals on her right anterior forearm. Her back had a positive dermatographism reaction. The rest of the skin examination was normal. There were no lesions at the pressure areas (Figs. 1.4–1.8).

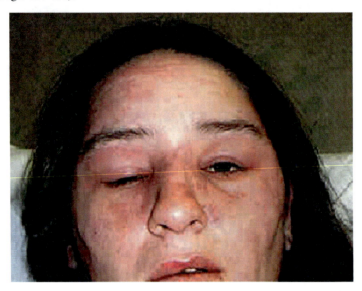

Fig. 1.4 Edematous and erythematous lesions with periorbital edema

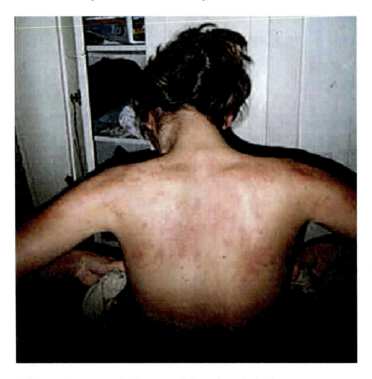

Fig. 1.5 Diffuse erythematous wheals scattered throughout the back

1 Urticaria

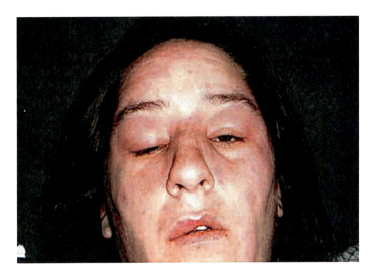

Fig. 1.6 Edematous and erythematous lesions with periorbital edema

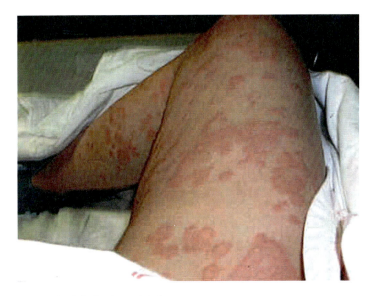

Fig. 1.7 Large urticarial wheals on right leg

With the Presented Data What Is Your Working Diagnosis

The working diagnosis was chronic urticaria and angioedema. This is because the patient has had the lesions over 4 years. There may be multiple types of urticarias occurring in this patient.

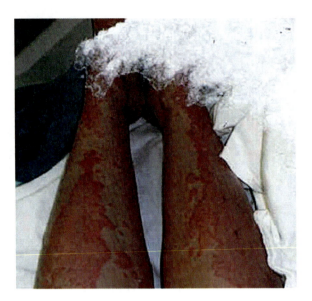

Fig. 1.8 Large urticarial wheals on bilateral lower legs

Differential Diagnosis

Chronic idiopathic urticaria, delayed pressure urticaria, progesterone autoimmune dermatitis, estrogen autoimmune dermatitis.

Workup

1. As discussed earlier, a detailed history is imperative to determine more information about her urticaria. A very thorough history was performed. When asked about birth control, she states that she had received a medroxyprogesterone injection for contraception approximately 4 years ago just prior to when these wheals developed. She believes that her hives are worse during her menstrual period and seem to almost completely subside after her menses. This also improved while she was pregnant, but had a severe flare after delivery.
2. CBC and CMP were normal. Hepatitis C was negative and ANA was 1:160. The remainder of the ANA profile was negative. Thyroid studies were normal. C3 was slightly low, but the rest of the complement profile was normal. RAST was only reactive to dust mites.
3. Intradermal testing with 0.01 mL of aqueous progesterone suspension (50 mg/mL) yielded a positive test within 30 min.

1 Urticaria

What Is Your Diagnosis and Why?

The diagnosis is autoimmune progesterone dermatitis. The intradermal testing with aqueous progesterone as well as the clinical history is indicative of autoimmune progesterone dermatitis. The fact that this developed after medroxyprogesterone injection, got better with pregnancy, worse after delivery, and flares during the luteal phase of menses also helped us to come up with our final diagnosis.

Management and Follow-Up

Autoimmune progesterone dermatitis is autoimmunity against the patient's own progesterone mediated by TH-1 cytokines. Patients respond to anovulatory agents or oophorectomy. The patient was given the options of treatment and elected to be treated with oral contraceptive pills (OCP). She is doing well on an OCP, and has only had an occasional wheal with no flares. No episodes of angioedema have occurred in 2 years of being on OCPs.

Questions

1. Which of the following statements are true?

    (a) Roughly half of patients with urticaria have an associated angioedema.
    (b) Angioedema cannot occur without urticarial lesions.
    (c) Angioedema is often an effect of beta-blockers.
    (d) Angioedema related to food usually occurs without wheals.

2. Which sentence is incorrect?

    (a) Chronic urticaria is defined as lesions lasting longer than 6 weeks.
    (b) Angioedema may have a hereditary link.
    (c) Acute urticaria most often occurs in children.
    (d) Degranulation of mast cells occurs only in type I and type II hypersensitivity reactions.

3. Symptomatic dermatographism is _____.

    (a) Usually caused by bugs or drugs.
    (b) The most common type of physical urticaria.
    (c) A linear wheal that typically lasts less than 30–60 s.
    (d) Mucosal surfaces are typically involved.

4. The main precipitator of itch in urticaria is _____.

   (a) Prostaglandins.
   (b) Cytokines.
   (c) Histamine.
   (d) Heparin.

5. Cholinergic urticaria could be triggered by all of the following except _____.

   (a) Sitting in the sauna at the health spa.
   (b) Moderate exercise.
   (c) Applying a heat pack to a sore shoulder.
   (d) A recent divorce from a spouse.

Answers: 1(a), 2(d), 3(b), 4(c), 5(c)

Discussion

Definition

Urticaria, also known as hives or the nettle rash, classically is defined as the whealing of the skin. Today, the word urticaria is used in a broader sense. It may refer to the wheal, angioedema, or both. The wheal is defined as localized vasodilatation of the superficial dermis. This vasodilatation creates increased vascular permeability, blood flow, redness, and swelling. Itch will then ensue secondary to this phenomenon. Angioedema is similar to a wheal except that it is a more expansive process. The vasodilatation is greater and occurs deeper into the dermis, extending into the subcutaneous tissues.

Over time urticaria has been divided into two main groups, chronic and acute "ordinary" urticaria and physical urticarias. Acute "ordinary" urticaria is defined as lesions that last less than 6 weeks and occur at random without any local physical trigger. It becomes chronic if these lesions prevail for 6 weeks or greater. Physical urticaria is defined as wheals and or angioedema that result as a response to external physical stimuli (1).

Brief History

Urticaria has been described since the times of Hippocrates. It developed its current name around the eighteenth century. It was named after the skin reaction that ensued after contact with the stinging nettle (*Urtica dioica*) (1).

Prevalence of Urticaria

Urticaria affects the lives of many people globally. Urticaria is part of the 20 most common skin diseases. It is a skin disease that affects anywhere from 1 to 20% of the world's population (2). These rates vary widely based upon different published literature. The most frequent types of urticarias are the acute form. The acute urticaria typically lasts for a few days to a few weeks and then resolve. Approximately 50% of patients with urticaria have an associated angioedema, 40% do not, and 10% have just angioedema (2).

Acute urticaria is more often seen in children and has been estimated that up to 20% of children are affected before adolescents (2). Children under ages of 6 months are rarely affected by angioedema and urticaria, but cases have been reported in newborns. Chronic urticaria is more notably prevalent in middle-aged female adults with a ratio of 2:1 (2, 3).

Pathophysiology

Simply put, urticaria results from the release of vasoactive substances such as histamine, bradykinin, leukotrienes (LT) C_4, D_4, or E_4, and prostaglandin (PG) D_2 from mast cells and basophils. These substances cause vasodilatation with subsequent extravasation of fluid into the dermis forming an urticarial lesion. The release of histamine is what drives the intense itch that is present with urticarial lesions.

Urticarial lesions have several different etiologies. They can be broken down into three major categories: idiopathic, immunologic, and nonimmunologic. Immunologic can be subdivided into autoimmune, IgE-dependent, immune complex, and complement- and kinin-dependent. Nonimmunologic is broken down into direct mast cell-releasing agents, vasoactive stimuli, aspirin/nonsteroidal antiinflammatory drug (NSAID), and angiotensin-converting enzyme (ACE) inhibitors (3, 4).

The driving force behind the majority of urticarial reactions is the improper activation of the mast cell. There are other important players in the pathogenesis of urticaria but none play a role as large as the mast cell. Situations may arise where an urticarial reaction occurs mast cell independently. These are due to C1 inhibitor deficiency, angiotension-converting enzyme inhibitor-induced urticaria, or prostaglandin nonimmunologic contact urticaria (3).

Mast cells are located throughout the body but differ in reaction to stimuli based on their location. They are the chief cell to initiate type I hypersensitivity reactions. Mast cells can activate and release different mediators, such as histamine, by both IgE-dependent and IgE-independent stimuli. Dermal mast cells are located throughout the dermis but have preference for appendages such as pilosebaceous follicles, nerve fibers, and blood vessels (3, 4). Mast cells are classified into two major types based on protease content. The first are those with the neutral proteases tryptase and chymase (MC_{TC}), and the second are those with only tryptase (MC_T). MC_{TC} make up the majority of skin and intestinal submucosa mast cells. MC_T predominates in bowel mucosa, alveolar wall, and nasal mucosa (3).

Degranulation of mast cells can be caused by several different mechanisms. It can be triggered by type I, type II, or type III hypersensitivity reactions. The urticarial reaction can also occur through complement-mediated reaction, non-IgE-mediated mechanism, physical stimuli, and idiopathically. Degranulation ensues when two or more high affinity IgE receptors (FcεR1) crosslink on the mast cell, physical stimuli induce a neoantigen which stimulates IgE antibody production, or stimulation of cholinergic sympathetic innovation of sweat gland (4). In type I hypersensitivity reactions, crosslinking of receptor-bound IgE by a specific antigen triggers degranulation. Various other immunologic stimuli work through the IgE receptor to cause granulation. For example, in autoimmune urticaria, activation occurs with IgG antihigh affinity IgE receptor (FcεR1) (4). Other nonimmunologic stimuli can cause degranulation of mast cells by binding to specific receptors. Substances such as opiates, C5a anaphylatoxin, stem cell factor, and substance P are all capable of degranulation (1, 3).

The mast cell degranulation activation stimulus may differ, but the resulting degranulation reaction is essentially identical. Proinflammatory mediators are released by the mast cell upon degranulation. These mediators include cytokines (IL-3, -4, -5, -6, -8, -13, GM-CSF, TNF-α), proteases (chymase, tryptase, and granzyme B), eicosanoids (prostaglandins D2, leukotriene C4, D4, E4), histamine, heparin, and platelet-activating factor (1, 3, 4). Upon release of these substances, binding occurs on the postcapillary venules. A subsequent vasodilatation and increased vascular permeability develops. Inflammatory cells migrate to the urticarial lesions secondary to the release of histamine, TNF-α, and IL-8 release from the mast cell.

Histamine is not only largely in charge of the vascular changes that occur during urticaria, but is also the major precipitator of the itch. Activation of histamine receptors (H1, H3, and H4) triggers a local pruritic response which generally lacks a central component (4).

Clinical Manifestations

Urticaria can be classified in different ways. Probably, the most prevalent method is based upon the clinical characteristics. Urticaria is divided into six groups: ordinary urticaria, physical urticaria, contact urticaria, angioedema without wheals, urticarial vasculitis, and urticarial syndromes.

Ordinary Urticaria

"Ordinary urticaria" can be further subdivided into acute and chronic urticaria. All urticarial reactions develop as acute lesions, but if they persist 6 weeks or greater they become labeled as chronic. Spontaneous wheals develop daily or close to daily, last 2–24 h, and then fade. There is a predilection for developing the lesions at night, but they may occur at anytime throughout the day (5). Angioedema may also be present and often occurs with an acute urticarial episode (1). If systemic symptoms are present, a suspicion for urticarial vasculitis or an urticarial syndrome should be contemplated (1, 3).

An association between chronic urticaria and *Helicobacter pylori* has been made. Treatment of *H. pylori* seems to improve the urticaria (1, 3, 4). Parasitic infections, where endemic, can be a cause of urticaria.

Physical Urticaria

Physical urticarias are classified based on the evoking stimulus (2–4). The different categories include: mechanical trauma, temperature change, exercise-induced, adrenergic, solar, and aquagenic. The majority of physical urticarias develops within minutes of the stimulus and subsides within 2 h (1). The wheals are typically located at the stimulated area, but a systemic effect may occur. This is seen more often in cholinergic urticaria (CU), food-induced, and exercise-induced urticaria.

Urticaria due to Mechanical Stimuli

Dermographism

Dermographism refers to "skin writing." Dermographism can be divided into simple and symptomatic. Simple occurs in approximately 5% of the population from firm stroking of the skin with subsequent erythema and a wheal (3). Symptomatic dermographism is the most common physical urticaria (1). Whealing and erythema develops at the site of friction. These wheals are often linear and subside within approximately 30–60 min. Mucosal surfaces are not involved. Most cases of dermographism are idiopathic but have been known to be caused by different factors such as drugs and bugs (3). Dermographism can last months to years. Other forms of dermographism, such as delayed dermographism, red dermographism, localized dermographism, white dermographism, and cholinergic dermographism, exist.

Immediate Pressure Urticaria

Immediate pressure urticaria is wheals that develop within minutes of a perpendicular pressure stimulus applied to the skin (6). Wheals develop within minutes of driving, sitting in a chair, or another direct pressure stimulus.

Delayed Pressure Urticaria

Delayed pressure urticaria (DPU) is a distressing disorder. It is often difficult to treat and can interfere with every-day activities. DPU has deep erythematous swellings that develop at sites of sustained pressure on the skin, after a delay of at least 30 min. DPU typically occurs in conjunction with chronic ordinary urticaria. The lesions are typically painful, pruritic, and persistent. They may last for days. Systemic manifestations, such as malaise, arthralgias, myalgias, and even leukocytosis, are sometimes present (7).

Vibratory Angioedema

Vibratory angioedema can occur in two forms: autosomal dominant form and an acquired form (6). Vibratory angioedema is a rare type of urticaria that develops after a vibratory stimulus triggers localized swelling and erythema. This typically develops within minutes of any vibratory stimulus and last a few hours or less.

Temperature Change Urticaria

Heat Urticaria

Heat urticaria is subdivided into CU and localized heat contact urticaria.

CU presents with small 1–3 mm wheals that may coalesce to form much larger wheals. CU develops secondary to a cholinergic stimulus such as sweating, an increase in core body temperature, or an emotional stressor. The wheals appear within 15 min of the stimulus and tend to persist for minutes to 2 h (3, 6). CU most frequently occurs in young adults and is distributed symmetrically on the top half of the body with the risk of angioedema (3).

Localized heat contact urticaria is a very rare form of urticaria and occurs when heat is applied to the skin (3). Erythema and whealing ensue within minutes of the contact of the heat source. The whealing occurs only at the site of the heat application whether it is from warm water or radiant heat such as sunshine. The lesions usually last an hour. Systemic symptoms, such as flushing, headache, nausea, wheezing, and syncope, have been reported (6). It is often confused with solar urticaria or CU and must be distinguished from these two entities.

Cold Urticaria

Cold urticaria is characterized by whealing within minutes of cold exposure. Cold urticaria can be from a primary contact, secondary contact, reflex, or familial inherited. Refer to Chap. 2 for more detail.

Exercise-Induced Anaphylaxis

Exercise-Induced Anaphylaxis (EIA) is characterized by anaphylactic symptoms that occur after exercise. The majority of these patients develop EIA after exercise that is preceded with ingestion of a specific food or heavy meal within 4 h of exercise (3). Not all EIA cases are preceded by food ingestion. It is more commonly seen in young adults and has been known to occur in children and is induced by moderate exercise, usually jogging (6). Itching develops which is preceded by urticaria with or without angioedema lasting for minutes to hours (6). Systemic symptoms may follow, including decreased pulmonary function, nausea, vomiting, abdominal pain, and collapse. The most commonly implicated products are food, aspirin/NSAIDS, and alcohol (8).

Solar Urticaria

Pruritus, erythema, and wheals develop within minutes of exposure to ultraviolet (UV) light and last less than 2 h. Typically, it occurs in the UV spectrum of 300–500 nm. Solar urticaria can affect anyone but is favored in young adults. The most commonly affected areas are the upper chest, shoulders, and arms. The face and the dorsal hands are spared due to photohardening. UV radiation through clothing, windows, fluorescent bulb may be significant enough to produce solar urticaria. The amount of exposure is directly linked to the severity of the urticaria. Systemic symptoms, such as headache, flushing, and angioedema, are known to occur (9).

Aquagenic Urticaria

Contact with any temperature of water induces small pruritic wheals usually on the upper half of the body. It most often affects young adults and lasts for less than 1 h. The water carries an epidermal antigen to the mast cell which causes degranulation and the histamine reaction (6).

Contact Urticaria

Contact urticaria is the development of wheals, where an external substance comes into contact with the skin producing a wheal and flare. Most often the reaction is limited to just the area of contact and appears within minutes to hours of contact (9). Contact urticaria can be subgrouped into an IgE–allergen interaction and a nonallergic IgE-independent group. The IgE group is usually caused by exposure to allergens such as grass, latex, food, animals, etc. Atopic children are at highest risk for developing the IgE-dependent type. IgE-dependent can be complicated by anaphylaxis (1).

Angioedema Without Wheals

Angioedma without wheals is most often idiopathic, but may occur with drug reactions or in patients who possess a C1 esterase inhibitor deficiency. NSAIDS, aspirin, and ACE inhibitors are the most common implicated drugs. C1 esterase inhibitor deficiency should be considered if there is significant family history, recurrent larengeal edema, or abdominal pain (3).

Urticarial Vasculitis

Urticarial vasculitis clinically resembles chronic urticaria. The lesions are often indistinguishable. Urticarial vasculitis wheals last greater than 24 h and have an associated burning sensation as well as the itch (10). The lesions are often confused with delayed pressure urticaria as they occur often at pressure point sites. Petechiae and purpura are usually present, but this is thought to occur more secondary to the intense scratching by the patient (1). Histologic examination demonstrates a leukocytoclastic vasculitis. When urticarial vasculitis is present an associated disorder, such as systemic lupus, hypocomplementemic urticarial vasculitis syndrome, hepatitis, Sjögren syndrome, mixed cryoglobulinemia, or hematologic malignant disorder, exists as well (3).

Urticarial Syndromes

Muckle–Wells Syndrome

Muckle–Wells syndrome (MWS) is an autosomal dominant autoinflammatory disorder that is characterized by an urticarial-like eruption with systemic symptoms such as chills, arthralgia, malaise, sensorineural deafness, and amyloidosis (1). Renal failure often develops secondary to the amyloidosis. The classic triad of MWS is rash, deafness, and amyloidosis.

Pruritic Urticarial Papules and Plaques of Pregnancy

Pruritic urticarial papules and plaques of pregnancy (PUPPP) is the most common dermatoses of pregnancy. PUPPP primarily occurs in primiparous women and is thought to be associated with rapid and excessive weight gain during the third trimester of pregnancy. Urticarial papules and plaques develop within the abdominal striae, but are periumbilical sparing. The lesions are usually rapidly self-resolving postpartum (1).

Schnitzler Syndrome

Schnitzler syndrome is a rare chronic nonpruritic urticaria with an IgM gammopathy. An associated recurrent fever, arthralgias, bone pain, and osteosclerosis may occur as well. Lab findings may include an elevated white blood count (WBC) and elevated erythrocyte sedimentation rate (ESR). Skin findings consist of sharply dermarcated, maculopapular erythematous lesions located mainly on the lower extremities and abdomen. The wheals last several hours to 1 week (1).

Autoimmune Progesterone Dermatitis

Autoimmune progesterone dermatitis is an eruption that consists of cyclic episodes of dermatitis that coincide with the luteal phase of the menstrual cycle. Lesions can vary from urticarial lesions to eczematous to an erythema multiforme-like lesions. The lesions are a result of the increase in progesterone levels and typically improve or resolve after menses (11).

Diagnostic Procedures

History-Taking

History-taking is key to the diagnosis of the different forms of urticaria. Studies have demonstrated that a detailed patient history is usually sufficient to diagnose chronic urticaria (1). It is important to first establish whether the patient has an urticarial wheal or a lesion that mimics urticaria. Once this is determined, the lesions must be deemed acute or chronic. If there are daily wheals for more than 6 weeks, it is considered chronic, and less than 6 weeks as acute. The location of the wheals, severity, duration, triggers, environment, occupation, whether angioedema is present, prescription and over-the-counter medications taken, past medical history, and familial history are just some of the questions that must be asked to make a correct diagnosis. Food is often implicated by patients as the cause of their urticaria. While food does cause urticaria, it is not the culprit the majority of the time. Food induces a reaction within minutes to hours of ingestion. Many cases of chronic urticaria are often due to a physical urticaria or a combination of a physical urticaria with ordinary urticaria (12).

Table 1.1 Challenge test for physical/cholinergic urticarias

Physical/cholinergic urticaria	Clinical test	Time read after provocation
Symptomatic dermatographism	Moderate stroking of the skin with a blunt smooth object on upper back or volar arm	10 min
Delayed pressure urticaria	Suspension of weights over shoulder for 15 min (7 kg with a 3 cm strap)	6 h
Heat contact urticaria	Heat source of 45°C on volar forearm for 5 min	10 min
Cold contact urticaria	Melting ice cube in thin plastic bag for 5 min on volar arm or abdomen	10 min
Solar urticaria	UVA 6 J/cm^2 & UVB 60 mJ/cm^2 irradiation on the buttocks	10 min
Aquagenic urticaria	Wetting the skin with water at any temperature	Immediately and at 10 min
Vibratory urticaria/angioedema	Vortex vibrator for 10 min at 1,000 rpm on the volar forearm	10 min
Cholinergic urticaria	Exercise on machine to point of sweating, then continue for 15 min or 42° batch for 15 min after body temperature has increased by >1°C over baseline	Immediately and 10 min after
Autoimmune progesterone dermatitis	Intradermal testing with 0.01 ml of an aqueous suspension (50 mg/ml) of progesterone	30 min, 24 h, 48 h

Table derived from (12, 17).

Laboratory Test

Based on history, laboratory test may be appropriate. An ESR, WBC, TSH, *H. pylori*, C4 levels, skin biopsy, and autologous serum skin test (ASST) should be considered (1). The ASST is helpful in distinguishing chronic autoimmune urticaria from chronic idiopathic urticaria (13). The patient's serum is collected during a flare. It is then injected intradermally into the uninvolved forearm. Controls are injected with saline and histamine at the same time. If the bleb is 1.5 mm greater than the saline bleb, it is considered a positive test for autoimmunity (1). This should be confirmed by in vitro testing as the ASST has a 65–81% sensitivity and a 71–78% specificity (14).

Challenge test may be used to differentiate among the physical urticarias. See Table 1.1 for details.

Treatment

The first step in treating urticaria is to avoid or remove the provoking stimulus. This will prevent flares as well as diminish the need for any pharmacotherapy. The treatment of urticaria can be broken down into first-, second-, and third-line therapies (1, 3).

First-line therapies consist of patient education and nondrug approaches. These therapies include the avoidance of aggravating factors such as alcohol, stress, overheating, and cooling lotions such as 1% menthol in aqueous cream or calamine (13). The mainstay of therapy has always been antihistamines. Even though practically all urticarial patients are placed on some type of antihistamines, only 40% of these will clear or almost clear on treatment in a tertiary care center (3).

Antihistamines are classified as first-generation, second-generation, and H_2 antagonists. First-generation antihistamines like the second-generation antihistamines are reverse agonists at H_1 receptors. This prevents the production of many important inflammatory mediators such as P-selectin, intercellular adhesion molecule-1, vascular cell adhesion molecule-1, inducible nitric oxide synthase, IL-1ß, IL-6, TNF-α, and GM-CSF (1). Antihistamines also inhibit histamine release, therefore preventing basophil and mast cell degranulation. They are generally more effective if taken on a daily basis (3, 13).

First-generation antihistamines are rarely used as monotherapy secondary to their side effects of drowsiness and anticholinergic effects. They prove to be very beneficial at night when sleep disturbance is a problem (13).

Second-generation antihistamines were developed to diminish the sedating, CNS, and anticholinergic effects of the first generation antihistamines (1). Two of the second-generation antihistamines, cetirizine and levocetirizine, have antiinflammatory properties. Second-generation antihistamines are prescribed as first line therapy. If there is little to no response after increasing the dose of the second-generation antihistamine, a H_2 antagonist is prescribed.

H_2 antagonists have been shown to be effective with H_1 antihistamines in some patients. This is most likely due to the fact that 15% of the histamine receptors in the skin are H_2 receptors (1). H_2 antagonists should not be used as monotherapy.

For patients who do not respond to first-line treatment with general measures and antihistamines, second-line agents may be used. Lots of different drugs and treatments have been used but there are no high levels of evidence to support these different modalities.

Doxepin is a tricyclic antidepressant that has robust H_1 and H_2 receptor antagonist activity (3). It is very effective but its use is limited by its sedating qualities. It is often used at night time in a dose of 10–50 mg. The dose of 25 mg has demonstrated to suppress a histamine-induced flare for 6 days (15).

Oral steroids are often needed to control the disease in the short term, but they are not recommended for the long-term treatment secondary to the numerous side effects that are associated with their use. If they are needed for long-term use, it is crucial that the lowest dose necessary is used (16). Higher doses of first-generation antihistamines, up to four times a day, are preferred over the utilization of oral steroids.

Leukotriene receptor antagonists are inhibitors of the strong inflammatory mediators C4, D4, and E4. They were originally developed for asthma, but have proven to be effective in urticaria. Leukotriene antagonists are used in combination with antihistamines. Evidence shows success in CIU as well as aspirin/NSAID-induced chronic urticaria (1, 3).

Nifedipine is a calcium channel blocker that has been used with mixed success (16). The mechanism of action is the alteration of calcium influx into cutaneous mast cells impeding degranulation (1). Lack of clinical success has diminished its use, but it is a reasonable addition to antihistamines when patients have urticaria as well as hypertension (3).

If a primarily neutrophilic infiltrate or urticarial vasculitis is present, colchicine and dapsone may be two options to try.

Sulfasalazine may be useful in chronic urticaria where delayed pressure urticaria symptoms are present (3). CBC and hepatic enzymes must be monitored and avoided if glucose-6-phosphate dehydrogenase deficient or aspirin sensitive.

Phototherapy with psoralens plus UVA have had mixed studies. UVA and narrowband have been used to control the pruritus associated with urticaria (3).

Third-line agents for the treatment of urticaria are used when the patient is nonresponsive to first- or second-line therapies. Immunomodulatory agents such as cyclosporine, tacrolimus, cyclophosphamide, methotrexate, mycophenolate mofetil, and intravenous immunoglobulins have been used with some success. Other therapies such as plasmapheresis, hydroxychloroquine, warfarin, terbutaline, tranexamic acid, and albuterol have all been utilized (1, 3).

Conclusion

Urticaria can have multiple presentations that occur from numerous etiologies. The key to treatment is identifying the etiology. This is done by clinical presentation, laboratory findings, thorough history, and physical examination. Most acute urticarial cases have an identifiable cause; chronic urticaria is often deemed idiopathic. Treatment usually consists of the removal of trigger as well as the use of an antihistamine. Combination of therapies, both topical and oral, may be needed. Urticaria can be a difficult disease to control and often a recipe treatment is not sufficient.

References

1. Poonawalla T, Kelly B. Urticaria: a review. Am J Clin Dermatol 2009; 10(1): 9–21.
2. Ring J, Cifuentes L, Möhrenschlager M. In: Kaplan A, Greaves M, editors. Urticaria and Angioedema. New York: Informa Healthcare USA, 2009: 15–25.
3. Grattan C, Black AK. Urticaria and Angioedema. In: Bolognia JL, Jorrizo JL, Rapini RP, editors. Dermatology. Vol. 1. London: Elsevier, 2003: 287–302.
4. Sabroe R, Graves M. What is Urticaria? Anatomical, Physiological, and Histological Considerations and Classification. In: Kaplan A, Greaves M, editors. Urticaria and Angioedema. New York: Informa Healthcare USA, 2009: 1–14.
5. Zuberbier T, Greaves MW, Juhlin L, et al. Definition, classification, and routine diagnosis of urticaria: a consensus report. J Invest Dermatol Symp Proc 2001; 6:123–127.
6. Black A. Physical and Cholinergic Urticaria. In: Kaplan A, Greaves M, editors. Urticaria and Angioedema. New York: Informa Healthcare USA, 2009: 181–216.

7. Lawlor F, Black AK. Delayed pressure urticaria. Immunol Allergy Clinics North Am 2004; 24: 247–258.
8. Harada S, Horikawa T, Ashida M, et al. Aspirin enhances the induction of type I allergic symptoms when combined with food and exercise in patient with food-dependent exercise induced anaphylaxis. Br J Dermatol 2001; 145: 336–339.
9. Botto NC, Warshaw EM. Solar urticaria. J Am Acad Dermatol 2009; 60(5): 877.
10. Wisnieski J. Urticarial vasculitis. Curr Opin Rheumatol 2000; 12(1): 24–31.
11. Herzberj AJ, Strohmeyer CR, Cirillo-Hyland VA. Autoimmune progesterone dermatitis. J Am Acad Dermatol 1995; 32(2): 333–338.
12. Greaves M, Kaplan A, Grattan C. Diagnostic Techniques for Urticaria and Angioedema. In: Kaplan A, Greaves M, editors. Urticaria and Angioedema. New York: Informa Healthcare USA, 2009: 141–150.
13. Grattan C, Powell S, Humphreys F, et al. Management and diagnostic guidelines for urticaria and angio-edema. Br J Dermatol 2001; 144: 708–714.
14. Greaves MW. Chronic idiopathic urticaria. Curr Opin Allergy Clin Immunol 2003; 3: 363–368.
15. Sabroe RA, Kennedy CT, Archer CB. The effects of topical doxepin on response to histamine, substance P and Prostaglandin E2 in human skin. Br J Dermatol 1997; 137(3): 386–390.
16. Kaplan A. Treatment of Chronic Urticaria: Approaches Other Than Antihistamines. In: Kaplan A, Greaves M, editors. Urticaria and Angioedema. New York: Informa Healthcare USA, 2009: 365–390.
17. Magerl M, Borzova E, Giménez-Arnau A, et al. Review article. The definition and diagnostic testing of physical and cholinergic urticarias – EAACI/GA^{2}LEN/EDF/UNEV consensus panel recommendations. Allergy 2009; 64: 1715–1721.

Chapter 2
Cold Urticaria

Grace Peace Yu, Alan A. Wanderer, and Massoud Mahmoudi

Abstract Cold urticaria is a physical urticaria in which patients experience urticaria, angioedema, or both in response to direct contact with cold environments, the ingestion of cold beverages or foods, and the handling of cold objects. In this chapter, we present two challenging cases of cold urticaria that highlight the diagnostic evaluation and treatment options for these patients.

Keywords Urticaria • Cold urticaria • Cold stimulation time test

Case 1

An 10-year-old Caucasian boy with a history of asthma presented to your clinic 2 years ago with a 7-month history of hand swelling on contact with cold objects, and an episode of diffuse angioedema and mild hypotension after immersion in the ocean. Prior to the onset of his symptoms, he neither took any medications nor experienced any insect stings.

We recommended the following treatment regimen: avoidance of cold environments, including swimming in cold water to prevent drowning; Medic-Alert bracelet; EpiPen for life-threatening symptoms; and cetirizine at 10 mg daily. His mother refused additional medications because of concern of side effects. The patient returned every 3 months for follow-up and remained stable until approximately 2.5 years after symptom onset when his symptoms worsened. Specifically, he developed difficulty in breathing, wheezing, urticaria, and angioedema every day after coming out of a warm shower and into a 70°F room. We recommended the following:

1. Discontinuation of cetirizine,
2. Cyproheptadine 4 mg three times a day,

G. Peace Yu (✉)
Stanford University School of Medicine, Department of Pediatrics,
Division of Allergy and Immunology, Stanford, CA, USA
e-mail: graceyu@stanford.edu

3. Levocetirizine 5 mg daily,
4. Loratadine 10 mg daily,
5. Ranitidine 150 mg twice daily,
6. Montelukast 10 mg nightly,
7. Albuterol as needed for difficulty in breathing,
8. Diphenhydramine 50 mg as needed for urticaria and angioedema.

Despite the above regimen, his symptoms persisted. At the same time, his asthma had significantly worsened with asthma exacerbations requiring emergency room visits and oral steroid bursts every week. Prior attempts to initiate controller medications had been unsuccessful because of the mother's concern about steroid side effects.

He was also evaluated by the Pediatric Infectious Disease, Rheumatology, and Gastroenterology clinics for a 2-month history of low-grade fevers in the 99–100°F range, intermittent headaches, arthralgias, abdominal pain, and rectal bleeding. He did not have any ocular symptoms, weight loss, night sweats, or fatigue. Family history was significant for the mother having allergic rhinoconjunctivitis but no family members being affected with urticaria or angioedema.

On examination, he appeared healthy and well-developed. His weight was at the 99th percentile and his height was at the 90th percentile. He had mild expiratory wheezing, mild tenderness to palpation over his bilateral maxillary sinuses associated with pale inferior turbinates that obstructed approximately 70% of his nasal passageways, as well as hypermobility of his joints. The rest of his examination was normal including no joint swelling, tenderness, or erythema. He did not have any rashes, swelling, lymphadenopathy, organomegaly, or abdominal pain.

With the Presented Data, What Is Your Working Diagnosis?

A 10-year-old boy presented with a 2.5-year history of urticaria and angioedema after exposure to cold environments and handling cold objects. His working diagnosis is cold urticaria of unknown etiology.

Differential Diagnosis

1. Acquired cold urticaria (ACU)

    Primary ACU
    Secondary ACU
      Cryoglobulinemia
      Infectious diseases
      Leukocytoclastic vasculitis
      Hypothyroidism
      Miscellaneous: insect stings, drugs, malignancy

2. Familial cold auto-inflammatory syndrome

Work-Up

A 5-min cold stimulation time test (CSTT) over the volar aspect of his forearm and hand led to urticarial wheals and diffuse swelling of his forearm, hands, and digits.

Laboratories:

1. CBC with differential, serum electrolytes, liver function tests, erythrocyte sedimentation rate, anti-nuclear antibody, and rheumatoid factor: normal.
2. Epstein–Barr virus IgM and IgG: negative.
3. No mutations detected in Exon 3 of the cold-induced auto-inflammatory syndrome (*CIAS1*) gene.
4. Total IgE: 1,913 kU/L (normal <100 kU/L).
5. Extensive aeroallergen IgE testing yielded only cat IgE 2.9 kU/L and cockroach IgE 1.8 kU/L (normal <0.35 kU/L) (Skin prick tests could not be performed as the patient was on antihistamines).
6. Stool occult blood samples ×3: negative.
7. Stool *Campylobacter*, *Salmonella*, *Escherichia coli* toxin, *Shigella* toxin, and ova and parasites: negative.
8. Inflammatory bowel disease panel consisting of anti-neutrophil cytoplasmic antibody (pANCA) and anti-*Saccharomyces cerevisiae* antibody (ASCA): negative.

Studies:

1. Pulmonary function tests showed reversible small airway obstruction.
2. Sinus CT showed mild opacification of the left posterior ethmoid, left sphenoid, and maxillary sinuses.
3. Chest CT was normal.
4. Abdominal and pelvic CT scan was normal.

What Is Your Diagnosis and Why?

The clinical history of urticaria and angioedema upon cold exposure and the positive CSTT suggest primary ACU. The patient underwent a work-up for secondary causes of ACU, including an infectious disease work-up as noted above. He had evidence of chronic sinusitis that was treated with 3 weeks of amoxicillin–clavulanic acid. This led to resolution of his low-grade fevers and headache, but his symptoms of cold-induced urticaria and angioedema persisted.

Follow-up

A pediatric rheumatologist diagnosed him with hypermobility syndrome as the cause of his arthralgias. The gastroenterology work-up did not yield the cause of his intermittent abdominal pain and rectal bleeding. However, neither an upper or lower endoscopy was performed. (Occasionally, severe chronic histamine release in cold urticaria is associated with hyperacidity and peptic ulcers.) His abdominal pain and rectal bleeding resolved gradually without specific diagnosis or treatment.

Given the worsening of his severe persistent allergic asthma, his mother was eventually convinced to start him on combination inhaled steroid and long-acting beta-agonist therapy. However, despite maximal doses of this therapy plus additional inhaled steroid therapy, his asthma continued to worsen. As a result, he was started on the anti-IgE monoclonal antibody omalizumab (Xolair) (375 mg SQ every 2 weeks) after special informed consent was obtained from his parent. A case report of a 12-year-old girl with idiopathic cold urticaria who had complete resolution of her urticaria with omalizumab highlighted that this could also be an effective treatment for his cold urticaria (1). However, it was unclear whether her symptoms resolved because of omalizumab or because of the natural history of her disease. After our patient's first dose of omalizumab, his asthma symptoms significantly improved and he no longer had daily symptoms of cold urticaria. Currently, he suffers cold urticaria and angioedema symptoms only with accidental immersion in cold water or after evaporative cooling after exercise. His current medications consist of omalizumab, levocetirizine (10 mg twice daily), montelukast (10 mg nightly), ranitidine (150 mg twice daily), and self-injectable intramuscular epinephrine (as needed for life-threatening reactions).

Case 2

A 17-year-old girl presented to our office with a 7-year history of syncopal and near-syncopal events after exposure to cold environments, angioedema of the tongue and oropharynx after ingestion of cold beverages and foods, and swelling of the hands and urticaria after handling cold objects.

She first presented at 10 years of age after having daily syncopal and near-syncopal events after awakening in the morning in her unheated bedroom. One year later, she had a near-drowning after jumping into a swimming pool. Other symptoms included the following:

1. After washing her hands in cold water -> hand swelling and urticaria.
2. After eating ice cream -> tongue and throat swelling.
3. After exposure to cold air -> periorbital swelling, chest tightness, and cough not relieved by albuterol.
4. After exposure to cold environments -> mild to moderate severity bitemporal headaches that improved after taking a hot shower.
5. Unknown trigger -> abdominal pain associated with mild non-bloody diarrhea a couple of times per week.

The patient denies any urticaria or angioedema associated with any other physical stimuli, including pressure, exercise, heat, sun, or warm water. She has never used self-injectable epinephrine, which she currently carries with her. She denies fevers, conjunctivitis, difficulty hearing, or arthralgias.

Her symptom frequency decreased from daily to once a month upon treatment with cetirizine (10 mg daily) and cyproheptadine (12 mg qhs). Treatment side effects include morning drowsiness and dry mouth. She had three episodes of a flat, erythematous, pruritic rash on her inner thighs associated with a painful sensation located on the skin overlying her spleen. Her rheumatologist treated her with dexamethasone 4 mg daily for 3 days with resolution of her symptoms. The parents also moved from Washington State to California to enable her to live in a warmer climate. However, her parents feel that her overall symptoms have been gradually worsening. Last winter, they set the temperature in their home at 72–74°F to prevent her symptoms, but now the heat needs to be set at 74–76°F to prevent episodes of urticaria. They also felt that she had difficulty last summer when their home was being cooled by ceiling fans. The patient's mother has food allergies and the father has allergic rhinoconjunctivitis and asthma. No family members have urticaria, angioedema, or rash upon cold exposure.

The patient was previously followed by a pediatric rheumatologist but with a recent change in insurance, they are now seeing us for continued care. Her physical examination revealed a well-appearing young woman. Her lungs were clear, abdominal examination was benign, skin was clear, and musculoskeletal examination showed no abnormalities.

Cyproheptadine and cetirizine were discontinued and she was started on doxepin at 10 mg nightly which was gradually increased to 25 mg twice daily with marked improvement in her symptoms. We reviewed an action plan for emergency treatment of her symptoms. We also recommended purchase of an electrically heated warming jacket, continued avoidance of swimming to prevent drowning, and purchase of a Medic-Alert bracelet.

A few months after her initial evaluation, she developed acute sinusitis and marked worsening of her symptoms with abdominal pain and intermittent vomiting upon awakening every morning that gradually resolved after a warm shower. She was treated with a 4-week course of amoxicillin–clavulanic acid with resolution of her sinusitis symptoms. Her doxepin was increased to 75 mg nightly and she was started on levocetirizine 5 mg daily, montelukast 10 mg nightly, and ranitidine 150 mg twice daily with near-complete resolution of her symptoms.

Unfortunately, she subsequently developed a systemic reaction after being exposed to a 64°F environment for 7 h. Her symptoms included near-syncope, disorientation, headache, and abdominal pain. She was treated with intramuscular epinephrine and 911 was called. In the emergency room, she was tachycardic but normotensive and was treated with diphenhydramine 50 mg intramuscular, methylprednisolone 2 mg/kg IV, 2 L of warmed IV fluids, and a Bair Hugger® rewarming blanket with gradual resolution of her symptoms. Upon discharge from the emergency room, her doxepin was increased to 150 mg nightly. At this dose of doxepin, she had only mild anticholinergic side effects of dry mouth. She has had complete resolution of her symptoms on her current treatment regimen for the last 5 months.

With the Presented Data, What Is Your Working Diagnosis?

A 17-year-old girl with a 7-year history of urticaria and angioedema upon exposure to cold environments, ingestion of cold beverages and foods, as well as near-drowning after swimming. Most likely diagnosis is cold urticaria of unknown etiology.

Differential Diagnosis

1. Acquired cold urticaria (ACU)

    Primary ACU
    Secondary ACU
      Cryoglobulinemia
      Infectious diseases
      Leukocytoclastic vasculitis
      Hypothyroidism
      Miscellaneous: insect stings, drugs, malignancy
2. Familial cold auto-inflammatory syndrome

Work-Up

A CSTT over the volar aspect of her forearm for 5 min led to an urticarial wheal.

Laboratories:

1. Infectious disease testing:
    (a) CBC with differential: normal.
    (b) C-reactive protein and erythrocyte sedimentation rate: normal.
    (c) Urinalysis: normal.
    (d) Serum electrolytes, renal function tests, and liver function tests: normal.
    (e) Epstein–Barr virus viral capsid antigen IgM and IgG, and Epstein–Barr nuclear antigen: negative.
    (f) Hepatitis B and C serologies: negative.
    (g) VDRL: negative.
2. Rheumatology testing:
    (a) Anti-nuclear antibody and rheumatoid factor: negative.
    (b) CH50, C3, and C4 levels: normal.
    (c) Anti-Smith, anti-RNP, anti-SSA, anti-SSB, and anti-SCL70 antibodies: negative.

(d) Serum cryoprecipitin levels at 24 and 48 h: normal.
(e) Dilute Russell's viper venom time screen: normal*.
(f) Beta-2 glycoprotein-1 IgG, IgM, and IgA: negative**.
(g) Phosphatidic acid IgG, IgM, and IgA autoantibodies: negative**.
(h) Cardiolipin IgA: negative**.
   * Test to detect lupus anticoagulant.
   **Tests to evaluate for antiphospholipid syndrome.

3. Other:

   (a) No mutations detected in Exon 3 of the *CIAS1* gene.
   (b) C1 inhibitor protein: normal.
   (c) C1 inhibitor functional level: normal.
   (d) FcɛRI autoantibody: negative.
   (e) Total IgE: 187 kU/L (normal <100 kU/L).
   (f) Aeroallergen screening panel showed rye grass IgE 0.42 kU/L, Timothy grass 0.41 kU/L, and dust mite 0.93 kU/L (normal < 0.35 kU/L).
   (g) Food allergen screening panel: negative.

What Is Your Diagnosis and Why?

Primary ACU. The clinical history of urticaria and angioedema upon cold exposure as well as the positive CSTT point toward this diagnosis. Evaluation for secondary causes of cold urticaria, including infection, cryoglobulinemia, and vasculitis, was negative. The patient does not have the typical presenting features of familial cold auto-inflammatory syndrome (FCAS), including onset before 6 months of age or fever, conjunctivitis, and arthralgias after cold exposure. Testing for mutations in the *CIAS1* gene known to cause FCAS was also negative.

Discussion

Definition

Primary ACU is an idiopathic physical urticaria in which patients suffer from urticaria, angioedema, or both after direct contact with cold, ingestion of cold beverages or foods, handling cold objects, or exposure to environmental cold. The diagnosis depends on a compatible history and physical examination, no evidence of underlying disease demonstrated by a normal panel of laboratory tests (i.e., complete blood count with differential, erythrocyte sedimentation rate, anti-nuclear antibody, infectious mononucleosis serology, syphilis testing, total complement, and cryoglobulin level), and positive CSTT (2).

Differential Diagnosis

When evaluating a patient for cold urticaria, it is important to keep the differential diagnosis in mind as cold urticaria syndromes are heterogeneous and have differing etiologies and treatments. Cold urticaria syndromes can be classified as either acquired or familial (Table 2.1) (2).

Acquired forms are either primary (idiopathic) or secondary (associated with or caused by cryoglobulinemia, an infectious disease, malignancy, hypothyroidism, drugs, insects stings, or leukocytoclastic vasculitis) (2). The best described infectious disease associated with the onset of cold urticaria is infectious mononucleosis (3, 4) but case reports have also described syphilis, rubeola, varicella, hepatitis, and respiratory viral infections (2). Hypothyroidism has also been associated with cold urticaria (5).

Atypical ACU is atypical because of negative CSTT. However, under unique circumstances cold exposure can cause urticaria:

1. Systemic ACU: symptoms of urticaria, angioedema, and/or hypotension develop in unique cold environments, such as cold humid air.
2. Cold-dependent dermatographism: only pre-cooled skin exhibits dermatographism.
3. Cold-induced cholinergic urticaria: exercise in cold environments causes punctate urticaria which does not occur in warm environments.
4. Delayed cold urticaria: urticaria develops 12–48 h after cold exposure.
5. Localized cold reflex: urticarial response at a skin location distant (i.e., 5–8 cm) from the site of cold exposure.

Familial forms include familial delayed cold urticaria, FCAS, and a newly described familial atypical cold urticaria (FACU) (6, 7). Familial delayed cold urticaria is

Table 2.1 Cold-induced urticaria syndrome classification

Acquired cold urticaria (ACU) with positive cold stimulation time test (CSTT)
Primary ACU
Secondary ACU
Cryoglobulinemia
Infectious diseases
Leukocytoclastic vasculitis
Hypothyroidism
Miscellaneous: insect stings, drugs, malignancy
Atypical ACU: atypical responses to CSTT
Systemic ACU
Cold-dependent dermatographism
Cold-induced cholinergic urticaria
Delayed cold urticaria
Localized cold reflex
Familial types: negative response to CSTT
Familial delayed cold urticaria
Familial cold auto-inflammatory syndrome
Familial atypical cold urticaria

autosomal dominant and manifests as pruritic urticaria-like lesions that occur 9–18 h after cold exposure (8). FCAS is caused by dominantly inherited or de novo mutations in *CIAS1*, a gene that encodes a protein called cryopyrin (9). Cryopyrin is part of a multiprotein complex termed the inflammasome that activates caspase 1, allowing for the cleavage of pro-interleukin(IL)-1β into its mature form (10). IL-1 mediates inflammation, and mutations in *CIAS1* may lead to constitutive activity of cryopyrin and release of IL-1. It is hypothesized that this leads to the symptoms of fever, arthralgias, conjunctivitis, and atypical urticarial rash with neutrophilic infiltration that is characteristic of these patients after generalized cold exposure (9). Indeed, FDA-approved IL-1 targeted therapies such as Anakinra (Kineret) and Rilonacept (Arcalyst) have been used successfully in the treatment of FCAS (11).

Diagnostic criteria for FCAS have been proposed based on the clinical features of 45 patients with this syndrome and are shown in Table 2.2 (9).

Profuse sweating, extreme thirst, headache, drowsiness, and nausea have also been seen after cold exposure in a significant percentage of affected FCAS patients vs. non-affected family members. Amyloidosis has also been reported with FCAS (9). In a cohort of 137 patients with the clinical diagnosis of FCAS, 135 had mutations in the *CIAS1* gene (12).

Finally, a newly described autosomal dominant form of cold-induced urticaria called FACU was recently described in three families (6). This disorder differs from FCAS because skin biopsies show that the rash appears to be mast cell mediated. Furthermore, patients with this disorder do not experience the fevers, chills, prolonged rash, or arthralgias that FCAS patients experience. Proposed diagnostic criteria for FACU are shown in Table 2.3.

All 20 of the affected patients in the study met all six criteria mentioned above. Evaporative cooling tests (described below) were positive.

Table 2.2 Proposed diagnostic criteria for Familial Cold Auto-Inflammatory syndrome

1. Recurrent intermittent episodes of fever and rash that primarily follow natural, experimental, or both types of generalized cold exposures.
2. Autosomal dominant pattern of disease inheritance.
3. Age of onset <6 months of age[a].
4. Duration of most attacks <24 h.
5. Presence of conjunctivitis associated with attacks.
6. Absence of deafness, periorbital edema, lymphadenopathy, and serositis[b].

[a]Of the patients presented, 95% were less than 6 months of age (range 2 days to 10 years old).
[b]This criterion is used to differentiate FCAS from other periodic fever syndromes, such as Muckle–Wells syndrome which is characterized by late-onset sensorineural deafness.

Table 2.3 Proposed diagnostic criteria for Familial Atypical Cold Urticaria (FACU)

1. Rash: localized pruritic erythema after cold exposure with urticaria, angioedema, or both
2. Autosomal dominant pattern of disease inheritance
3. Rash resolution usually <1 h after rewarming
4. Absence of fever, chills, or joint complaints
5. Age of onset in childhood with lifelong duration of symptoms
6. Negative CSTT result (no wheal formation)

Pathophysiology

The pathophysiology of primary ACU is thought to be secondary to anti-IgE, IgG, or IgM autoantibodies (13), possibly induced by an antigenic stimulus such as a viral infection preceding the cold urticaria. The antibodies formed could then attach to cell-bound IgE and, following cold-induced physico-chemical alteration of the complexes, lead to histamine and other vasoactive mediator release from mast cells. Others have suggested that a putative skin antigen could induce IgE, which together with cold exposure causes cold urticaria (14). The primary target cells are skin mast cells (15) that release histamine, platelet-activating factor, prostaglandin D_2, eosinophilic chemotactic protein, and neutrophilic chemotactic factor (2).

Presentation

Primary ACU is the most common cold urticaria syndrome. Its onset ranges from 3 months to 74 years of age, with the mean age of onset ranging from 7 to 25 years (16, 17). Symptoms occur abruptly and affect males and females equally (16, 17).

The clinical manifestations are diverse and may involve multiple organ systems (2):

- Skin: nonpseudopodic wheals.
- Oropharynx: swelling of the lips, tongue, and pharynx.
- Lower respiratory tract: hoarseness, and wheezing.
- Cardiovascular system: hypotension, and tachycardia.
- Gastrointestinal system: abdominal pain, hyperacidity, ulcers, and diarrhea.
- Reproductive system: uterine contractions.
- Central nervous system: headaches, and disorientation.

A proposed classification for symptom severity is shown below (16):

Type I – localized urticaria and/or angioedema
Type II – generalized urticaria and/or angioedema without hypotensive or respiratory symptoms
Type III – severe systemic reactions with ≥ 1 episode suggestive of respiratory distress (such as wheezing or shortness of breath) or hypotension (such as dizziness, sensation of fainting, disorientation, or shock)

Spontaneous resolution can occur after 1–2 years (2, 17). However, symptoms can persist for more than 20 years (2). Mean duration of symptoms was 4.1–9.3 years in several studies (2, 16, 17), but these studies are limited by their retrospective design and lack of long-term follow-up.

Work-Up

A thorough history and physical examination are essential to the work-up and help guide diagnostic testing (18, 19). Please see below for suggested questions for the history, areas to focus on during the physical examination, and diagnostic tests and studies. The history questions are targeted toward patients with symptoms of cold urticaria. They also, however, include additional questions to ensure that the history is comprehensive and does not miss other causes of urticaria and angioedema.

1. History questions

    - Do you think you are experiencing hives, swelling, or both?
    - How long have you had the symptoms?
    - How old were you when the symptoms first started?
    - What time of day do your symptoms occur?
        - Daytime?
        - Nighttime?
        - Both?
    - How often do the symptoms occur?
        - Daily?
        - Weekly? Number of times per week?
        - Monthly? Number of times per week?
        - Less than monthly? # times__every__months?
    - What medications were you taking when your symptoms first started? What medications were you taking during the month prior to the onset of your symptoms? What medications were discontinued after the onset of your symptoms? These should include all prescription and over-the-counter medications as well as herbs, vitamins, and health supplements.
    - Were you stung by any insects when your symptoms first started?
    - Were you sick in any way prior to the start of your symptoms? For example, did you have any cold symptoms, liver or spleen problems, swelling of your lymph nodes, fatigue, or weight gain?
    - Do your symptoms occur more frequently during a particular season?
        - Winter?
        - Spring?
        - Summer?
        - Fall?
    - What triggers your symptoms?
        - Ingestion of cold foods or beverages?
        - Cold environments?
        - Swimming in cold water?
        - Direct contact with cold (e.g., washing hands in cold water)?
        - Exercising in cold weather?
    - How soon after cold exposure do your symptoms develop?
    - What part of your body is affected first?
    - What symptoms have you had in the past?

CNS

- Disorientation?
- Dizziness?
- Near-fainting?
- Fainting?
- Headaches?
- Blurry vision?

ENT

- Swelling around your eyes? Lips? Face? Tongue? Throat?
- Hoarseness?
- Runny nose?
- Sneezing?

CV

- Fast heart rate?
- Pale skin?
- Blue skin?

Respiratory

- Shortness of breath?
- Difficulty in breathing?
- Coughing?
- Wheezing?
- Did you take any asthma medications or inhalers such as albuterol?
- If so, did it help?

Abdominal

- Nausea?
- Vomiting?
- Abdominal pain?
- Diarrhea?

Skin

- Was the rash red? Flat? Raised? Burning? Itchy?
- Did the rash leave behind any darkening of skin?
- Did the rash and/or swelling occur only where there was cold exposure or did the rash and swelling spread to other parts of your body?

- How severe were the symptoms?
- Are the symptoms activity related?
- Are your symptoms related to your menstrual cycle?
- Have you been tested for the cause of your symptoms?
- If so, what have you been tested for?
- What have you used to treat the symptoms?

- How effective have your previous treatments been?
- What side effects have you had from your treatments?
- Are there any other situations that produce symptoms similar to those due to cold exposure, such as heat exposure, vibration, pressure, sunlight, exercise, or warm water?
- Do you suspect that foods, animal or plant exposures, drugs, chemicals, latex, or personal care products (e.g., cosmetics and shampoos) may be causing your symptoms?
- Have you experienced symptoms during or up to 8 h after intercourse?
- Do you have other allergies such as asthma? Hayfever? Eczema? Food Allergies?
- Have you had any major infections such as pneumonia, sinusitis, hepatitis, ear infections, skin infections, or meningitis?
- Have you had any sexually transmitted diseases such as syphilis, gonorrhea, or HIV (AIDS)?
- Do you have any risk factors for sexually transmitted diseases such as IV drug use, blood transfusions, or sexual activities outside of a monogamous relationship?
- Do you have any sores on your genital region?
- Have you had any history of thyroid disease?
- Have you had a previous diagnosis of cancer?
- Do you have any autoimmune conditions such as lupus or rheumatoid arthritis?
- Have you traveled to a foreign country within 2 years prior to the onset of your symptoms? If so, which countries and when?
    - Have you experienced diarrhea or vomiting since your foreign travel?
    - Have you ingested water from a well, river, pond, lake, or other unpurified water source within 1 year prior to the onset of your symptoms?
    - Have you received any injections or transfusions in a foreign country?
- Have you had any surgeries?
- Do you have any symptoms such as anxiety, mood swings, panic reactions, or depression?
- Do stressful situations cause hives?
- Do you have family members who have similar symptoms?
- Have you had family members who have died of drowning?
- Do you have family members with asthma, hayfever, or food allergies?
- In your opinion, have your symptoms changed since they started?
    - Worsened?
    - Unchanged?
    - Improved?

Review of systems:

- Fever?
- Chills?
- Fatigue?

- Weight loss?
- Weight gain?
- Night sweats?
- Dry eyes?
- Puffiness around eyes?
- Prominence of eyes?
- Conjunctivitis?
- Cold sores?
- Painful teeth or gum disease?
- Dry mouth?
- Tenderness over face?
- Discolored nasal drainage?
- Sore throat, difficulty in swallowing, or hoarseness?
- Recent mass or lump on skin or beneath skin?
- Swelling of the thyroid gland (located in the front of the neck below the Adam's apple)?
- Chronic cough?
- Abdominal swelling or tenderness?
- Blood in stool?
- Increased or decreased frequency of urination?
- Pain or urgency with urination?
- Blood in urine?
- Irregular menstrual cycle?
- Joint pain, swelling, or redness?
- Bone pain or fractures?
- Muscle weakness or pain?
- Tremors?
- Profuse sweating?
- Thirst?
- Drowsiness?
- Loss of hearing?
- Dry skin?
- Easy bruising or bleeding?
- Unusual hair loss?

2. Thorough physical examination, including evaluation for the following:

- Hypertension
- Hepatosplenomegaly
- Lymphadenopathy
- Rash
- Swelling
- Musculoskeletal abnormalities

Patients can present to the office with no objective signs or symptoms of urticaria or angioedema. Also patients can think they are experiencing urticaria or angioedema when in fact their rash or swelling represents an entirely different medical condition

2 Cold Urticaria

such as erythema multiforme. As a result, it is important to confirm the symptoms by having the patient come into the office at the time of symptoms. If this is not feasible, having them take high resolution photographs of their affected skin at the onset of symptoms and at the time the symptoms disappear will help to confirm the diagnosis.

3. CSTT: defined as the minimum time of cold contact stimulation required to induce an immediate coalescent wheal.

    (a) Procedure: **1.** A cold (0–4°C) stimulus (e.g., ice cube in a plastic bag) is applied to the volar aspect of the forearm for 5 min followed by rewarming over 5–10 min. The test is interpreted as positive when a coalescent wheal develops at the site of ice cube administration. If positive, repeat the test with the ice cube on different sites on the forearm at 1 min decrements to determine the shortest interval of time that can elicit a positive test. If the test is negative at 5 min, repeat the test with application of an ice cube in 1 min increments up to 10 min at different sites. If no wheal develops after 5–10 min of rewarming, the test is interpreted as negative.

4. If CSTT is negative, consider immersion of extremity (e.g., hand or forearm) in cold (4–15°C) water for 5 min.

    (a) Caution must be taken in performing this test as systemic reactions, including hypotension, have occurred.

5. If the above tests are negative, consider specific tests that would elicit symptoms:

    (a) In cold-induced dermatographism, stroking pre-cooled skin.
    (b) In FACU one can try evaporative cooling tests such as placing room temperature water on the skin and covering the skin for 10 min (6). Subsequent exposure of the droplet and surrounding skin to cool air can produce erythema and limited urticaria.

6. Complete blood count with differential, erythrocyte sedimentation rate, antinuclear antibody, syphilis serology, infectious mononucleosis serology, total complement, and serum cryoglobulin level to evaluate for secondary causes of cold urticaria.

7. Further testing if clinical history indicates the following:

    (a) Rheumatoid factor
    (b) Total complement and C3 and C4 levels
    (c) Cold agglutinin level
    (d) Serum cryoprecipitin level
    (e) Serum chemistries (e.g., liver function and renal function tests)
    (f) Hepatitis A, B, and C serologic testing
    (g) Thyroid stimulating hormone, free T4 level, and anti-thyroid peroxidase and anti-thyroglobulin antibodies
    (h) C1 esterase inhibitor level and function, C1q
    (i) Serum protein electrophoresis

(j) Immunophenotyping of peripheral blood lymphocytes to evaluate for malignant B cells
(k) T and B cell gene rearrangements with PCR amplification to detect occult T and B cell neoplasms
(l) Serum immunoglobulins (IgG, IgA, and IgM)

8. Studies as clinical history and physical examination indicate

   (a) CT sinus
   (b) CT chest, abdomen, and pelvis to evaluate for lymphoma or other neoplasm
   (c) Skin biopsy

9. If history is compatible with FCAS, testing for mutations in the *CIAS1* gene.

Treatment

Treatment of primary ACU is directed at education, avoidance of cold environments, and medications as shown in Table 2.4.

Medications can effectively suppress the symptoms of cold urticaria. Cyproheptadine was the first H1 antihistamine to be shown to be effective in cold urticaria in a double-blind study. Doxepin has both H1 and H2 receptor antagonist activity and is also effective in cold urticaria. Cyproheptadine and doxepin should be titrated to allow for maximal benefit while minimizing side effects such as sedation and weight gain. Cyproheptadine can be started at 2 mg/day and gradually increased to 2–4 mg three times daily (2). Doxepin can be started at 10 mg nightly and gradually increased to 150 mg nightly (personal unpublished data). Doxepin should not be used concurrently with monoamine oxidase inhibitors and also in patients with glaucoma, urinary retention, or congestive heart failure.

The efficacy of ketotifen, a mast cell stabilizer, at 1 mg twice daily has also been demonstrated in a double-blind study. The second-generation non-sedating H2 blockers have also been found to be effective in reducing symptoms with a recent study showing that 20 mg/day of desloratadine significantly improved objective symptoms of ACU compared to the standard dose of 5 mg/day without an increase in adverse events (20). Case reports of combination H1 and H2 receptor antagonists, montelukast alone, zafirlukast with cetirizine, and omalizumab have also been used in cold urticaria.

If patients participate in aquatic activities, they should take prophylactic medications, swim in a heated pool, swim with a friend, and carry self-injectable intramuscular epinephrine with them (2). If surgery is necessary, the operating room temperature should be increased to prevent symptoms (2).

In response to emergency situations where respiratory or cardiovascular compromise has occurred secondary to ACU, basic and advanced pediatric or adult cardiac life support treatment is indicated. In addition, patients should be placed in a recumbent position, intramuscular epinephrine should be administered, 911 called, and intramuscular, intravenous, or oral antihistamines should be given. Emergency medical

Table 2.4 Treatment of primary acquired cold urticaria

A. *Education*
   a. Description of the disease, pathophysiology, treatment options, and prognosis
   b. Action plan for what to do in case of systemic reaction
   c. Training and demonstration of self-injectable intramuscular epinephrine
   d. Medic-Alert bracelet
B. *Avoidance*
   a. Avoidance of immersion in cold water to prevent drowning
   b. Avoidance of cold environments (e.g., ski resorts)
   c. Avoidance of cold food or beverage ingestion
   d. Moving to warmer climate
   e. Electrical warming vest (can be purchased through warmgear.com and other vendors)
C. *Medications*
   a. Antihistamines
      i. Diphenhydramine
      ii. Cyproheptadine
      iii. Doxepin
      iv. Ketotifen
      v. Second-generation non-sedating H2 blockers
         1. Levocetirizine
         2. Cetirizine
         3. Loratadine
         4. Desloratadine
         5. Fenofexadine
      vi. H1 blockers
         1. Ranitidine
         2. Famotidine
         3. Cimetidine
   b. Other
      i. Montelukast
      ii. Zafirlukast
      iii. Omalizumab

services include rewarming with prewarmed (37°F) IV fluids and using a warming device such as a Bair Hugger®. Warm, humidified oxygen, and ipratropium bromide and albuterol can be used for respiratory symptoms. Steroids can be given to prevent a late-phase response, although this is controversial (2). Steroids are not effective as treatment for acute onset of cold-induced hives or cold-induced systemic reaction.

Repeating the CSTT during the course of therapy can allow for an objective measure of symptom control. If the test is positive at less than 3 min, this makes it more likely that the patient will have a life-threatening type III reaction upon cold exposure. Also, the CSST can be used when a patient is off all medications to test for spontaneous resolution of symptoms.

Overall, the goal of therapy is to allow patients to lead as productive and fulfilling lives as possible through education, avoidance of cold exposures, and medications to suppress symptoms.

Questions

1. What symptoms can be associated with cold urticaria?

    (a) Dizziness
    (b) Urticaria
    (c) Angioedema
    (d) Abdominal pain
    (e) All of the above

2. What signs and symptoms distinguish FCAS from primary ACU?

    (a) Fevers, chills, conjunctivitis, and arthralgias
    (b) Loss of hearing
    (c) Lymphadenopathy and splenomegaly
    (d) Delayed onset of symptoms
    (e) None of the above

3. What is the mode of inheritance for FCAS?

    (a) Autosomal dominant
    (b) Autosomal recessive
    (c) Compound heterozygote
    (d) Mitochondrial
    (e) Dominant negative

4. What are the treatment options for FCAS?

    (a) Steroids
    (b) Recombinant IL-1 receptor antagonist
    (c) Non-steroidal anti-inflammatory drugs
    (d) a and b
    (e) All of the above

5. What are the treatment options for primary ACU?

    (a) H1 receptor antagonists
    (b) H2 receptor antagonists
    (c) Leukotriene receptor antagonists
    (d) Omalizumab
    (e) All of the above

6. Tests that can be used to evaluate for underlying causes of cold urticaria are as follows:

    (a) Complete blood count with differential
    (b) Erythrocyte sedimentation rate
    (c) Serum cryoglobulin level
    (d) C3 and C4
    (e) All of the above

7. Which infections have been associated with cold urticaria?

    (a) Infectious mononucleosis
    (b) Varicella
    (c) Syphilis
    (d) a and b
    (e) All of the above

8. What gene has been shown to be mutated in FCAS?

    (a) CIAIS1
    (b) SERPING1
    (c) c-kit
    (d) F12
    (e) None of the above

9. Biopsy of the rash of a patient with FCAS will show infiltration by what cell type?

    (a) Eosinophils
    (b) Neutrophils
    (c) Mast cells
    (d) T lymphocytes
    (e) Macrophages

10. Diagnostic criteria for FACU include the following:

    (a) Autosomal dominant pattern of disease inheritance
    (b) Rash resolution usually <1 h after rewarming
    (c) Absence of fever, chills, or joint complaints
    (d) Negative CSTT result (no wheal formation)
    (e) All of the above

Answer key: 1. (e), 2. (a), 3. (a), 4. (e), 5. (e), 6. (e), 7. (e), 8. (a), 9. (b), 10. (e)

References

1. Boyce JA. Successful treatment of cold-induced urticaria/anaphylaxis with anti-IgE. *J Allergy Clin Immunol* 2006; **117**(6): 1415–8.
2. Wanderer AA, Hoffman HM. The spectrum of acquired and familial cold-induced urticaria/urticaria-like syndromes. *Immunol Allergy Clin North Am* 2004; **24**(2): 259–86, vii.
3. Lemanske RF Jr., Bush RK. Cold urticaria in infectious mononucleosis. *JAMA* 1982; **247**(11): 1604.
4. Anderson RH. Cold urticaria with infectious mononucleosis: case report. *Va Med* 1983; **110**(9): 549–50.
5. Mahmoudi M, Naguwa S. Cold-induced urticaria associated with hypothyroidism. *J Am Osteopath Assoc* 1999; **99**(8): 394.
6. Gandhi C, Healy C, Wanderer AA, Hoffman HM. Familial atypical cold urticaria: description of a new hereditary disease. *J Allergy Clin Immunol* 2009; **124**(6): 1245–50.
7. Hoffman HM, Mueller JL, Broide DH, Wanderer AA, Kolodner RD. Mutation of a new gene encoding a putative pyrin-like protein causes familial cold autoinflammatory syndrome and Muckle-Wells syndrome. *Nat Genet* 2001; **29**(3): 301–5.

8. Soter NA, Joshi NP, Twarog FJ, Zeiger RS, Rothman PM, Colten HR. Delayed cold-induced urticaria: a dominantly inherited disorder. *J Allergy Clin Immunol* 1977; **59**(4): 294–7.
9. Hoffman HM, Wanderer AA, Broide DH. Familial cold autoinflammatory syndrome: phenotype and genotype of an autosomal dominant periodic fever. *J Allergy Clin Immunol* 2001; **108**(4): 615–20.
10. Martinon F, Burns K, Tschopp J. The inflammasome: a molecular platform triggering activation of inflammatory caspases and processing of proIL-beta. *Mol Cell* 2002; **10**(2): 417–26.
11. Hoffman HM. Therapy of autoinflammatory syndromes. *J Allergy Clin Immunol* 2009; **124**(6): 1129–38; quiz 1139–40.
12. Aksentijevich I, D Putnam C, Remmers EF, Mueller JL, Le J, Kolodner RD *et al*. The clinical continuum of cryopyrinopathies: novel CIAS1 mutations in North American patients and a new cryopyrin model. *Arthritis Rheum* 2007; **56**(4): 1273–85.
13. Gruber BL, Baeza ML, Marchese MJ, Agnello V, Kaplan AP. Prevalence and functional role of anti-IgE autoantibodies in urticarial syndromes. *J Invest Dermatol* 1988; **90**(2): 213–7.
14. Kaplan AP, Garofalo J, Sigler R, Hauber T. Idiopathic cold urticaria: in vitro demonstration of histamine release upon challenge of skin biopsies. *N Engl J Med* 1981; **305**(18): 1074–7.
15. Keahey TM, Indrisano J, Kaliner MA. A case study on the induction of clinical tolerance in cold urticaria. *J Allergy Clin Immunol* 1988; **82**(2): 256–61.
16. Wanderer AA, Grandel KE, Wasserman SI, Farr RS. Clinical characteristics of cold-induced systemic reactions in acquired cold urticaria syndromes: recommendations for prevention of this complication and a proposal for a diagnostic classification of cold urticaria. *J Allergy Clin Immunol* 1986; **78**(3 Pt 1): 417–23.
17. Alangari AA, Twarog FJ, Shih MC, Schneider LC. Clinical features and anaphylaxis in children with cold urticaria. *Pediatrics* 2004; **113**(4): e313–7.
18. Mahmoudi M. Cold-induced urticaria. *J Am Osteopath Assoc* 2001; **101**(5 Suppl): S1–4.
19. Wanderer AA. Hives: The Road to Diagnosis and Treatment of Urticaria. AnsonPublishing LLC, Bozeman; Montana 2007.
20. Siebenhaar F, Degener F, Zuberbier T, Martus P, Maurer M. High-dose desloratadine decreases wheal volume and improves cold provocation thresholds compared with standard-dose treatment in patients with acquired cold urticaria: a randomized, placebo-controlled, crossover study. *J Allergy Clin Immunol* 2009; **123**(3): 672–9.

Chapter 3
Contact Urticaria Syndrome

Zack Thompson and Howard I. Maibach

Abstract Contact urticaria syndrome (CUS) consists of a heterogeneous group of vascular and inflammatory reactions that occur within minutes to an hour of contact with a causative agent. Reactions can vary from a localized wheal and flare, to more systemic aspects – asthma, anaphylaxis, and even death – depending upon the agent and patient response. The breadth of eliciting agents and incidence of CUS has been growing as awareness of the syndrome has developed, although the true scope of the syndrome in the general population remains uncertain due to a lack of epidemiological information. Diagnosis has historically been and remains difficult, as reactions typically disappear within hours and before patients even meet with a healthcare worker. As a result, detailed patient histories and immediate type allergy testing are the primary modes of diagnosis. Treatment consists primarily of awareness and agent avoidance. Extreme cases may require patients to wear a bracelet detailing their allergies, and possibly carry antihistamines or self-administered epinephrine.

Keywords Urticaria • Contact urticaria

Introduction

Case 1

Chief Complaint

The patient is a tall and otherwise healthy 36-year-old Caucasian male surgeon who runs and lifts weights regularly. He has a moderately severe, treatment-resistant hand eczema that was not successfully managed either by himself or by his referring dermatologist.

Z. Thompson (✉)
University of California San Francisco, 2901 Cityplace West Blvd., Apt. 442,
Dallas, TX 75204-0360, USA
e-mail: zackt@alumuni.princeton.edu

History of Present Illness

The dermatitis started out as a relatively mild discomfort with a transient redness, typically clearing on the weekend when he was not operating. Therapy consisted of topical corticosteroids and moisturizers. At first this appeared adequate; over time, the dermatitis became sufficiently severe that he was no longer able to operate.

On direct questioning, he stated that he noted exacerbation of burning, stinging, and itching within the first half hour of donning latex gloves. On this basis, he empirically switched from brand-to-brand without significant resolution.

Past Medical History

He had allergic rhinitis controlled by oral antihistamines, and flexural eczema as a child, which was now clear. He had not worn surgical latex gloves for 3 months.

Physical Examination

A comprehensive dermatological examination revealed normal skin with no lesions, ecchymosis, rashes, or dermatitis. Physical examination of the hands – his area of chief complaint – appeared within normal limits.

Differential Diagnosis

Differential diagnosis included endogenous and exogenous dermatitis, and immunologic contact urticaria (ICU).

Impression and Follow-Up

Our impression was ICU to latex protein in his surgical gloves.

Diagnostic patch testing with the routine series of the North American Contact Dermatitis Group (NACDG) (1), and utilizing the International Contact Dermatitis Research Group (ICDRG) scoring methodology (2), revealed no clinically relevant positives at 96 h.

As he had no signs or symptoms other than skin involvement, testing to produce an immediate response to an allergen (i.e., immediate type testing, which typically is immunoglobulin E, or IgE, mediated and consists of a wheal and flare) in the form of a use test – a test that mimics the situation in which the response was initially produced – was performed with a glove from his hospital's operating room. The latex glove was used on one hand and a vinyl glove (a control) was used on the other.

At 30 min, he noticed burning, stinging, and itching. Examination of the vinyl gloved hand was negative. The latex hand had splotchy redness and numerous wheals; thus, prick testing was not necessary.

He returned to surgery utilizing low-content latex protein gloves for surgery, and vinyl gloves for other purposes.

He was asymptomatic 2 years after the above regimen.

Case 2

Chief Complaint

This 45-year-old Hispanic woman had a 20-year history of manageable atopic dermatitis. In the last 6 months, she required up to 80 mg of prednisone daily to maintain a reasonable skin function and comfort.

History of Present Illness

This atopic individual had learned to live with low-grade chronic dermatitis. She and her referring dermatologist requested consultation because of the exacerbations requiring high-dose systemic corticoid therapy. She had gained 30 pounds, presumably due to the prednisone therapy. She is also hypertensive and diabetic.

Family History

Family history was not remarkable.

Review of Systems

Not otherwise remarkable.

Social History

She was accustomed to hosting networking and business gatherings at home for her husband's business, but was no longer able to perform this function.

Physical Examination

Redness, swelling, scaling, and thickening (lichenification) were observed. Nearly 30% of the skin on her body was involved, with the face, neck, dorsal hands, and forearms most affected.

Differential Diagnosis

Differential diagnosis included endogenous and exogenous dermatitis, and ICU.

Impression and Follow-Up

Because of the dramatic exacerbation of symptoms which were not well-controlled on topical and high-dose systemic corticosteroids, we suspected an intervening exogenous factor.

Our working diagnosis was ICU, as she related on direct questioning that she noted burning, stinging, and itching when handling uncooked foods. We suspected that the contact urticaria might be due to one or more of the foods that she handled while cooking.

Diagnostic patch testing with the routine series of the NACDG (1) and utilizing the ICDRG scoring methodology (2) revealed no clinically relevant positives.

Because of the extent and severity of the dermatitis, she was admitted to the hospital and was almost completely clear in 5 days with the application of triamcinolone cream 0.05%, and a plastic occlusive suit for 8 of each 24 h.

Immediate type testing via a use test – in this case, placing fresh food she had been handling prior to the reaction directly on her skin – on slightly dermatitic skin revealed extensive wheals and flares. These responses appeared within 20 min of contact with wheat, rice, and turkey, and were negative to numerous other foods. Ten controls to the reacting foods were negative.

Avoidance of these fresh foods in her cooking permitted an almost complete long-term (i.e., last follow-up at 2 years) return to her normal existence.

Discussion

History

Descriptions of symptoms related to urticaria have been discovered as far back as the time of Hippocrates (3). Causal relationships between these reactions and contact with foods, spices, and a variety of other substances have been acknowledged for over a century. For example, urticarial reactions documented during the last century include the first reported case of allergy to vanilla in 1893, and reactions to nettles and hairy caterpillars (e.g., *Thaumetopoea pityocampa*) (4). However, the heterogeneity of urticarial signs and symptoms was not recognized until fairly recently.

The term contact urticaria was first introduced by Fisher in 1973 (4). Contact urticaria syndrome (CUS) was defined as a biological entity by Maibach and Johnson in 1975, in a study analyzing immediate-type hypersensitivity to the insect repellent diethyltoluamide, or DEET (5). Early studies in Hawaii (Elpern 1985a, b, 1986), Poland (Rudzk et al. 1985), Sweden (Nilsson 1985), Denmark (Veien et al. 1987), Finland (Turjanmaa 1987), and Switzerland (Weissenbach et al. 1988) indicated that immediate contact reactions are common. Despite an increasing variety of studies, much of the subsequent research has focused on a single urticaria-eliciting agent in an occupational setting. Since most studies have not analyzed incidences of contact urticaria in the general population brought about by a range of eliciting agents, the epidemiology remains inadequately documented.

Prevalence

As noted above, epidemiologic data on contact urticaria are limited, since the primary focus of most research has been on occupational studies of CUS. Bashir and Maibach observed that if the demographic profile of the occupations studied deviates from that of the general population, this may lead to skewing of the reported etiologies (6). The majority of studies performed to date have focused on a relatively small number of verticals, primarily in food services/preparation, medical services, and husbandry. Given the limited nature of these populations, any extrapolation of this data could lead to inaccurate assessments regarding incidence, severity, and other factors affecting diagnosis and treatment.

The most comprehensive epidemiologic data on occupational contact urticaria in USA relate to contact with natural rubber latex, beginning with Nutter's work in 1979 (7). Since usage of latex gloves represents only one cause of contact urticaria and is skewed toward the population of people in only a few professions (e.g., health care workers, and hairdressers), it is does not provide a good basis for extrapolation. Research in other US occupations is somewhat more limited in scope. Thus, it is difficult to assess the prevalence of contact urticaria in USA based on domestic studies.

On the contrary, Finland maintains one of the best occupational disease documentation systems in the world. From 1990 to 1994, there were 2,759 cases of allergic contact dermatitis reported to the Finnish Register of Occupational Diseases, of which 815 (29.5%) were contact urticaria and 1,994 (70.5%) were allergic contact dermatitis. Contact urticaria was most prevalent among those in occupations related to food and health care (Table 3.1) (8). While the data from Finland are obviously influenced by geography, culture, and regional occupational

Table 3.1 Prevalence ranking among the professions (7)

S. no	Occupations	Number per 100k workers	Total number
1.	Bakers	140.5	53
2.	Preparers of processed food	101.8	4
3.	Dental assistants	95.5	28
4.	Veterinary surgeons	72.5	3
5.	Domestic animal attendants	69.1	61
6.	Farmers, silviculturalists	57.7	341
7.	Chefs, cooks, cold buffet managers	38.5	40
8.	Dairy workers	37.9	5
9.	Horticultural supervisors	37.8	6
10.	Laboratory technicians, radiographers	35.6	9
11.	Physicians	33.0	20
12.	Butchers and sausage makers	28.9	7
13.	Laboratory assistants	24.6	15
14.	Dentists	23.4	5
15.	Nurses	21.2	42
16.	Waiters in cafes and snack bars	15.1	9
17.	Kitchen assistants, restaurant workers	13.6	16
18.	Hairdressers, beauticians, bath attendants	11.8	9
19.	Housekeeping managers, snack bar managers	11.5	9
20.	Packers	11.2	8
21.	Horticultural workers	10.7	5
22.	Assistant nurses, hospital attendants	10.2	14
23.	Industrial sewers	9.1	4
24.	Cleaners	6.7	21
25.	Electrical and teletechnical equipment assemblers	6.6	3
26.	Homemakers, home help (municipal)	6.2	5
27.	Technical nursing assistants	4.2	5
28.	Machine and engine mechanics	3.9	7
29.	Shop assistants, shop cashiers	2.1	9
	Total	3.7	815

weightings, the data weighted by incidence per 100,000 workers provide a good background for an epidemiologic understanding of the disease across other countries.

Studies of occupational and nonoccupational contact urticaria have generally demonstrated little-to-no correlation between incidence and race, age, or gender. Elpern's Hawaiian demographic study found no racial disparity among the White, Asian Filipino, Asian Japanese, Hawaiian, and part-Hawaiian participants. Furthermore, Elpern found that the incidence was comparatively stable from the ages of 20–80. While some exceptions exist – such as the tendency of children with spina bifida to show latex sensitization/allergy at a younger age, and some age-related variation in the degree of sensitivity by location on the body – the lack of correlation between contact urticaria incidence and age generally holds (6). Finally, the aforementioned Finnish study showed only a slight increase in frequency among women, demonstrating gender is also not much of a determining factor (7).

Pathophysiology

The mechanisms underlying CUS are broadly grouped into two categories: ICU and nonimmunologic contact urticaria (NICU). ICU and NICU are differentiated by a variety of factors, including: prior sensitization, elicitation time, systemic features, common causes, main mediators, inhibitors, and diagnostic tools (Table 3.2) (4).

NICU, also referred to as immediate-type irritancy, is the more commonly seen form of contact urticaria, and occurs without prior sensitization to the eliciting agent, usually within 45–60 min of exposure. The intensity of the reaction can vary based on the concentration, manner of exposure, area of skin affected, and the material itself. Generally, the reactions remain localized and are characterized by a wheal and flare appearance (Fig. 3.1) (6, 9). Highly sensitive skin areas, such as the face (particularly the eyelids and perioral areas) and neck, are more reactive than less sensitive areas like the back and extensor sides of the upper extremities, which are still more reactive than the rougher skin of the soles and palms.

Substances that have been thoroughly studied and tend to produce NICU reactions include benzoic acid and sodium benzoate (often used as preservatives in cosmetics), sorbic acid (a food preservative), cinnamic aldehyde (the chemical compound that gives cinnamon its flavor and odor), cinnamic acid (primarily used in perfumes), and nicotinic acid esters (often used as a chemopreventive agent). The appearance of these responses can vary widely based on the concentration of the irritant. For example, cinnamic aldehyde is used at low doses in chewing gum and mouthwashes to produce a pleasant tingly feeling in the mouth, but it can produce significant lip swelling at higher concentrations (5).

Table 3.2 Differences between immunologic contact urticaria (ICU) and nonimmunologic contact urticaria (NICU) (7)

	ICU	NICU
Prior sensitization	Yes	No
Elicitation time (open skin test)	10–20 min	<45 min
Systemic features	Occasionally	No
Common causes	Proteins	Simple chemicals
Main mediator	Histamine	Ecosanoids?
Inhibitors	Antihistamines, capsaicin (flare)	NSAIDs
Diagnosis	Skin prick test Specific IgE assay	Open/closed application test

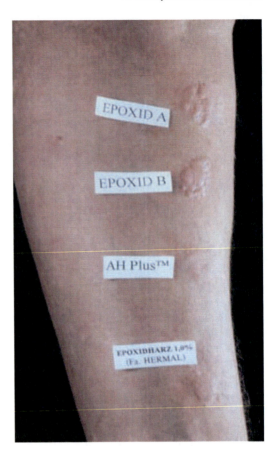

Fig. 3.1 Urticarial reactions to epoxy (epoxid) resins at test sites after 20 min (9)

The precise mechanism of NICU is open to question. In the past, it was believed that the release of histamine from mast cells in response to the eliciting agent might be the mechanism. However, subsequent studies suggest otherwise, as antihistamines have failed to block reactions to many known eliciting agents. The current consensus is that the mechanism is prostaglandin metabolism inhibition, as studies show that nonsteroidal anti-inflammatory drugs (NSAIDs) like aspirin can inhibit typical NICU reactions to known causative agents (7).

Conversely, ICU is the less common form of contact urticaria and typically appears faster than NICU, within 15–20 min of introduction. ICU requires prior sensitization, or the production of IgE antibodies specific to the eliciting substance. This sensitization can occur via many routes, including the skin, mucous membranes, respiratory and gastrointestinal tracts, or other organs. Unlike NICU, ICU can spread beyond a localized area, progressing to generalized urticaria (Fig. 3.2). This progression to higher stages (see Clinical Manifestations below) can lead to more severe reactions, with the potential to become life threatening (5).

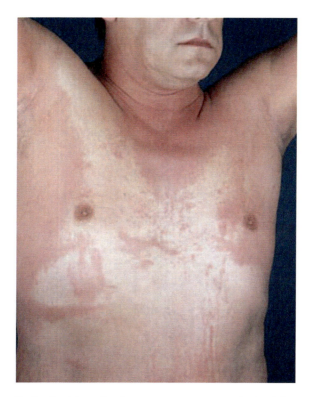

Fig. 3.2 Generalized urticarial reaction from exposure to epoxy resins involving the limbs, trunk, neck, and face. Reproduced with permission from Katie B. Wade and Dr. Harald Löffler, ref. (9) © Wiley-Blackwell

Clinical Presentation, Testing, and Diagnosis

One of the principal difficulties in diagnosing contact urticaria is that by definition the lesions disappear within hours, so they are not often present by the time patients meet with healthcare workers. Thus, a thorough patient history is often necessary to help diagnose contact urticaria, with a focus on understanding the following: association of the symptoms with a specific substance, details of employment and possible relation of the reaction to work exposure, identification of activities being performed at the time of onset, and a personal or family history. Maibach and Amin have created a staging system that, when combined with a patient history and available test methods, helps lead to a diagnosis (Table 3.3) (5).

Skin presentations can range from localized redness and swelling, eczema or itching, tingling, and burning, to the more generalized urticaria typically associated with ICU. Depending on the severity of the reactions, extracutaneous symptoms may present, such as wheezing, runny nose, watery eyes, lip swelling, hoarseness,

Table 3.3 Staging of contact urticaria syndrome (7)

Cutaneous (skin) reactions only:	
Stage 1	Localized urticaria (redness and swelling) Dermatitis (eczema)
	Nonspecific symptoms (itching, tingling, or burning)
Stage 2	Generalized urticaria
Extracutaneous reactions:	
Stage 3	Bronchial asthma (wheezing)
	Rhinitis, conjunctivitis (runny nose, and watery eyes)
	Orolarngeal symptoms (lip swelling, hoarseness, and difficulty in swallowing)
	Gastrointestinal symptoms (nausea, vomiting, diarrhea, and cramps)
Stage 4	Anaphylactoid reactions (shock)
Stage 5	Death

difficulty in swallowing, nausea, vomiting, cramps, and diarrhea. Extreme reactions can result in anaphylaxis and even death.

The most common in vivo test methods used for both ICU and NICU include the prick test, scratch test, chamber test, and chamber prick test. Other commonly used tests include the open application test (open test), use test, and RAST test. Control tests – namely, positive (histamine, 1 mg/mL) and negative (normal saline) – are an important part of interpreting the results of these tests.

The open test is believed to pose the lowest risk of anaphylaxis due to the small amount of exposure to the allergen. The open test involves spreading 0.1 mL of the testing agents over 3 cm × 3 cm areas of skin. Addition of propylene glycol (alcohol) to the test vehicle can enhance the sensitivity of the test, though care should be taken and intensity of the reaction should be considered. Again, test sites are normally examined every 15–20 min for 1 h.

If the results of the open test are negative, a prick or scratch test may be required. Prick and scratch tests are essentially administered in the same manner. Drops of diluted test allergens are applied to the test area – usually the volar aspects of the forearm. The allergens are introduced by scratching or piercing the skin with a lancet. Test sites are generally read every 15–20 min for 1 h. Positive reactions involve a wheal with a diameter of at least 3 mm and at least half that of the histamine control (10).

The chamber and chamber prick tests are administered similarly, with the only difference being the addition of the puncture in the latter. These tests are primarily used for testing foods when proven commercial allergens are unavailable. Small aluminum containers holding the causative agents are attached to the skin via a porous tape and held for 15 min, with results typically observed 5 min after removal.

If no reaction is elicited, a use test can be employed to mimic the activity that initially triggered the symptoms. Due to the risk of anaphylaxis from this method in particular, it is important to proceed cautiously and make facilities for resuscitation available. Serial dilutions are also an effective means of preventing anaphylaxis with this test. For example, dilution series that have been used in alcohol vehicles are 250, 125, 62, and 31 mmol/L for benzoic acid; and 50, 10, 2, and 0.5 mmol/L for methyl nicotinate (6).

A RAST (radioallergosorbent test) measures circulating antibodies present in serum. RAST can be a useful in vitro test for investigating cross-allergies, or when the patient has a history of anaphylaxis. One drawback is that a positive RAST test may be less specific than a positive open test.

Studies have shown that the following can generate false negatives: recent ingestion of NSAIDs, antihistamines, or capsaicin; prolonged exposure to ultraviolet A or B light over the prior 2 weeks; and tachyphylaxis caused by repeated use of the same site for testing (7). Thus, it is important to communicate this information to patients, and to avoid over testing any one site.

Treatment

Treatment for both ICU and NICU begins with understanding the eliciting agents through testing. The form of testing employed depends on the severity of the reaction, as mentioned above.

After the scope and severity of the triggers are understood, prevention and education are the primary treatment. Depending on the causative agent(s), avoidance will consist of some combination of dietary, activity, and occupational restrictions. Special consideration should be taken to note food extracts that may be used in other substances (e.g., the use of certain fruits and vegetables in cosmetics). Restricted activities may be as simple as avoiding a ranching environment in the event of a reaction to cow dander, or may create an occupational restriction if a response to shellfish is elicited in a cook.

In extreme cases of ICU, it may be necessary to wear a bracelet listing the patient's allergies. Table 3.4 provides a representative, but not exhaustive, list of agents known to cause contact urticaria. Carrying antihistamines and possibly self-administered epinephrine may also be indicated.

Table 3.4 Agents producing contact urticaria (5)

	Agents producing Immunologic contact urticaria (ICU)	Nonimmunologic contact urticaria (NICU)
Animals/animal products	Cockroaches Dander Hair Liver Locust Spider mite	Arthropods Caterpillars Corals Jellyfish Moths Sea anemones
Foods	Dairy Banana Wheat Chicken Shrimp	Cayenne pepper Cow's milk Fish Mustard Thyme

(continued)

Table 3.4 (continued)

	Agents producing Immunologic contact urticaria (ICU)	Agents producing Nonimmunologic contact urticaria (NICU)
Fragrances & flavorings	Balsam of Peru Menthol Vanillin	Balsam of Peru Benzaldehyde Cassia (cinnamon oil)
Medicaments	Antibiotics Benzocaine Clobetasol 17-propionate Dinitrochlorobenzene Mechlorethamine Phenothiazines Pyrazolones	Alcohols Benzocaine Chloroform Iodine Myrrh Tar extracts Witch hazel
Metals	Copper Nickel Platinum	Cobalt
Plants/plant products	Algae Birch Garlic Latex rubber Mahogany	Nettles Seaweed
Preservatives and disinfectants	Benzoic acid	Acetic acid Formaldehyde
Miscellaneous	Ammonia Lanolin alcohols Nylon Plastic	Pine oil Sulfur Turpentine

Questions

1. Which of the following is highly correlated to incidence and severity of contact urticaria?

   (a) Race
   (b) Age
   (c) Gender
   (d) None of the above

2. A white 60-year-old male office worker arrives for testing after an anaphylactic reaction to cat dander. Which of the following tests should be administered?

   (a) Open test
   (b) Chamber test
   (c) Chamber scratch test
   (d) Patch test for type IV hypersensitivity

3 Contact Urticaria Syndrome

3. Which of the following occupations typically does not experience a relatively high incidence of contact urticaria?

    (a) Nurse
    (b) Office worker
    (c) Chef
    (d) Hairdresser

4. Contact urticaria lesions typically disappear within what time frame?

    (a) 3 days
    (b) 2 weeks
    (c) 2–3 h
    (d) 1 week

5. A 33-year-old female hairdresser of Hawaiian decent presents with a NICU reaction to cobalt – a known NICU-producing agent. Which of the following would be most effective if administered?

    (a) Aspirin
    (b) Claritin
    (c) Capsaicin
    (d) Atarax

6. The best available epidemiologic data on occupational contact urticaria in USA are from which of the following?

    (a) Latex glove usage
    (b) Exposure to shellfish
    (c) Hairdressing chemicals
    (d) Farming

7. Which of the following is most likely the mechanism in NICU?

    (a) IgE
    (b) Histamine
    (c) Prostaglandins
    (d) None of the above

8. ICU typically presents in what time frame?

    (a) Almost immediately after contact
    (b) 15–20 min
    (c) <45 min
    (d) Around 1 h

9. A positive prick test typically involves a wheal of at least what diameter?

    (a) 3 cm
    (b) 1.5 cm
    (c) 1.5 mm
    (d) 3 mm

10. How often are test sites generally read during scratch testing?

    (a) Every 10 min
    (b) Every 15–20 min
    (c) Every 30 min
    (d) Every hour

Answers: 1. (d), 2. (a), 3. (b), 4. (c), 5. (a), 6. (a), 7. (c), 8. (b), 9. (d), 10. (b)

References

1. Warshaw E, Furda L, et al; Angiogenital Dermatitis in Patients Referred for Patch Testing. Retrospective Analysis of Cross-Sectional Data from the North American Contact Dermatitis Group, 1994-2004. Arch Dermatol. June 2008;144(6):749–755.
2. Lachapelle JM, Maibach HI. The Methodology of Patch Testing. In: Lachapelle JM, Maibach HI, eds. Patch Testing and Prick Testing. A Practical Guide. Germany: Springer. 2003:46–50.
3. Zuberbier T, Maurer M. Urticaria: Current Opinions about Etiology, Diagnosis and Therapy. Acta Derm Venereol. 2007;(87):196–205.
4. Wakelin SH. Clin Exp Dermatol. March 2001;26(2):132–136.
5. Amin S, Lahti A, Maibach H. Contact Urticaria and Contact Urticaria Syndrome (Immediate Contact Reactions). In: Zhai H, Wilhelm K-P, Maibach H, eds. Marzulli and Maibach's Dermatoxicology, 7th Edition. 2008:525–536.
6. Urticaria, Contact Syndrome: Follow-Up. http://emedicine.medscape.com/article/1050166-followup. Article updated Feb 11, 2009.
7. Boukhman M, Levin C, Maibach H. Contact Urticaria Syndrome. Occupational Hazards. Clinics in Occupational and Environmental Medicine. February 2001;1(1):13–33.
8. Kanerva L, Toikkanen J, Jolanki R, Estlander T. Finnish Institute of Occupational Health, Helsinki, Finland. Statistical data on occupational contact urticaria. Contact Derm. 1996,35(4):229–233.
9. Stutz N, Hertl M, Löffler H. Anaphylaxis Caused by Contact Urticaria Because of Epoxy Resins: An Extraordinary Emergency. Contact Derm. May 2008;58(5):307–309.
10. Levin C, Warshaw E. From Dermatitis: http://www.medscape.com/viewarticle/580843?src=rss. Article published 10/20/2008.

Chapter 4
Idiopathic Angioedema

Cristina J. Ramos-Romey and Timothy J. Craig

Abstract Idiopathic angioedema is characterized by recurrent episodes of swelling involving the deep dermis and subcutaneous tissue. Idiopathic angioedema is a diagnosis of exclusion, and a thorough evaluation is warranted to exclude underling conditions that may clinically present with angioedema. Here, we present two challenging cases of idiopathic angioedema.

Keywords Idiopathic angioedema • Angioedema

Case 1

Our patient MC is a 27-year-old female who was referred to our clinic due to recurrent facial and throat swelling for the last 18 months. She presented initially with a generalized red, pruritic rash, as well as lip and facial swelling. The skin rash resolved but the lip and facial swelling persisted. The swelling episodes are associated with throat tightness and shortness of breath. She has been hospitalized on three occasions due to severe swelling and airway compromise. These episodes are not related to any kind of activity or food ingestion. She has always had irregular menstrual cycles, but she has not noticed any correlation between her cycles and her symptoms. At the time of evaluation, she was not sexually active; but in high school she used oral contraceptive pills without any adverse effects. At the time the swelling episode started, she was not using over-the-counter or prescription medications. She was initially prescribed cetirizine without benefit. Hydroxyzine was partially effective, with mild improvement of the lip and facial swelling. Her throat swelling and shortness of breath responds to IM epinephrine. She has autoinjectable epinephrine at home and uses it at least twice a month. She had been taking prednisone

---

T.J. Craig (✉)
Section of Allergy and Immunology, Penn State Milton S. Hershey College of Medicine, Penn State University, Hershey, PA, USA
e-mail: craig@psu.edu

60 mg daily for 5 months, and with dose tapering she would have recurrence of the swelling requiring the use of IM epinephrine. During her initial clinic visits, she developed visible lip swelling with throat tightness.

Medications: Prednisone 40 mg daily orally, hydroxyzine 50 mg every 6 h orally, ranitidine 150 mg twice daily orally, fluoxetine 40 mg daily orally, montelukast 10 mg daily orally, and epinephrine 0.3 mg IM as needed. Past medical history includes a nonfunctional pituitary tumor which has not grown in 3 years and a history of childhood asthma. She has no known drug or food allergies.

Family history: Mother with a history of diabetes mellitus, high blood pressure, and coronary artery disease. Her father is deceased with a history of a heart condition. She has three siblings one with a history of hypoglycemia. No family history of autoimmune disease, recurrent swelling episodes, or unexplained abdominal pain.

Social and environmental history: She is single and lives with her mother in a 5-year-old home. She has a cat but did not have any pets at the time her symptoms started. No infestations with cockroaches or other insects in her home. No mold or water damage. They have carpets, gas-fueled central heating and cooling. She does not drink, smoke, use illegal drugs, and is not exposed to secondhand smoke. She worked at a veterinary office as a receptionist and assistant, and at present is receiving disability benefits.

Review of system: She reports weight gain, depression, and anxiety due to her illness. She denies fever, chills, weight loss, headache, ear pain, sore throat, chest pain, syncope, palpitations, abdominal pain, gastric reflux symptoms, stool changes, eczema, snoring, mouth breathing, joint complaints, seizures, or hearing problems. All other systems were negative.

Physical examination: Blood pressure was 120/62 mmHg, heart rate was 75 beats/min, and respiratory rate was 20 per min. Her general appearance was of a very pleasant female, morbidly obese, in no acute distress. HEENT examination revealed a normocephalic, atraumatic head, with buffalo hump and moon facies. Her conjunctiva was pink without erythema. Tympanic membranes were intact without any erythema or effusions. Nasal mucosa was pink, and turbinates were normal, without any rhinorrhea. There was no sinus tenderness or polyps. She had evidence of lip swelling and was unable to fully open her mouth (refer to Fig. 4.1). Oropharynx was clear without postnasal discharge and normal tonsils. Her thyroid gland was normal to palpation, and no masses were palpated. She had no cervical or supraclavicular adenopathy. Breath sounds were clear bilaterally. Cardiovascular examination revealed regular rate and rhythm, without murmurs. Her abdomen was globous, with positive bowel sounds, no tenderness, or distention. No masses or organomegaly were noted. Examination of her extremities showed strong pulses bilaterally in upper and lower extremities, and had adequate perfusion. She had pitting edema 2+ bilateral, without any clubbing, or cyanosis. Skin: violaceous striae, no evidence of urticaria, rash, or eczema. Muscle strength and tone was 5/5 in upper and lower extremities (Fig. 4.2).

Diagnostic testing. Medical history and medication review were unremarkable. Physical examination revealed facial angioedema and chronic changes due to chronic high dose corticosteroids. Patient brought initial evaluation done by primary

4 Idiopathic Angioedema

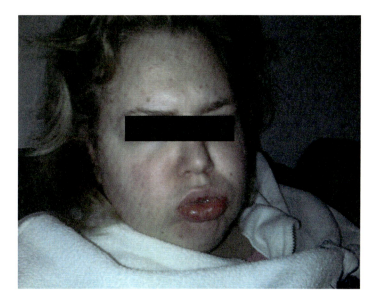

Fig. 4.1 Picture of a patient with swelling of the face

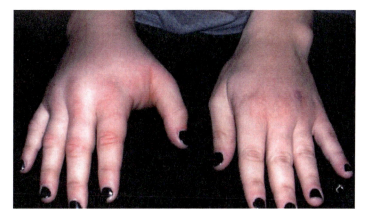

Fig. 4.2 Picture of a patient with swelling of the hands

physician. A complete blood count with differential and a comprehensive metabolic panel were all within normal range. Results are displayed in Table 4.1. Additional laboratory evaluation results were all within normal range.

Impression. Chronic angioedema without urticaria of unknown etiology.

Plan. During her clinic visit, she developed visible worsening of the facial swelling, throat tightness, and shortness of breath. She was given 0.3 mg of 1:1,000 epinephrine IM by autoinjector. She was taken to the emergency department and was admitted to our institution for the treatment of angioedema with upper airway involvement. She was hospitalized for 5 days at which time an extensive workup was performed.

Table 4.1 Initial laboratory evaluation

Tests	Results	Reference values
WBC (K/uL)	10	4.8–10.8
Hgb (g/dL)	13.0	12–16
Plts (K/uL)	114	140–340
Neut, abs (K/uL)	6.9	1.7–7.7
Lymph abs (K/uL)	2.3	1.2–4.9
Eos, abs (K/uL)	1	0.0–0.7
Na (mmol/L)	141	137–145
K (K/uL)	4.9	3.5–5.1
Cl (K/uL)	103	96–107
HCO_3 (K/uL)	31	22–30
Bun (mg/dL)	24	7–20
Cret (mg/dL)	0.7	0.6–1
Glu (mg/dL)	101	70–106
Ca (mg/dL)	9.3	8.4–10.2
Protein (g/dL)	7.2	6.5–8.3
Albumin (g/dL)	3.9	3.5–5.5
AST (unit/L)	33	10–40
ALT (unit/L)	74	13–69
ALk Phos (unit/L)	64	38–120
T Bili (mg/dL)	0.5	0.2–1.3

With the Presented Data, What is Your Working Diagnosis?

This is a 27-year-old female who presented to our clinic with recurrent swelling of her lips, face, and larynx unresponsive to antihistamines. Initial evaluation with complete medical history, medication review, physical examination, and basic laboratory evaluation did not reveal a clear cause for her symptoms. At this point, we suspected hereditary angioedema.

Differential diagnosis. The major differential diagnosis includes allergic and nonallergic angioedema. Allergic angioedema may be caused by medication or food allergy. Nonallergic angioedema include hereditary angioedema, acquired angioedema, autoimmune disease, infection, or malignancy.

Workup

During her hospitalization, a complete blood count with differential and a comprehensive metabolic panel was repeated, and results were all within normal range. We requested TSH, antithyroid antibodies, tryptase levels, CRP and total IgE. We also obtained complement levels along with C1 esterase inhibitor levels and function. Again this evaluation did not reveal any abnormalities. We then proceeded to order C1 q levels and C1 q binding essay. A CT scan of the chest and neck, which did not reveal any abnormal findings, was performed (Table 4.2).

Table 4.2 Laboratory results

Test	Results	Reference values
CRP (mg/dL)	<0.5	<0.5
C4 (mg/dL)	26	14–44
C1 inhibitor level (mg/dL)	24	11–26
C1 inhibitor function (%)	100	>65
C1q level (mg/dL)	5.9	5–8.6
C1q binding essay (mcg/mL)	>1.2	<4.4
Tryptase (ng/mL)	<1	2–10
IgE (IU/mL)	12.5	<115
TSH (uIU/mL)	0.56	0.3–5
Anti-TPO (IU/mL)	0	<35
ThyroglobulinAb (IU/mL)	0	<40

What is Your Diagnosis and Why?

Medication-induced angioedema. Our patient was not taking any medications when her angioedema started; therefore, medication-induced angioedema such as that seen with angiotensin converting enzyme (ACE) inhibitors is unlikely.

Food allergy. She was unable to correlate the angioedema episodes with a particular food. The prolonged duration of symptoms and the absence of urticaria make the diagnosis of food allergy unlikely.

Hereditary angioedema (HAE). The patient does not have a family history of recurrent angioedema, and laboratory evaluation showed normal C4, C1 inhibitor levels and C1 inhibitor functional assay within normal range, making HAE types I and II unlikely. Hereditary angioedema type III is also unlikely; her episodes do not correlate with her menses and did not manifest symptoms when she was on oral contraceptive pills. The lack of family history also argues against this diagnosis.

Acquired angioedema. Our patient had normal C1q, C4, and C1 inhibitor levels and lacks evidence of a lymphoproliferative disorder, infection, or autoimmune disease, therefore acquired angioedema would be unlikely.

Our patient underwent an extensive evaluation of her angioedema and after reviewing her medical history and laboratory evaluation, no etiology was found. She was diagnosed with chronic idiopathic angioedema without urticaria. In the past, she has responded well to prednisone but symptoms recurred when attempts to taper the dose were made. She also developed multiple complications from long-term high-dose prednisone, such as obesity, glucose intolerance, moon facies, buffalo hump, striae, myopathy, and adrenal suppression. Due to the severe corticosteroid side effects, steroid sparing therapy was considered. After obtaining baseline values for complete blood count, liver enzymes, BUN, creatinine, lipid profile, urinalysis, and uric acid levels, she was placed on high-dose H1 blockers with cetirizine 10 mg daily and hydroxyzine 50 mg every 6 h; ranitidine 150 mg twice daily, and cyclosporine 200 mg twice daily. She continued prednisone 60 mg daily with the plan to taper as tolerated and epinephrine autoinjector to be used as needed. On her next outpatient follow-up, the dose of prednisone was successfully tapered to 10 mg daily.

She remained without symptoms on 10 mg of prednisone for 2 weeks. She then reported waking up with swelling around her right eyelid and increased swelling in her face and neck which required the use of autoinjectable epinephrine. Symptoms rapidly improved and did not require emergency care. Upon further investigation, it was discovered that her primary care physician started lisinopril for high blood pressure 1 week earlier. After the lisinopril was discontinued, her angioedema again improved.

Case 2

CC is an 18-year-old female who consulted to our service by the emergency department physician due to facial swelling and throat tightness. She has suffered from recurrent angioedema for 6 years. She reports mild episodes with swelling of her extremities and torso once a week. She also reports severe episodes once a month with swelling of face, shortness of breath, and abdominal discomfort. She denies urticaria associated with the angioedema. The patient notes that her attacks of angioedema have worsened during this spring and summer. She has also noticed that pressure and vibration can trigger an attack, but she often has similar attacks without these triggers. She noted in the past that while on an oral contraceptive, containing drosperinone and ethinyl estradiol, she had more frequent angioedema episodes and they correlated with her menstrual cycle. After being changed to another oral contraceptive containing ethinyl estradiol and norgestrel, her symptoms decreased in frequency and she did not notice any correlation with her menstrual cycle. She reports having episodes of angioedema since 12 years of age, well before she was on oral contraceptive pill. She uses doxepin 25 mg as needed for episodes of angioedema. For this last episode, she was treated in the emergency room with IV methylprednisolone as well as epinephrine with the improvement of her symptoms. Past medical and surgical history was unremarkable.

Medications: Doxepin 25 mg as needed.

Allergies: The patient developed rash with sulfa-derived drug, no known allergies to food or insect venom.

Family history: Her mother has a history of food allergies as well as seasonal allergies, and her father has hypertension. There is no family history of angioedema, recurrent unexplained swelling, or autoimmune disorders.

Social history: She starts university in the fall, and worked at a chocolate store for the summer. She lives with her parents in a new home. They have carpets, gas-fueled heating and cooling. They have one dog at home. No mold or water damage in the home, and no infestations with cockroaches or insects. She denies tobacco, alcohol or illicit drug use. She is not exposed to secondhand smoke.

Review of system: She is able to perform normal activities without fatigue. No anxiety, fever, chills, weight loss, headache, ear pain, sore throat, chest pain, syncope, palpitations, abdominal pain, gastric reflux symptoms, stool changes, eczema, pruritus, urticaria, snoring, mouth breathing, joint complaints, seizures, or hearing problems. All other systems were negative.

Physical examination: Blood pressure was 114/76 mmHg, heart rate was 67 beats per min, and respiratory rate was 18 per min. Her general appearance was of a young female, in no acute distress. HEENT examination revealed a normocephalic, atraumatic head. Her conjunctiva was pink without erythema. Tympanic membranes were intact without any erythema or effusions. Nasal mucosa was pink, turbinates were normal, without any rhinorrhea. There was no sinus tenderness or polyps. Oropharynx was clear without postnasal discharge and normal tonsils. Her thyroid gland was normal to palpation, and no masses palpated. She had no cervical or supraclavicular adenopathy. Breath sounds were clear bilaterally. Cardiovascular examination revealed regular rate and rhythm, without murmurs. Her abdomen had violaceous striae, with positive bowel sounds, no tenderness, or distension. No masses or organomegaly were noted. Examination revealed an area of erythema, warm to the touch and swelling on her hip and left foot. She also had swelling and erythema of her left elbow. Skin was clear without evidence of urticaria, rash, or eczema. Muscle strength and tone was 5/5 in upper and lower extremities.

Diagnostic testing. Complete blood count with differential and comprehensive metabolic panel was normal. By patient's report, she had undergone testing at her physician's office and was found to have normal C1 esterase inhibitor levels and function. She has also been skin tested and demonstrated no sensitivities to aeroallergens or foods.

Impression. Chronic angioedema without urticaria of unknown etiology.

Plan. After her evaluation in the emergency room, she was started on fexofenadine 180 mg twice daily, ranitidine 150 mg twice daily, diphenhydramine 25 mg as needed, and epinephrine autoinjector to use if needed. During her hospital stay, she continued to have swelling episodes, fexofenadine was increased to 180 mg three times a day, and montelukast 10 mg daily was added to her regimen. She had significant improvement and was discharged home. A comprehensive evaluation was obtained before discharge.

With Presented Data, What Is Your Working Diagnosis?

This 18-year-old female presents with recurrent swelling affecting her face, extremities, and abdomen for 6 years. Based on the medical history and physical examination, she was diagnosed with chronic angioedema.

Differential diagnosis. The differential diagnosis includes hereditary angioedema (HAE), acquired angioedema due to autoimmune disease, idiopathic angioedema, and medication-induced angioedema.

Workup

CC brought her initial evaluation done by primary physician to her follow-up visit, and it included a CBC and metabolic panel which were normal. During the visit, her medical history and medication review were unremarkable. Physical examination

Table 4.3 Laboratory evaluation

Test	Results	Reference range
ESR (mm/h)	5	0–20
C4 (mg/dL)	29	14–44
C1 inhibitor level	24	11–26
C1 inhibitor function (%)	100	>65
C1q level (mg/dL)	13	5–8.6
Tryptase (ng/mL)	1	2–10
TSH (uIU/mL)	1.27	0.3–5
Anti-TPO (IU/mL)	<10	<40
ThyroglobulinAb (IU/mL)	<20	<35

revealed angioedema involving her elbow and extremities without the evidence of urticaria. Results of additional laboratory tests obtained for further evaluation are presented in Table 4.3.

Our evaluation consisted of a comprehensive laboratory evaluation at the emergency department with the presence of symptoms. This evaluation consisted of TSH, antithyroid antibodies, C4, C2, and C3 levels, C1 esterase inhibitor levels, erythrocyte sedimentation rate, and tryptase levels. Initial TSH level was elevated at 5.35 uIU/mL. TSH level was repeated and was found to be within normal range at 1.14 uIU/mL. All other laboratory results were within normal range.

What Is Your Diagnosis and Why?

Hereditary angioedema. Our patient started suffering from angioedema around the onset of puberty, which is common in HAE, but our laboratory evaluation does not support this diagnosis since she has normal C4 levels, which is the best screening test, and normal C1 esterase inhibitor levels and adequate function.

HAE type III could be considered since she had an increase in the frequency and severity of her angioedema attacks with the use of estrogen OCPs. The fact that she developed angioedema before the use of OCPs and the lack of a family history do not support this diagnosis.

Acquired angioedema. Autoimmune disease or lymphoma, which are associated with acquired C1 esterase inhibitor deficiency were also considered. Her medical history, review of systems, and physical examination did not reveal any findings to suggest this diagnosis. In addition, acquired angioedema usually presents later in life, and we did not have historic or physical evidence of an autoimmune process or lymphoproliferative disease, making this diagnosis unlikely.

Medication-induced angioedema. At the time that our patient presented with angioedema, she was not on any medications, this would exclude this diagnosis.

Our patient's history, physical examination, and normal laboratory evaluation did not identify an etiology for the angioedema. This led us to the diagnosis of chronic idiopathic angioedema. She failed treatment with zileuton, cetirizine, and doxepin.

She was started on a regimen consisting of fexofenadine three times daily, ranitidine 150 mg twice a day, and montelukast 10 mg daily. We also recommended that she take prednisone 40 mg × 5 days at the onset of severe symptoms and use her epinephrine autoinjector for life-threatening reactions. Since we could not exclude type III HAE, we requested that she discontinue her estrogen-containing oral contraceptive pill and replace it with a progestin-only contraceptive. She was content with her current contraceptive method and did not want to make any changes. Despite therapy, she continued to have significant angioedema episodes about two times per month. Nevertheless, she was content with current control of symptoms and refused treatment with immunomodulators.

Discussion

Angioedema is defined as swelling involving the deep dermis and subcutaneous tissue. It usually affects nondependant areas and can affect any body part, but most often the lips, tongue, pharynx, extremities, penis, and scrotum. Angioedema may also involve the abdomen viscera presenting as unexplained abdominal pain, nausea, and vomiting. The swelling is typically asymmetrical, nonpitting, and when unaccompanied by urticaria, it is nonpruritic. Some patients describe the swelling as being painful, burning, or a pressure-like sensation. The affected areas may be erythematous, poorly demarcated, and warm to the touch. The swelling usually progresses slowly ranging from hours to days, and resolves spontaneously in 24–72 h or earlier with appropriate therapy.

Angioedema presents with urticaria in 40–50% of patients, and occurs alone in 11% of patients (1). This distinction is important since the differential diagnosis varies in those with isolated angioedema or angioedema associated with urticaria. The prevalence of angioedema without urticaria has not been well described, and idiopathic angioedema is thought to be the most common cause of chronic angioedema (2). The differential diagnosis of angioedema without urticaria includes ACE-inhibitor-induced, ASA-induced, hereditary angioedema, acquired angioedema, and idiopathic angioedema. In addition, angioedema can be divided into acute and chronic angioedema. Chronic angioedema is defined as recurrent subcutaneous swelling lasting for more than 6 week. It has also been defined as three or more exacerbations occurring over 6–12 months (3, 4). The natural history of the disease has not been well described and difficult to predict since it varies by the underlying etiology if discovered.

Multiple inflammatory mediators have been implicated in the pathogenesis of angioedema, and multiple enzymatic pathways are activated and contribute to subcutaneous swelling. The principal mechanisms thought to be involved in angioedema are activation of the complement and kinin systems; crosslinking of IgE receptors on the surface of mast cells; the release of histamine, tryptase, prostaglandin D, leukotrienes C and D, and platelet activating factor; non-IgE-mediated activation of mast cells; and the release of vasoactive substances such as leukotrienes with aspirin sensitivity. The release of these vasoactive substances results in an increase in vascular permeability, and vasodilation, presenting clinically as edema and erythema. The complement cascade has also been implicated in the pathogenesis of angioedema. Activation of complement produces anaphylatoxins: C3a, C4a, and C5a, which contribute to histamine release and increased vascular permeability. Disruption of vascular endothelium leads to the release of Hageman factor (XIIa), which activates the kinin-kallikrein system. Prekallikrein, after activation by factor XIIa, converts kininogen to bradykinin. Bradykinin production results in increased vascular permeability and vasodilation (5).

Multiple triggers can lead to activation of above described pathways and produce angioedema. Crosslinking of IgE receptors by antigen, such as foods, medications, insect venom, etc., can activate mast cells, eosinophils, and basophils and cause the release of their mediators. Autoantibodies to IgE or to the high affinity receptor (FcεRI) on mast cells can also cause the release of inflammatory mediators. Physical stimuli such as pressure, cold, heat, water, and sunlight can produce non-IgE-mediated histamine release; however, these physical urticarias are usually accompanied by urticaria and are discussed in Chaps. 2 and 3. In hereditary C1 inhibitor (INH) deficiency, low levels or decreased function of C1 INH, a key regulatory protein of the complement and kinin-kallikrein system, can also produce angioedema. Acquired C1 INH deficiency associated with malignancy, autoimmune disease, or infection can also result in angioedema by depleting C-1-INH and the increased levels of bradykinin. ACE inactivates bradykinin, blockade of ACE by ACE inhibitors results in the increased production of bradykinin, and mimics the angioedema seen in HAE (5). Aspirin and other nonselective cyclooxygenase 1 (COX 1) inhibitors, such as nonsteroidal anti-inflammatory drugs (NSAIDs), have also been implicated in angioedema. With ASA the inhibition of COX leads to an increase in the production of cysteinyl leukotriene which induces angioedema (6). The pathogenesis of idiopathic angioedema is elusive and the diagnosis is of exclusion.

Evaluation

Workup

The initial evaluation of patients who present with chronic angioedema requires an extensive and detailed medical and family history, medication review, review of systems, and physical examination. A thorough evaluation would help identify precipitating factors, such as medications, allergies or associated medical condition that may trigger episodes of angioedema. Family history is also essential since a positive family history for angioedema would suggest HAE. If this evaluation fails to elucidate a cause, a laboratory evaluation is warranted. Most experts suggest, but there are little data to support that testing is essential, that the evaluation should include complete blood count with differential, comprehensive metabolic panel, erythrocyte sedimentation rate, antithyroglobulin and antimicrosomal antibodies, and a urinalysis. Levels of C4

4 Idiopathic Angioedema

Table. 4.4 Abnormal laboratory findings and mediators involved in angioedema

Diagnosis	C4 levels	C1 INH level	C1 INH function	C1q	Mediator
Idiopathic	Normal	Normal	Normal	Normal	Histamine
Allergic	Normal	Normal	Normal	Normal	Histamine
Aspirin induced	Normal	Normal	Normal	Normal	Leukotrienes
ACE-Inhibitor induced	Normal	Normal	Normal	Normal	Bradykinin
HAE type I	Low	Low	Low	Normal	Bradykinin
HAE type II	Low	Normal	Low	Normal	Bradykinin
HAE type III (estrogen-dependnt)	Normal	Normal	Normal	Normal	Bradykinin
Acquired C1 INH-deficiency	Low	Low	Low	Low	Bradykinin

should also be obtained to rule out hereditary or acquired C1 inhibitor deficiency (7). Further workup, to include a biopsy among others, should be directed based upon the history, examination, and initial laboratory screen (Table 4.4).

Management

Treatment of chronic idiopathic angioedema consists of symptom control. Nonsedating antihistamines are considered first-line treatment in idiopathic angioedema. If patients have partial but not complete resolution with standard dosing, studies have shown improvement with higher off-label doses of antihistamines. Dosing schedules of up to three times daily have been used with good results and minimal side effects. The addition of a sedating antihistamine at night time in combination with a nonsedating antihistamine in the morning has also been adopted in clinical practice, but randomized placebo controlled trails are lacking to support management. Limited data exists for the use of sedating antihistamines, but a small number of studies have shown effectiveness in angioedema. If sedating antihistamines are used in clinical practice, side effects should be anticipated and doses increased as tolerated. The use of H2 blockers is an area of debate; recent recommendations for the treatment of chronic urticaria and angioedema, suggest a trail of H2 blockers, and if no benefit is observed, they should be discontinued (8). The majority of patients respond well to oral corticosteroids, but systemic side effects limit their use. Treatment with oral corticosteroid should not be used frequently and should be limited to a short therapeutic course to decrease systemic symptoms. Patients with infrequent attacks of angioedema may benefit from the treatment with a short course of oral corticosteroids when symptoms occur. In patients who do not respond to antihistamines or in those who require frequent courses with corticosteroids, immunomodulatory drugs should be considered. A small number of studies have shown improvement with sulfasalazine, hydroxychloroquine, dapsone, and cyclosporine (8–10). These medications have potentially serious side effects which should be discussed with the patient before starting treatment. They also require regular monitoring of side effects after starting treatment. Recent reports of the off-label use of omalizumab (anti-IgE antibody) suggest some benefit in refractory angioedema and urticaria (11). Although it is infrequent for a patient with idiopathic angioedema to develop laryngeal edema, patients with history of upper airway symptoms should have autoinjectable epinephrine available at all times. Administration of epinephrine should not be delayed if there is upper airway involvement. Patients with idiopathic angioedema should avoid the treatment with ACE inhibitors as well as NSAIDs since they can precipitate or aggravate episodes of angioedema. A medical alert bracelet is also recommended for these patients.

Questions

1. What percentage of patient with angioedema also present with urticaria?

    (a) 10%
    (b) 90%
    (c) 20%
    (d) 40%

2. Which of the following is the most common cause of chronic angioedema?

    (a) Medication-induced angioedema
    (b) Idiopathic angioedema
    (c) Hereditary angioedema
    (d) Acquired angioedema

3. What mediators are thought to be involved in Aspirin-induced angioedema?

    (a) Leukotrienes
    (b) Bradykinin
    (c) Histamine
    (d) Kinin

4. Which medical condition has not been associated with angioedema?

    (a) Infection
    (b) Systemic erythematous lupus
    (c) Asthma
    (d) Leukemia

5. Which inflammatory cell is not involved in the pathogenesis of angioedema?

    (a) Eosinophils
    (b) Mast cells
    (c) Basophils
    (d) Neutrophils

6. The initial evaluation of a patient presenting with chronic angioedema should consist of:

(a) CBC and differential
   (b) Biopsy
   (c) Complete medical history
   (d) Antithyroid antibodies

7. The first-line treatment for chronic idiopathic angioedema is:

   (a) Montelukast
   (b) Second-generation antihistamines
   (c) Prednisone
   (d) H2 blockers

8. The differential diagnosis of chronic angioedema without urticaria includes which of the following?

   (a) Food allergy
   (b) Physical stimuli
   (c) Hereditary angioedema
   (d) Vasculitis

9. What laboratory abnormality would you expect to find in patients with chronic idiopathic angioedema?

   (a) Low levels of C4
   (b) Elevated levels of C1 esterase INH
   (c) Low levels of C1q
   (d) None of the above

10. Which of the following medications should be avoided in patients with idiopathic angioedema?

    (a) Acetaminophen
    (b) ACE inhibitors
    (c) Penicillin
    (d) Hydroxyzine

Answer key: 1(d), 2(b), 3(a), 4(c), 5(d), 6(c), 7(b), 8(c), 9(d), 10(b)

References

1. Kaplan AP, Greaves MW. Angioedema. J Am Acad Dermatol. 2005;53(3):373–388.
2. Banerji A, Sheffer AL. The spectrum of chronic angioedema. Allergy Asthma Proc. 2009; 30(1):11–16.
3. Ferdman R. Urticaria and angioedema. Clin Ped Emerg Med. 2007;8(2):72–80.
4. Frigas E, Park M. Idiopathic recurrent angioedema. Immunol Allergy Clin North Am. 2006;26(4):739–751.
5. Agostoni A, Aygoren-Pürsün E, et al. Hereditary and Hereditary and acquired angioedema: Problems and progress: Proceedings of the third C1 esterase inhibitor deficiency workshop and beyond. J Allergy Clin Immunol 2004;114:S51–S131.

6. Jenneck C, Juergens U, et al. Pathogenesis, diagnosis, and treatment of aspirin intolerance. Ann Allergy Asthma Immunol. 2007;99:13–21.
7. Kaplan AP. Chronic urticaria and angioedema. N Engl J Med. 2002;346:175–179.
8. Kaplan AP. Chronic urticaria: pathogenesis and treatment. J Allergy Clin Immunol. 2004;114(3):465–474.
9. Bernstein JA, Garramone SM, Lower EG. Successful treatment of autoimmune chronic idiopathic urticaria with intravenous cyclophosphamide. Ann Allergy Asthma Immunol. 2002;89(2):212–214.
10. Gonzalez P, Soriano V, Caballero T, Niveiro E. Idiopatic angioedema treated with dapsone. Allergol Immunopathol (Madr). 2005;33(1):54–56.
11. Dreyfus DH. Observations on the mechanism of omalizumab as a steroid-sparing agent in autoimmune or chronic idiopathic urticaria and angioedema. Ann Allergy Asthma Immunol. 2008;100(6):624–625.

Chapter 5
Hereditary Angioedema

Michael J. Prematta and Timothy J. Craig

Abstract Hereditary angioedema is a relatively rare genetic disease with an autosomal dominant inheritance pattern. It is caused by a quantitative or qualitative deficiency of Complement 1 inhibitor (C1-INH). Patients develop episodes of angioedema under the skin, cramping abdominal pain, or laryngeal edema, which can be fatal. The disease does not typically respond to antihistamine, corticosteroid, or epinephrine treatments. The following two cases in this chapter will illustrate the presentation, diagnosis, and management of the disease.

Keywords Angioedema • Hereditary angioedema

Case 1

Our patient is a 51-year-old Caucasian male who presented to the emergency department with epigastric pain. He says his pain started as "crampy" abdominal pain about 16 h before presenting to the emergency department and progressed to very severe crampy pain, and, later, he developed multiple episodes of nausea and vomiting. He reports having had similar problems in the past – some episodes as long as 20 years ago, but usually it is not this severe and resolves within 2–5 days. His medications include hyocyamine for a diagnosis of irritable bowel syndrome. He reports occasional use of ibuprofen for muscle aches related to exercise, and says he did take a few of these approximately 1 week ago.

T.J. Craig (✉)
Section of Allergy and Immunology,
Penn State Milton S. Hershey College of Medicine, Penn State University,
Hershey, PA, USA
e-mail: tcraigpsu@yahoo.com

His past medical history includes a diagnosis of irritable bowel syndrome due to frequent episodes of abdominal cramping, sometimes associated with nausea and vomiting. He has had two colonoscopies and two upper endoscopies in the past to evaluate his frequent gastrointestinal complaints and the studies were reported as normal. He had an appendectomy 10 years ago and a cholecystectomy 3 years ago.

He has no known drug allergies. Regarding family history, his father died hours after an emergency department visit years ago. He is married and has a son. He does not smoke, but drinks alcohol socially. He drinks city water, does not eat undercooked meat, has not had recent travel, and denies known work exposures.

On physical examination, his vital signs included a temperature of 37.8°C, blood pressure 135/98 mmHg, heart rate 105 beats per minute, and respiratory rate 16 breaths per minute. Generally, he appeared to be in moderate discomfort. He had mild conjunctival injection, normal tympanic membranes, and normal nasal mucosa. His heart had a regular rate and rhythm with no murmurs. His lungs were clear to auscultation. On abdominal examination, he had surgical scars present in right upper and right lower quadrant. He had increased bowel sounds and his abdomen was mildly distended with voluntary guarding and tenderness worse in the epigastric area. Extremities showed no clubbing, cyanosis, or edema, and he had a normal skin, neurologic, and mental status examination. The emergency department physicians performed several laboratory diagnostic tests that are presented in Table 5.1.

Table 5.1 Laboratory tests from the emergency department visit for the patient in Case 1

Test	Value	Normal range
WBC ($10^3/\mu L$)	13.8 H	4.8–10.8
Hemoglobin (g/dL)	13	12–16
Hematocrit (%)	39.5	37–47
Platelets ($10^3/\mu L$)	220	140–340
Neutrophils ($10^3/\mu L$)	11.8 H	1.7–7.7
Lymphocytes ($10^3/\mu L$)	1.8	1.2–4.9
Monocytes ($10^3/\mu L$)	0.4	0.0–1.1
Basophils ($10^3/\mu L$)	0.0	0.0–0.2
Eosinophils ($10^3/\mu L$)	0.2	0.0–0.7
Sodium (mmol/L)	140	135–145
Potassium (mmol/L)	4.3	3.5–5.0
Chloride (mmol/L)	106	98–110
Bicarbonate (mmol/L)	24	22–32
BUN (mg/dL)	12	8–22
Creatinine (mg/dL)	0.8	0.6–1.1
Calcium (mg/dL)	8.8	8.5–10.0
AST (SGOT) (U/L)	28	15–46
ALT (SGPT) (U/L)	25	10–50
Alkaline phosphatase (U/L)	182 H	40–110
Total bilirubin (mg/dL)	0.9	0.3–1.9
Lipase level (U/L)	523 H	0–160
Amylase level (U/L)	88	40–140

H denotes higher than normal

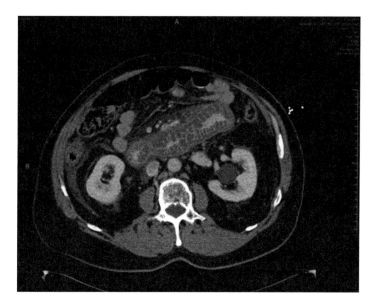

Fig. 5.1 Abdominal CT scan of the patient in Case 1 showing duodenal swelling

In the emergency department, he was given intravenous fluids and ondansetron (antiemetic, serotonin 5-HT3 receptor antagonist) with mild improvement of his nausea, but no improvement of his pain. He was then given morphine with slight improvement in his pain. Because he had persistent abdominal pain with a mildly elevated lipase level, an abdominal CT scan was obtained which showed "marked duodenal wall thickening/edema and heterogeneous enhancement, with adjacent stranding and ascites." This is shown in Fig. 5.1.

With the Above Data, What Is Your Working Diagnosis?

This 51-year-old gentleman presented with abdominal pain which may or may not be related to recurrent abdominal pain that he has experienced regularly for years. He has required abdominal surgeries in the past, including a cholecystectomy and appendectomy. He presented on this occasion with crampy abdominal pain, nausea, and vomiting. He was found to have a slightly elevated neutrophil count, alkaline phosphatase, and lipase levels, and he had duodenal wall thickening on CT scan.

At this point, a differential diagnosis of things that can cause abdominal pain, mildly elevated lipase, and duodenal wall thickening include peptic ulcer disease, Zollinger–Ellison Syndrome, Crohn's disease, acute or acute-on-chronic pancreatitis, duodenal ischemia, duodenal lymphoma, or adenocarcinoma.

Peptic ulcer disease (PUD) and Zollinger–Ellison syndrome leading to duodenitis or ulceration could explain some of his most recent symptoms.

PUD can cause duodenal swelling and abdominal pain, especially if he was recently taking ibuprofen; however, it would not necessarily explain his past episodes of abdominal pain with normal colonoscopies and endoscopies in the past.

Crohn's disease may be another possible cause of his symptoms, but he has been evaluated for Crohn's disease with two colonoscopies in the past, which were normal.

Pancreatitis could definitely be a cause for his symptoms. He does have a mildly elevated lipase level, elevated neutrophil count, and the CT scan showed thickening of the duodenum, which can happen due to its proximity to the pancreas. This could explain his acute symptoms, although it would not explain his 20-year history of abdominal pain unless he also has chronic pancreatitis, which was not evident on CT scan.

Duodenal ischemia is another potential cause of these symptoms. This would be consistent with the thickening of the duodenum. However, he is 51 years old without any history of coronary artery or other vascular disease. It could explain his most recent symptoms, but it is unlikely to have caused his long history of symptoms.

Duodenal lymphoma or adenocarcinoma is another potential cause of his most recent symptoms. This would be something that would need to be ruled out if he continued to have duodenal wall thickening on repeat imaging; however, the chronicity of his symptoms makes a neoplastic process unlikely.

The allergy service was eventually consulted at the request of the patient, who was concerned that a food allergy may have been causing some of his recurrent abdominal pain, nausea, and vomiting, although he could not think of any specific food that may have triggered this. We reviewed his past symptoms which helped us arrive at a final diagnosis.

According to the allergy service assessment, he had recurrent abdominal cramps, sometimes associated with nausea and vomiting, and each episode would last 2–5 days followed by remission of his symptoms. He said he felt well between episodes. These episodes occurred as often as twice per month, but he also had months without symptoms. Also, his father had died suddenly in his 30s. The patient says he was told that his father went to the emergency department for an issue of shortness of breath and was given epinephrine and discharged home. He apparently died later that same day. Our patient says that he was also told that his father had similar intermittent abdominal symptoms.

Work-Up

Given this history, we were very suspicious of hereditary angioedema (HAE). To evaluate for this, we ordered a Complement 4 (C4) level, a Complement 1 inhibitor (C1-INH) functional analysis, and a C1-INH quantitative level.

His C4 level was <10 mg/dL (normal is 14–45 mg/dL), his C1-INH level was 2 mg/dL (normal is 11–26 mg/dL), and his C1-INH functional assay was 24% (normal is >68%).

What Is Your Diagnosis and Why?

From these data and the history, we diagnosed our patient with HAE type I. This was diagnosed because he had a low C4 level and low C1 inhibitor level in the context of chronic abdominal pain with evidence of bowel wall edema. He was started on the androgen danazol 200 mg three times a day, and was then weaned to once a day, which decreased the frequency of his exacerbations.

Case 2

A 26-year-old Caucasian female was seen at an outside emergency department for a sensation of fullness in her throat. Over a 12-h period, the fullness progressed and she also experienced difficulty in swallowing, which worsened to the point of drooling. She was driven to our emergency department where she was found to have stridor, muffled voice, and drooling. She was administered intramuscular epinephrine with little or no response. Intubation was attempted several times, but was unsuccessful. She was then taken to the operating room for an emergency tracheostomy, which was successful. Most of the rest of her history was obtained from her sister.

Her sister informed us that the patient was previously healthy. She commented that the patient had never had any similar complaints before; however, the patient was complaining of back pain lately and her sister thought that she had been taking ibuprofen for the pain. The patient never had any surgeries before the day of presentation. She had an uncomplicated vaginal delivery 2 years ago. Her history was remarkable for penicillin allergy, but no chronic illnesses and no need for medications except a birth control pill. The patient lived in an apartment with her 2-year-old daughter. She smoked one half pack per day and drank alcohol occasionally. She was unemployed at the time of presentation. She had never used illegal drugs to her sister's knowledge.

Regarding her family history, her father died in his 30s after a tooth extraction, but her mother, sister, and daughter were all healthy.

Her home medications included an oral contraceptive pill, and she may have been taking ibuprofen recently for back pain. Her sister was unaware of any other medications.

The review of symptoms was obtained from her sister, and the only positives included the throat symptoms and recent back pain previously mentioned. The patient had also commented on a transient red rash and feeling fatigued the day before presentation.

Her physical examination was as follows: a tracheostomy was in place, and she was slightly sedated from the procedure. Her temperature was 37.5°C, heart rate was 102 beats per minute, blood pressure was 121/67 mmHg, respiratory rate was 12 breaths per minute, but it was reportedly 35 breaths per minute before the tracheostomy was performed, oxygen saturation was 100% on 50% FIO_2, and she

Table 5.2 Laboratory tests from the ICU for patient 2

Test	Value	Normal range
White blood cells ($10^3/\mu L$)	18.1 H	4.8–10.8
Hemoglobin (g/dL)	14.6	12–16
Hematocrit (%)	42.5	37–47
Platelets ($10^3/\mu L$)	159	140–340
Neutrophils ($10^3/\mu L$)	16.5	1.7–7.7
Lymphocytes ($10^3/\mu L$)	1.4	1.2–4.9
Monocytes ($10^3/\mu L$)	0.2	0.0–1.1
Basophils ($10^3/\mu L$)	0.0	0.0–0.2
Eosinophils ($10^3/\mu L$)	0.0	0.0–0.7
Sodium (mmol/L)	135	135–145
Potassium (mmol/L)	4.1	3.5–5.0
Chloride (mmol/L)	106	98–110
Bicarbonate (mmol/L)	21 L	22–32
BUN (mg/dL)	9	8–22
Creatinine (mg/dL)	0.6	0.6–1.1
Calcium (mg/dL)	8.4	8.5–10.0
AST (SGOT) (U/l)	17	15–46
ALT (SGPT) (U/l)	27	10–50
Alkaline phosphatase (U/L)	91	40–110

H denotes higher than normal

was receiving continuous positive airway pressure at 5 cm H_2O. The patient weighed 132 pounds. Her pupils were equal, round, and reactive to light. Her tongue was mildly swollen and protruded with minimal drooling. She had a tracheostomy in place with a small amount of bleeding and sutures to hold it in place. Her breath sounds were clear with equal breath sounds bilaterally. Her heart had a regular rate and rhythm, with a normal S1 and S2, and no murmurs. She had normal bowel sounds, and her abdomen was soft and nontender. She had no clubbing, cyanosis, or edema of her extremities. She also had no rashes while in the hospital.

The results of her laboratory work-up are presented in Table 5.2.

Chest X-ray revealed hypoventilatory changes in the lungs, worse in the lower lungs, and right middle lobe. It also showed blunting of both costophrenic angles, which most likely reflected atelectasis.

CT scan of the neck revealed "significant parapharyngeal soft tissue swelling and edema. There is thickening of the epiglottis and aryepiglottic folds with resultant narrowing of the subglottic airway. No evidence of abscess."

With These Presented Data What Is Your Working Diagnosis?

This 26-year-old female presented with fatigue and a nonspecific rash followed by throat fullness and swelling leading to shortness of breath, muffled voice, and drooling with failed intubation attempts, and ultimately required a tracheostomy.

5 Hereditary Angioedema

She had a chest X-ray showing atelectasis and a neck CT scan showing laryngeal swelling. The presented data and examination lead us to a diagnosis of laryngeal edema causing difficulty in swallowing and breathing.

The differential diagnosis includes angioedema due to a food allergy, angioedema related to a side effect of a medication, especially nonsteroidal anti-inflammatory agents, ACE inhibitor-induced angioedema, hypothyroidism causing angioedema, idiopathic angioedema, diphtheria, Streptococcal pharyngitis, epiglottitis from *Haemophilus influenza* type b infection, pharyngeal abscess, acquired angioedema, or HAE.

Work-Up

We called the patient's family doctor and confirmed that she was not taking an ACE inhibitor. We also obtained further blood work. Thyroid stimulating hormone (TSH) was 3.12 mU/L (normal range 0.5–5 mU/L) and free Thyroxine 4 (T4) was 1.13 ng/dL (normal range 0.7–1.48 ng/dL). Rapid Strep antigen test was negative. Blood and throat cultures were sent. C4 level was low at <10 mg/dL (normal level is 14–45 mg/dL). C1Q quantitative level was 5.9 mg/dL (normal range is 5.0–8.6 mg/dL).

Food allergy is a possible cause of laryngeal edema. Although she had no known history, a food allergy could develop at any time.

Nonsteroidal anti-inflammatory drugs (NSAIDs) such as ibuprofen can cause angioedema in certain patients, even though she has tolerated them before. If this were suspected, one would recommend strict avoidance of NSAIDs.

ACE inhibitors lead to increased bradykinin and can be a cause of angioedema, and should be avoided in any patient with a history of angioedema. This patient, however, was not taking an ACE inhibitor.

Hypothyroidism is a possible cause of angioedema; however, her thyroid tests were normal and the angioedema is usually peri-orbital and on the extremities.

Idiopathic angioedema would be the diagnosis in the majority who presented with recurrent angioedema with or without urticaria; however, it is a diagnosis of exclusion and would not likely be associated with a low C4 level.

An infection would be a possible cause. *Epiglottitis* could cause a scenario like this; however, it is a less common disease as the *H. influenza* type B vaccine is now administered to children. Severe Streptococcal pharyngitis or an infection with diphtheria is another possible cause, but both are unlikely by history.

Acquired angioedema is another possible etiology. This is usually associated with a lymphoproliferative disorder or SLE and is characterized by complement consumption or the presence of autoantibodies against the C1 inhibitor. This would be associated with low C4 levels as in this patient, but one would expect the C1Q level also to be low. This patient has no known history and no evidence of lymphoproliferative or autoimmune disease.

What Is Your Diagnosis and Why?

Hereditary angioedema is the most logical diagnosis for this presentation. This is a slightly late presentation for HAE, but is consistent with the low C4 levels and laryngeal edema. It is also consistent with the family history of the father dying after a tooth extraction. HAE is inherited in autosomal dominant fashion and, thus, her father likely died of an HAE attack. Our patient also had a nondescript rash and fatigue before this incident, and there are reports in the literature of prodromal symptoms including erythema marginatum-like rash or generalized fatigue before the onset of an HAE exacerbation.

To confirm the diagnosis of HAE, one would order a repeat C4 level, a C1-INH antigenic level, and a C1-INH functional assay. Our patient's C4 level was still less than 10 but C1-INH antigenic level was 30.2 (normal rage 7.8–23.4), which is actually high, excluding HAE type I which is associated with low C1-INH levels. However, her C1-INH functional assay was low at 38% (normal > 67%, abnormal if <41%), which confirms a diagnosis of HAE type II which is associated with normal or high levels of C1-INH that is functionally limited.

Discussion

HAE is a rare autosomal dominant inherited condition caused by a deficiency of C1 esterase inhibitor (C1-INH) quantity or function, and sometimes this condition is actually called C1 inhibitor deficiency. An estimated 85% of patients have HAE type I which is associated with a deficient amount of C1-INH, and the other 15% of patients have HAE type II which is caused by a functional defect in C1-INH. Together, the prevalence of HAE type I and II is estimated to be 1 in 50,000, with no race or gender predominance (1). More recently, a third type of HAE has been described that appears to be unrelated to C1-INH level or function and more commonly affects women (2). Some have called this HAE type III, although the work-up, treatment, and pathogenesis are different from what will be discussed further in this chapter, and it may be related to a mutation of the factor XII gene. HAE type III is more difficult to diagnose as it is associated with normal C4 and C1-INH levels. In the following description, the term HAE is used to describe HAE type I or II, but not HAE type III.

HAE is characterized by the onset of subcutaneous or submucosal swelling under any area of skin or any part of the respiratory or gastrointestinal tract. Typically, angioedema exacerbations begin to occur sometime during childhood or the second decade of life, but can begin at any age. A typical exacerbation or "attack" involves nonpitting edema with poorly defined margins that is not itchy, and it can affect one or more areas at a time and is usually asymmetric. Typical locations that patients develop angioedema include the hand, foot, leg, arm, face, or genital area. Figure 5.2 shows an example of an attack involving the hand.

5 Hereditary Angioedema

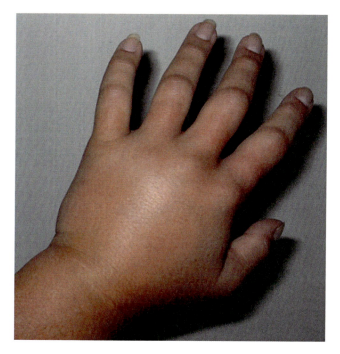

Fig. 5.2 An HAE exacerbation affecting the hand

Figure 5.3 shows an example of a facial exacerbation with lip and cheek swelling. The episodes can occur at times of generalized stress, after trauma (either external trauma or associated with a surgery), during an infection, or after prolonged pressure to a specific body area. Some women have more attacks during times of menstruation. Certain medications can also make a person more predisposed to an exacerbation, including oral contraceptives containing estrogen and angiotensin converting enzyme (ACE) inhibitors. The patient in Case 2 was taking an oral contraceptive pill, which may have made her more predisposed to an exacerbation. Despite the fact that the above conditions can increase the risk of developing an exacerbation, the majority of attacks have no recognizable trigger.

Another area that can be affected includes the gastrointestinal tract, as HAE exacerbations can lead to the development of swelling of the intestinal mucosa. This most commonly causes cramping abdominal pain, nausea, and vomiting, but also can be associated with constipation or diarrhea. Commonly, patients may have long histories of abdominal symptoms before being diagnosed with HAE, which may have led to misdiagnosis and unnecessary abdominal surgeries. The patient in Case 1 was diagnosed with irritable bowel syndrome and also had a cholecystectomy and appendectomy in the past. Often times, patients with HAE will undergo surgery for what is thought to be an acute abdominal surgical emergency, but the patient actually is having an abdominal HAE exacerbation. Often times, this is before patients are diagnosed, but can be a problem even for patients who are

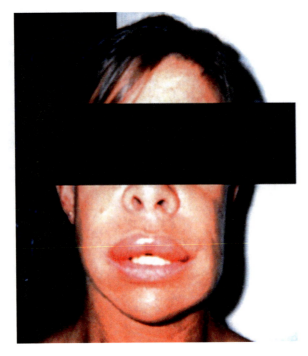

Fig. 5.3 An HAE exacerbation causing swelling of the face and cheeks

diagnosed with HAE as many surgeons and emergency physicians may not be familiar with this disease. However, certainly a patient with HAE can develop appendicitis, cholecystitis, or another acute abdominal problem, so one still has to consider these diagnoses in patients with known HAE, especially if symptoms do not improve with treatment.

Patients can also develop laryngeal swelling causing difficulty in swallowing or breathing, and drooling. Before any HAE treatments were available, the odds of an HAE patient dying from an HAE exacerbation were estimated to be approximately 30%, usually by asphyxiation. Both the patients in Cases I and II had histories of family members dying of unknown causes. This is frequently reported in the family history of patients with HAE, as years ago, patients were even less likely to be diagnosed. In the past, people with HAE may have died of asphyxiation due to laryngeal edema, and families may only report that the patient died suddenly of unknown causes. Laryngeal edema can happen spontaneously, but it is also a particularly feared complication of patients undergoing dental procedures. The father of the patient in Case 2 reportedly died suddenly after a tooth extraction. It is likely that he had HAE and may have died of laryngeal edema as an HAE exacerbation after his tooth extraction.

Angioedema episodes often develop slowly with 12–36 h of slowly increasing swelling, but can also develop more rapidly. The patient described in Case 2 had at least 12 h of sensation of a full throat and then progressed to worsening symptoms.

Typical angioedema "attacks" or exacerbations last 2–5 days without treatment, but can last longer. Abdominal exacerbations can linger for several days. The frequency of exacerbations varies considerably from patient to patient. Some patients can go several months or even years without an exacerbation, while others develop exacerbations multiple times per month. Little is known about why some patients develop more frequent exacerbations than others.

HAE exacerbations are often accompanied by a prodrome before the onset of symptoms. Several prodromes have been reported, including numbness or tingling of a specific area before the edema begins, an erythema marginatum-like rash, generalized fatigue, and muscle aches. Prodromes can occur for as long as 48 h before the onset of an HAE exacerbation, but usually occur within 12 h of the exacerbation (3). The patient in Case 2 had fatigue and a rash before the attack. Either of these symptoms may have been a prodrome. The rash most likely was an erythema marginatum-like rash, a described prodrome of HAE.

Pathophysiology

As mentioned above, HAE types I and II are caused by a quantitative or qualitative deficiency of C1-INH. C1-INH is the main regulator of the early steps of the classic complement pathway, and also inhibits the fibrinolytic and contact systems. C1-INH serves to regulate activation of the contact system, and it does this by inactivating plasma kallikrein and factor XIIa. By doing this, C1-INH prevents excessive generation of bradykinin. Elevated levels of bradykinin lead to increased vascular permeability, leading to extracellular fluid leakage and edema formation; therefore, bradykinin is thought to be the major mediator responsible for angioedema in these patients. While activation of the contact system seems to be the major cause of angioedema, C1-INH inhibits parts of the complement system, the contact system, and the fibrinolytic system, and consumption in these pathways may further consume the protein increasing the amount of bradykinin production. Therefore, activation of any of these systems may lead to further C1-INH depletion, making C1-INH less available to inhibit the contact system, and may predispose patients to an HAE attack (4).

Work-Up

It is important to consider HAE as a diagnosis in several types of patients. Patients who should be considered include any patient with episodes of swelling lasting greater than 24 h that are not associated with hives, and also patients with episodes of recurrent cramping or colicky abdominal pain that last at least 24 h, but often persist for days at a time. A family history of similar problems or sudden death may also increase the suspicion of this disease.

Table 5.3 Laboratory values associated with different types of angioedema

Angioedema type	C4 level	C1-INH level	C1-INH function	C1Q level
Idiopathic	Normal	Normal	Normal	Normal
HAE type I	Low	Low	Low	Normal
HAE type II	Low	Normal or high	Low	Normal
HAE type III	Normal	Normal	Normal	Normal
Acquired	Low	Normal or low	Low	Low

HAE hereditary angioedema, *C4* complement 4, *C1* complement 1, *INH* inhibitor

In a patient with suspected HAE, checking C4 level is the best single screening test. It is very important that this be sent to a facility that is accredited. One study demonstrated low C4 levels in 100% of patients with untreated HAE (5). This test must be performed while a patient is not receiving treatment including fresh frozen plasma, C1-INH infusions, danazol, or plasmin inhibitors for at least 1 week before laboratory tests are drawn. A very small percentage of patients may have only low C4 levels during an acute attack of angioedema, so if a patient has normal lab work, but there is still suspicion of an HAE, one should check C4 level at the time of angioedema to see if the level is reduced. One must also keep in mind that the reference ranges for C4 is not well defined for patients less than 1 year old, so it may be more difficult to exclude a diagnosis in this subset of patients. If the C4 level is low, the next step would be to recheck the C4 level and also test C1 inhibitor level and function. It is also important to perform these tests at an accredited laboratory. Patients with low C4 levels can also have acquired angioedema caused by autoantibodies against C1-INH or consumption of C1-INH by immune complexes. This can be associated with SLE or lymphomas, and these patients should also have low C1-INH function and usually low C1-INH antigen levels. This can be diagnosed by checking the C1Q level, which would be expected to be low in acquired but not HAE. Table 5.3 summarizes expected laboratory abnormalities in idiopathic, hereditary, and acquired angioedema.

Management and Treatment

The prevention of HAE attacks should begin with practical measures, which include avoidance of trauma and use of prophylactic medication before surgeries. Also, medications that can exacerbate HAE should also be avoided – these include estrogens, which specifically can exacerbate HAE, and ACE inhibitors, which can exacerbate any type of angioedema. Patients are also likely to do better if conditions like gastritis and *Helicobacter pylori* infections are treated (6). Long-term prophylaxis for patients with HAE has been achieved in some cases with antifibrinolytics, attenuated androgens, and plasma-purified C1-INH. Plasma-purified C1-INH, attenuated androgens, and off-label use of fresh frozen plasma have all been used with success for short-term prophylaxis before and after surgeries, especially oral surgeries. Treatment for acute HAE attacks is mainly supportive with no approved treatment in the US; however, there are several off-label treatments including C1-INH concentrate infusions, fresh frozen plasma, and danazol treatment.

Epsilon-aminocaproic acid (EACA) is an antifibrinolytic agent used off-label to treat HAE as a long-term prophylactic agent, and doses of 8–10 g per day have been shown to reduce frequency and severity of HAE attacks. Side effects of this medication include muscle discomfort, postural hypotension, sedative properties, and menstrual discomfort caused by the clotting of menstrual blood. In addition to these side effects is the theoretical risk of thrombophilia (7). A contraindication to the use of EACA is a history of thrombosis or epilepsy. In countries outside the USA, tranexamic acid has also been used as prophylaxis, but is not approved for use in the USA.

As noted above, attenuated androgens are used for both long- and short-term prophylaxis for HAE, and have even been used off label for acute HAE attack treatment; however, they are unlikely to have efficacy for acute treatment. Danazol is the attenuated androgen that is most often prescribed to treat HAE, and is approved for adults at doses of 50–200 mg one to three times daily and in some cases every other day therapy is effective. Once it has been initiated, the dose should be titrated down slowly as tolerated to the least effective dose in order to minimize its side effects. Some of these side effects include masculinization, acne, voice deepening, hirsutism, weight gain, and anxiety. This medication can also affect the liver, so liver function tests should be monitored. Additionally, danazol can alter growth in children and it is relatively contraindicated in children. It is contraindicated during pregnancy due to the possibility of masculinization of a female fetus. While attenuated androgens have been shown to be an effective agent, they do have significant dose-related side effects that can limit their use (8).

Recently, C1-INH has been approved by the US Food and Drug Administration for use for the prophylactic treatment of HAE with semi-weekly intravenous infusions of 1,000 units. In many countries, C1-INH has been used for the treatment of acute HAE attacks for over 20 years; however, C1-INH is not yet approved in the USA for acute attacks, although it is sometimes used in the USA as an off-label treatment for acute attacks. Several studies and reports show that the symptoms of acute HAE attacks begin to improve within 30 min of treatment with plasma-purified C1-INH infusion.

Where C1-INH concentrate is unavailable, fresh frozen plasma (FFP) has also been used as an off-label treatment with success for prophylaxis and to treat acute attacks of angioedema. However, because FFP also contains other substrates, including kininogens, there is a potential to worsen some acute attacks of HAE. Despite this potential risk, several groups still treat acute attacks of HAE with FFP when C1-INH concentrate is unavailable, with the knowledge that the benefit and adverse effect profile of C1-INH is superior to FFP (9).

Several other products are being studied in clinical trials that may soon be available. One such product is a recombinant human C1-INH (rhC1-INH) called Rhucin (Pharming, Netherlands). This is similar to human plasma-purified C1-INH, but polysaccharide groups added to the protein cause the half life to be significantly shortened. This results in an effective treatment for acute HAE exacerbations, but probably limits its role as a prophylactic agent.

Other medications are also being developed. Ecallantide (DX-88) (Dyax, Cambridge, MA) is a kallikrein inhibitor and is effective for the acute treatment of HAE, with the advantage of being a subcutaneous injection. Another product being studied for aborting acute attacks of HAE is icatibant. Icatibant (Shire, Germany) is similar in structure to bradykinin and acts as a selective bradykinin-2 receptor antagonist (10).

With the new advances discussed above, the quality of life for patients with HAE is increasing significantly. Nonetheless, the disease is still under-recognized and under-diagnosed. Patients frequently go many years and see many doctors before being diagnosed. The new advances are effective only if the disease is diagnosed and therapy properly instituted. The future for HAE patients will be far brighter than that faced by their parents and ancestors.

Questions

1. Which one of the following is the single best screening test for HAE?

    (a) C2 level
    (b) C3 level
    (c) C4 level
    (d) C1-INH level
    (e) C1-INH functional assay

2. Which of the following laboratory findings would be associated with acquired angioedema, but not HAE?

    (a) Low C1-INH level
    (b) Low C1-INH function
    (c) Low C4 level
    (d) Low C2 level
    (e) Low C1Q level

3. What is thought to be the major mediator causing angioedema in patients with HAE?

    (a) Bradykinin
    (b) C4
    (c) C2
    (d) Kallikrein
    (e) Plasminogen

4. Which one of the following is most likely to be effective for an acute HAE exacerbation?

    (a) Epinephrine

(b) C1-INH infusion
(c) Diphenhydramine
(d) Prednisone
(e) Ranitidine

5. What is the mode of inheritance for HAE?

    (a) X-linked dominant
    (b) X-linked recessive
    (c) Autosomal dominant
    (d) Autosomal recessive

6. Which of the following medications may cause more frequent HAE exacerbations?

    (a) ACE inhibitors
    (b) Beta-blockers
    (c) Estrogens
    (d) Penicillin
    (e) A and C

7. What is the typical length of an untreated HAE exacerbation?

    (a) 30–60 min.
    (b) 1–6 h
    (c) 8–24 h
    (d) 24–48 h
    (e) 48–120 h

8. Which of the following is not likely to be associated with HAE?

    (a) Presence of tingling before episodes of angioedema.
    (b) Itching or hives
    (c) Abdominal pain
    (d) Laryngeal edema
    (e) Limb swelling

9. Which of the following conditions would likely be associated with both normal C4 levels and C1-INH levels?

    (a) HAE type I
    (b) HAE type II
    (c) HAE type III
    (d) Acquired angioedema
    (e) Idiopathic angioedema
    (f) C and E

10. Which of the following treatments may make a person with HAE appear to have a normal C4 level?

    (a) Danazol treatment

(b) Fresh frozen plasma infusion
(c) C1-INH infusions
(d) All of the above

Answers: 1(c), 2(e), 3(a), 4(b), 5(c), 6(e), 7(e), 8(b), 9(f), 10(d)

References

1. Gompels MM, Lock RJ, Abinun M, et al. C1 inhibitor deficiency: consensus document. *Clinical and Experimental Immunology.* 2005; 139: 389–394.
2. Bork K, Gul D, Hardt J, Dewald G. Hereditary angioedema with normal C1 inhibitor: clinical symptoms and course. *The American Journal of Medicine.* 2007; 120: 987–992.
3. Prematta MJ, Kemp JG, Gibbs JG, Mende, C, Rhoads C, Craig TJ. Frequency, timing, and type of prodromal symptoms associated with hereditary angioedema attacks. *Allergy and Asthma Proceedings.* 2009; 30: 506–511.
4. Davis AE III. The pathophysiology of hereditary angioedema. *Clinical Immunology.* 2005; 114: 3–9.
5. Gompels MM, Lock RJ, Morgan JE, et al. A multicentre evaluation of the diagnostic efficiency of serological investigations for C1 inhibitor deficiency. *Journal of Clinical Pathology.* 2002; 55: 145–147.
6. Visy B, Fust G, Bygum A, et al. Helicobacter pylori infection as a triggering factor of attacks in patients with hereditary angioedema. *Helicobacter.* 2007; 12: 251–257.
7. Frank MM, Gelfand JA, Atkinson JP. Hereditary angioedema: the clinical syndrome and its management. *Annals of Internal Medicine.* 1976; 84: 580–593.
8. Hosea SW, Santaella ML, Brown EJ, et al. Long-term therapy of hereditary angioedema with danazol. *Annals of Internal Medicine.* 1980; 93: 809–812.
9. Prematta M, Gibbs JG, Pratt EL, Stoughton TR, Craig TJ. Fresh frozen plasma for the treatment of hereditary angioedema. *Annals of Allergy, Asthma, & Immunology.* 2007; 98: 383–388.
10. Bernstein JA. Hereditary angioedema: a current state-of-the-art review, VIII: current status of emerging therapies. *Annals of Allergy, Asthma, & Immunology.* 2008; 100: S41–46.

Part II
Skin Manifestation of Drug Allergy

Chapter 6
Stevens–Johnson Syndrome/Toxic Epidermal Necrolysis

Satoshi Yoshida

Abstract Stevens–Johnson syndrome and toxic epidermal necrolysis are variants of a single disease because of their manifestations and pathomechanisms. Stevens–Johnson syndrome/toxic epidermal necrolysis is a severe condition within the spectrum of diseases, including erythema multiforme major, toxic epidermal necrolysis, and Stevens–Johnson syndrome, and it is characterized by extensive epidermal death and widespread blisters and erosive lesions. Two challenging cases of toxic and epidermal necrolysis and several case study questions of the Stevens–Johnson syndrome/toxic epidermal necrolysis disease spectrum are discussed.

Keywords Stevens–Johnson syndrome • Toxic epidermal necrolysis • Drug-induced hypersensitive syndrome • Erythema multiforme

Case 1

A 63-year-old man presented to our clinic with complaints of generalized itching rash and high fever. He had liver cirrhosis due to hepatitis C virus contracted 35 years earlier via a blood transfusion during lobectomy of the right lung for tuberculosis. He had also undergone surgery for esophageal varices and hepatocellular carcinoma, and had been treated with amlodipine besylate, atenolol, essential amino-acid granules, furosemide, spironolactone, and ursodeoxycholic acid. Three weeks before consultation, he had started treatment with allopurinol for hyperlithemia. Eighteen days after the start of allopurinol therapy, he developed fever and sore throat. Twenty-three days after the start of treatment, the patient complained of an itching rash on his chest. He was admitted to our hospital because of generalized erythema (Fig. 6.1).

S. Yoshida (✉)
Department of Allergy and Immunology, Johns Hopkins Medicine International,
Tokyo Midtown Medical Center, Tokyo, Japan
e-mail: syoshida-fjt@umin.ac.jp

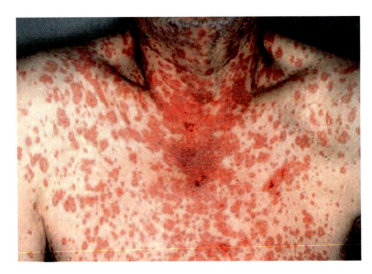

Fig. 6.1 Fingertip-sized areas of erythema with edema were diffusely distributed over the trunk and extremities

Fingertip-sized areas of erythema with edema were diffusely distributed over the trunk and extremities. Some of the lesions were flat, dark red erythema that formed a target-like pattern. No mucocutaneous lesions were identified except for a tiny erosive change on the lower lip. He had adenopathy in his neck, axillary, and groin regions. Body temperature was elevated to 38.8°C.

Data

Laboratory examinations revealed leukocytosis (13,200/μl), neutrophilia (10,620/μl), and atypical lymphocytes (334/μl). Serum levels of liver enzymes: ALT: 45 IU/L, AST: 45 IU/L, and LDH: 567 IU/L, were elevated. Renal function was also impaired (BUN 62.8 mg/dl; creatinine 2.2 mg/dl), and proteinuria was 1.6 g/day. Serum levels of gamma globulin (40.2%), IgG (3,430 mg/dl), and IgA (588 mg/dl) were elevated. Antinuclear antibody was negative and the CD4/CD8 ratio was within normal limits (1.21). The titer of IgG antibodies against human herpes virus-6 was less than 10× at the first visit and showed no increase 7 weeks later (IgG 20×; IgM < 10×). Titers of antibodies against other herpes viruses (cytomegalovirus, Epstein-Barr virus, herpes simplex virus, varicella-zoster virus) in paired serum samples remained unchanged. Antibodies against hepatitis type C virus were positive but those against hepatitis B or human immunodeficiency virus were negative.

Biopsy of a new erythematous lesion of the abdomen revealed panepidermal necrosis resulting from dermoepidermal gap formation (Fig. 6.2). Satellite cell necrosis was identified at junctions with uninvolved skin. Dermal infiltration of mononuclear cells was limited, but some dermal infiltrates stained with antigranzyme B antibody.

6 Stevens–Johnson Syndrome/Toxic Epidermal Necrolysis

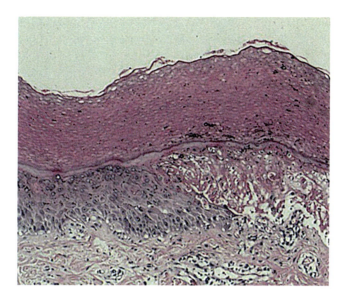

Fig. 6.2 Panepidermal necrosis resulting from dermoepidermal gap formation

Results of drug lymphocyte stimulation tests for allopurinol (320%) and oxypurinol (244%) were within normal limits (<180%).

Drug-induced hypersensitivity syndrome, Stevens–Johnson syndrome, and toxic epidermal necrolysis were suspected, and all drugs were discontinued immediately. Treatment with antihistamine and topical corticosteroids could not control the exanthema. The erythema rapidly spread, and resulted in painful erythroderma with elevation of body temperature to 40°C.

1. With the presented data, what is your diagnosis and why?
   (a) Drug-induced hypersensitive syndrome
   (b) Toxic epidermal necrolysis
   (c) Staphylococcal scalded skin syndrome
   (d) Pityriasis rosea

Answer: (b)

Histopathologically proven epidermal cell death has a diagnostic value equivalent to that of clinical detachment in a case with abortive skin manifestations. Immediate histological investigations are indispensable in drug-induced hypersensitivity syndrome. Also, the absence of extensive bloody blisters and erosive changes of the mucous membrane is not suggestive of Stevens–Johnson syndrome.

Staphylococcal scalded skin syndrome is induced by epidermolytic exotoxins (exfoliatin A and B), which are released by *Staphylococcal aureus* and cause detachment within the epidermal layer. One of the exotoxins is produced by the bacterial chromosome, while the other is produced by a plasmid, which is a piece of self-replicating DNA that often code for secondary characteristics, such as antibiotic resistance and toxin production. These exotoxins are proteases that cleave desmoglein-1, which normally holds the granulosum and spinosum layers together.

Pityriasis rosea is an acute, benign, self-limiting skin rash. Classically, it begins with a single "herald patch" lesion, followed in 1 or 2 weeks by a generalized body rash lasting about 6 weeks. Its etiology is unknown, though it is thought to involve viral infection. An upper respiratory tract infection may precede all other symptoms in as many as 68.8% of patients.

Discussion

First described in 1922, Stevens–Johnson syndrome is an immune-complex-mediated hypersensitivity complex that is a severe expression of erythema multiforme (1). It is known by some as erythema multiforme major, but disagreement exists in the literature. Stevens–Johnson syndrome and toxic epidermal necrolysis have been considered variants of a single disease. For that reason, many refer to the entity as Stevens–Johnson syndrome/toxic epidermal necrolysis. Stevens–Johnson syndrome/toxic epidermal necrolysis occurs with a worldwide distribution similar in etiology and occurrence to that in the United States. Cases tend to have a propensity for the early spring and winter. In Stevens–Johnson syndrome, the male-to-female ratio is 2:1. Most patients are in the second to fourth decade of their lives; however, cases in children as young as 3 months have been reported.

At the early stage, clinical presentations of Stevens–Johnson syndrome/toxic epidermal necrolysis are very similar to those of ordinary types of drug-induced skin reactions. As a consequence of this, diagnosis of Stevens–Johnson syndrome/toxic epidermal necrolysis is difficult, and the start of treatment is often delayed, resulting in the high mortality rates of Stevens–Johnson syndrome/toxic epidermal necrolysis. Lesions may continue to erupt in crops for as long as 2–3 weeks. An acute rash progresses toward widespread blisters and erosions of skin and mucous membranes. The rash can begin as macules that develop into papules, vesicles, bullae, urticarial plaques, or confluent erythema. The center of these lesions may be vesicular, purpuric, or necrotic. The typical lesion has the appearance of a target. The target is considered pathognomonic. However, in contrast to the typical erythema multiforme lesions, these lesions have only two zones of color. The core may be vesicular, purpuric, or necrotic; that zone is surrounded by macular erythema. Some have called these targetoid lesions. Lesions may become bullous and later rupture, leaving denuded skin. The skin becomes susceptible to secondary infection. Macules rapidly spread and coalesce, leading to epidermal blistering, necrosis, and sloughing. While minor presentations may occur, significant involvement of oral, nasal, eye, vaginal, urethral, gastrointestinal tract, and lower respiratory tract mucous membranes may develop in the course of the illness. Gastrointestinal tract and respiratory involvement may progress to necrosis. Mucosal pseudomembrane formation may lead to mucosal scarring and the loss of function of the involved organ system. Esophageal strictures may occur when extensive involvement of the esophagus exists. Mucosal shedding in the tracheobronchial tree may lead to respiratory failure. Ocular sequelae may include corneal ulceration and anterior uveitis. Blindness may develop secondary to severe keratitis or panophthalmitis in 3–10% of patients. Vaginal stenosis and penile scarring have been reported. Renal complications are rare.

The four etiologic categories are reported, such as (1) infectious, (2) drug-induced, (3) malignancy-related, and (4) idiopathic. More than half of the patients with Stevens–Johnson syndrome report a recent upper respiratory tract infection. Viral diseases that have been reported include herpes simplex virus, human immunodeficiency virus, coxsackie viral infections, influenza, hepatitis, mumps, mycoplasmal infection, lymphogranuloma venereum, rickettsial infections, and variola. Bacterial etiologies include group A beta streptococci, diphtheria, brucellosis, mycobacteria, Mycoplasma pneumoniae, tularemia, and typhoid. An "incomplete" case was recently reported after *Mycoplasma pneumoniae* infection (2). Coccidioidomycosis, dermatophytosis, and histoplasmosis are the fungal possibilities. Malaria and trichomoniasis have been reported as protozoal causes. In children, Epstein–Barr virus and enteroviruses have been identified. Drug etiologies include penicillins, antibacterial sulfonamides, oxicam nonsteroidal antiinflammatory drugs, nevirapine, or allopurinol. Anticonvulsants, including phenytoin, carbamazepine, valproic acid, lamotrigine, and barbiturates, have been implicated. Mockenhapupt et al. stressed that most anticonvulsant-induced Stevens–Johnson syndrome occurs in the first 60 days of use (3). In late 2002, the United States Food and Drug Administration (FDA) and the manufacturer Pharmacia noted that Stevens–Johnson syndrome had been reported in patients taking the cyclooxygenase-2 inhibitor valdecoxib. In 2007, the FDA reported Stevens–Johnson syndrome/toxic epidermal necrolysis in patients taking modafinil. Allopurinol has recently been implicated as the most common cause in Europe and Israel (4). Cocaine recently has been added to the list of drugs capable of producing the syndrome. Various carcinomas and lymphomas have been associated. Incidence and/ or severity of both disorders may be higher in bone-marrow transplant recipients, in *Pneumocystis jiroveci* (formerly *Pneumocystis carinii*) infected human immunodeficiency virus patients, and in patients with systemic lupus erythematosus. Stevens–Johnson syndrome is idiopathic in 25–50% of cases.

Diagnosis is usually obvious by the appearance of initial lesions and clinical syndrome. In up to half of cases, no specific etiology has been identified. Treatment is supportive care; corticosteroids, cyclophosphamide, and other drugs may be tried. Roujeau proposed the following criteria: the ratio of the detached area to the whole body surface was less than 10% for Stevens–Johnson syndrome, more than 30% for toxic epidermal necrolysis, and 10–30% for Stevens–Johnson syndrome/ toxic epidermal necrolysis overlap (5). This criteria has been well known as the commonly accepted definition named SCORTEN (a toxic epidermal necrolysis-specific illness severity score) (6). A skin biopsy may be performed. The recent diagnostic criteria for toxic epidermal necrolysis issued by the Japanese Ministry of Heath, Labor and Welfare are as follows: Toxic epidermal necrolysis is a mucocutaneous disorder involving more than 10% of the total body surface area, characterized by extensive erythema, blister, epidermal detachment, erosions, enanthema, and high fever. Pathologically, multiple keratinocyte death (apoptosis) results causing separation of the epidermis from the dermis. The death receptor, Fas, and its ligand, FasL, have been linked to the process. Some have also been thought to be linked inflammatory cytokines to the pathogenesis. Nevertheless, the pathomechanisms of these diseases are still not understood fully.

The cornerstone of treatment for toxic epidermal necrolysis and so called transitional Stevens–Johnson syndrome/toxic epidermal necrolysis is meticulous skin care, fluid replacement, nutritional support, and surveillance for and aggressive treatment of infection. The administration of systemic corticosteroids in the treatment of Stevens–Johnson syndrome and toxic epidermal necrolysis is contraversial. There are several open-label retrospectives published concerning the treatment of Stevens–Johnson syndrome/toxic epidermal necrolysis overlap or toxic epidermal necrolysis in adults and children with cyclosporine, plasmapheresis, corticosteroids, pentoxyfilline, mycophenolate mofetil, and cyclophosphamide.

Prognosis depends on how early the syndromes are diagnosed and treated; mortality may reach 40%. Stevens–Johnson syndrome and toxic epidermal necrolysis are clinically similar except for their distribution. Although they are rare diseases, as the disorders affect between 1 and 5 people/million, their mortality rates are determined primarily by the extent of skin sloughing. When body surface area sloughing is less than 10%, the mortality rate is approximately 1–5%. However, when more than 30% of body surface area sloughing is present, the mortality rate is between 25% and 35%. Immediate diagnosis and early application of appropriate treatment are essential.

In the present case, a 3-week history of treatment with allopurinol, fever, peripheral atypical lymphocytes, lymphadenopathy, and liver and renal involvement suggested drug-induced hypersensitivity at first. Serial polymerase chain reaction and antibody examination rules out reactivation of herpes virus, including human herpes virus 6. In addition, panepidermal death on histopathological examination excluded drug-induced hypersensitivity syndrome. The absence of extensive bloody blisters and erosive changes of the mucous membrane was not suggestive of Stevens–Johnson syndrome. Blisters and epidermal detachment were not apparent. However, this case was diagnosed as toxic epidermal necrolysis because of erythroderma with histopathologically proven parenchymal cell death, representing invisible epidermal detachment. Extensive death of the epidermis and mucous membrane triggers a cytokine and chemical mediator storm and occasionally results in severe liver, renal, and interstitial dysfunction. Skin manifestations and renal dysfunction in this patient responded well to oral prednisolone.

Drugs including antibiotics, nonsteroid antiinflammatory drugs, anticonvulsants, and allopurinol have been suspected to be the main causative agents of toxic epidermal necrolysis. The causative drug was not determined in the present case. However, 3 weeks of treatment with allopurinol and multiorgan involvement suggested that allopurinol should be the causative agent. Allopurinol is a major causative agent of drug-induced hypersensitivity syndrome, which was initially suspected in the present patient. Virological and serological investigations excluded drug-induced hypersensitivity syndrome, but clinically invisible epidermal detachment might cause toxic epidermal necrolysis to be overlooked. Rapid snap-frozen section diagnosis might be helpful for diagnosis. Therefore, immediate histological investigation is indispensable when drug-induced hypersensitivity syndrome, toxic epidermal necrolysis, and related diseases are suspected.

Case 2

A 67-year-old man presented with a severe cutaneous eruption that had begun 3 days after taking naproxen sodium. His medical history revealed a similar eruption three times after the intake of naproxen, in the last 5 years. Ten days before admission, he had received tobramycin ophthalmic solution for keratitis of the right eye and naproxen sodium for analgesia. After the use of these agents only once, an erythematous and bullous rash had started on his face and neck, which rapidly spread to his arms and legs. His past medical history included a 15-year history of insulin-dependent diabetes mellitus, glaucoma of the right eye, and peripheral arterial disease on both legs. He had suffered from a cerebrovascular event 2 years ago and had been taking piracetam 800 mg/day and ginkgo glycosides 9.6 mg/day since then.

On physical examination, he was found to have malaise and fever (37.5–38.6°C) and his general status was poor. Ophthalmologic assessment revealed abscess formation on the corneal and scleral tissues of the right eye, with prominent erythema and a dense purulent secretion. Dermatologic examination showed an erythematous and bullous eruption located mainly on the face, neck, upper chest, and the sun-exposed parts of the upper extremities. A few target lesions were scattered on the trunk (Fig. 6.3). The lesions showed a sharp demarcation at the collar line and on the arms not covered by shirt. On some areas, flaccid bullae and erosions were confluent. Nikolsky's sign was positive. The extent of involvement was approximately 30–40% of the body surface. In addition to skin lesions, he showed erosions on the buccal and palatal mucosa.

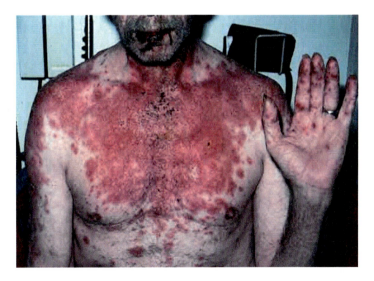

Fig. 6.3 Erythematous and bulbous eruptions located mainly on the face, neck, upper chest, and the sun-exposed parts of the upper extremities. A few target lesions were scattered on the trunk

Data

Skin biopsy revealed extensive epidermal necrosis (Fig. 6.4). The intact areas around the necrosis showed vacuolar degeneration of the layer, edema of the superficial dermis, melanophages, and a mild perivascular lymphocytic infiltration. Laboratory tests yielded the following pathological changes: erythrocyte sedimentation rate 80 mm/h, CRP 58.50 mg/dl, fibrinogen 532 mg/dl, creatinin 5.8 g/dl, LDH 1206 U/L, creatinin kinase 344 U/L, ALT 48 U/L, AST 18 U/L, gamma GTP 64 U/L, albumin 3.1 g/dl, total protein 6.4 g/dl, leukocytes $14.3 \times 103/\mu l$, neutrophils 88.7%, Hb 12.2 g/dl. Ht 36.5%, and thrombocytes $550 \times 103/\mu l$.

1. With the presented data what etiology do you consider in this patient?

    (a) Adverse interaction among prescribed medication
    (b) Viral infection
    (c) Autoimmune reaction
    (d) Photo-induced sensitivity

2. What is your diagnosis and how do you treat this patient?

    (a) Cutaneous phlegmon
    (b) Photoallergic contact dermatitis

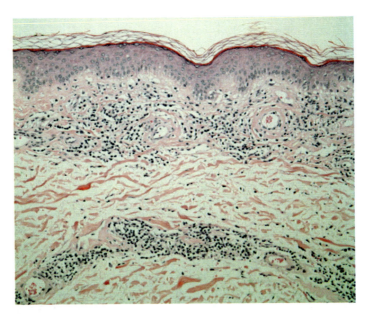

Fig. 6.4 Extensive epidermal necrosis with lymphocytes infiltration to the upper dermis

(c) Photo-induced toxic epidermal necrolysis
(d) Drug-induced lupus erythematosus

Answers: 1(d), 2(c)

Photoallergic contact dermatitis is an eczematous delayed-type hypersensitivity response of the skin when affected by a combination of allergen and ultraviolet light (mostly UVA; Ultraviolet A). Only previously sensitized persons can develop a photoallergic reaction. Common photoallergic agents include sunscreens, fragrances, antibacterial agents such as chlorhexidine, and drugs such as chlorpromazine and promethazine.

Drug-induced lupus erythematosus is an autoimmune disorder, similar to systemic lupus erythematosus, which is induced by the chronic use of certain drugs. These drugs cause an autoimmune response producing symptoms similar to those of systemic lupus erythematosus. There are 38 known medications that cause drug-induced lupus erythematosus, but there are three that report the highest number of cases: hydralazine, procainamide, and isoniazid. While the criteria for diagnosing drug-induced lupus erythematosus have not been thoroughly established, symptoms of drug-induced lupus erythematosus typically present as myalgia and arthralgia. Generally, the symptoms recede after discontinuing the use of the drugs, but there are reported cases of drug-induced lupus erythematosus that do not go away completely after the offending drug is removed. In patients with systemic lupus erythematosus, photosensitivity is frequently observed as well as in healthy subjects. In people with cutaneous lupus, photosensitivity affects 50% of those with discoid lupus and 70–90% of those with subacute cutaneous lupus. Its prevalence is significantly higher in systemic lupus erythematosus than in controls only when it is detected using the laboratory method.

Discussion

In some reported case of Stevens–Johnson syndrome and erythema multiforme, which are considered in the same spectrum of toxic epidermal necrolysis with a less severe clinical course, skin lesions were mainly located on sun-exposed areas. In some of the case reports, the lesions had developed after ingestion of clobazam, sulfasalazine, chloroquine, and sulfadoxine/pyrimethamine (7). In this case, a young female while treating with clobazam had developed lesions of toxic epidermal necrolysis in light exposed area. Patch and photopatch tests with clobazam were negative.

The pathogenesis of photo-induced erythema multiforme, Steven–Johnson syndrome, and toxic epidermal necrolysis is unknown. It is well known that erythema multiforme lesions may occur at skin sites of recent physical trauma or sunburn, and these reactions are usually assumed to be a recipient isomorphic (Koebner) phenomenon. In the photo-Koebner phenomenon of erythema multiforme, ultraviolet radiation is thought to induce the release of mediators that increase vascular permeability and promote the deposition of immune complexes in the skin. In the aforementioned cases of Stevens–Johnson syndrome/toxic epidermal necrolysis with photo-distributed lesions, the phototoxic effects of sulfonamides are speculated as inducing the lesions.

The role of ultraviolet light (UV) in photo-induced toxic epidermal necrolysis, although hypothetical, can be explained by the following mechanism. Recent studies showed a clear predominance of CD8+ T lymphocytes in the epidermis of toxic epidermal necrolysis (8). Cytotoxic T lymphocytes have a major role in epidermal damage, possibly by means of cytokine synthesis. Intracellular adhesion molecule 1 (ICAM-1) is thought to play a role in the trafficking of T lymphocytes to the epidermis. It is known that UVB induces tumor necrosis factor-alpha and interleukin-1 secretion by keratinocytes, and that these cytokines are capable of increasing the expression of ICAM-1. Thus, activated cytotoxic T lymphocytes present in the bloodstream are attracted by the death of these cells. As a result, UV has the potential to exaggerate the reaction, even though it is not the initiator.

Among the drugs responsible for toxic epidermal necrolysis, nonsteroidal antiinflammatory drugs, including naproxen, are usually the leading group. Naproxen is also well known for its phototoxic effect. We do not know the exact mechanisms involving the occurrence of toxic epidermal necrolysis lesions conflicted to sun-exposed areas in this patient. It may be speculated that the phototoxic potential of naproxen is responsible for this reaction. However, the previous and less severe eruptions because of naproxen may indicate an immunological mechanism. The rapid onset of lesions after only one dose of naproxen also seems to be in favor of an immune pathogenesis. In this case, the provocative photo test could not be performed, as the lesions were widespread, and the general status of the patient was poor.

Questions

A previously healthy 19-month-old girl with an upper respiratory infection was treated with ampicillin-sulbactam. Ten days later, she developed a rash that worsened, with a sore mouth, lips, and eyes and in another few days, erythema, malaise, intermittent pyrexia, photophobia, and dysuria (Figs. 6.5 and 6.6). She had no previously known drug allergies, and was on no medication except ampicillin-sulbactam. Her past medical and family histories were noncontributory.

Upon admission, she was in considerable pain from severe oropharyngeal, genital, and corneal ulcerations. She was unable to speak or to take fluids by month, and unable to open her eyes. Micturition was exceedingly painful. She had an extensive, generalized, maculopapular eruption, crusts, and blisters with separation of sheets of skin in areas where the blisters had become confluent, as well as bullous lesions with a positive Nikolsky's sign. We estimated that approximately 30% of her total body skin area was eroded. She had hemorrhagic erosions of lips, with the loss of epithelium from the oropharynx and from the vulva.

Laboratory evaluations found a leukocyte count of $7.4 \times 10^3/\mu l$ with 5% eosinophils, hemoglobin of 12.8 g/ml, and platelets of $109 \times 10^3/\mu l$. Urinalysis and serum chemistries

6 Stevens–Johnson Syndrome/Toxic Epidermal Necrolysis

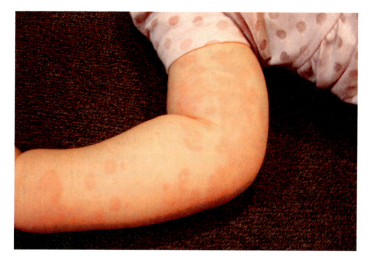

Fig. 6.5 Progressive multiple target-like erythema appeared in extremities

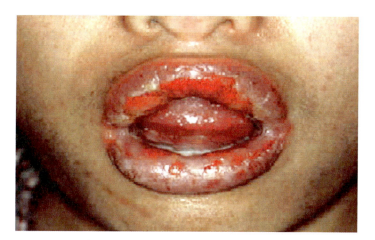

Fig. 6.6 Cheilmucositis around lips

were normal except for a slightly elevated liver function test results. Urine, blood, and serum chemistries were normal except for a slightly elevated liver function test results. Urine, blood, and sputum cultures were negative, and chest radiograph was within normal limits. Bacteriologic and virologic cultures of specimens collected from cutaneous lesions were negative. Serologic tests for varicella-zoster virus and herpes virus were negative. Biopsy of a new erythematous lesion of extremities revealed panepidermal necrosis (Fig. 6.7).

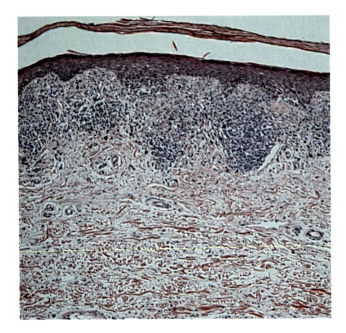

Fig. 6.7 Biopsy of a new erythematous lesion of extremities revealed panepidermal necrosis with lymphocytes infiltration as well as multiple keratinocyte apoptosis of the epidermis

1. What is your diagnosis and why?

    (a) Erythema multiforme
    (b) Stevens–Johnson syndrome
    (c) Toxic epidermal necrolysis
    (d) Stevens–Johnson syndrome/toxic epidermal necrolysis overlap

2. What is the appropriate therapy for this patient?

    (a) Antibiotics
    (b) Intravenous immunoglobulin therapy
    (c) Topical corticosteroid
    (d) Hemodialysis

Answers: 1. (d), 2. (b)

The primary clinical differentiation in children has to be made from staphylococcal scalded skin syndrome, which follows an infection by group 2 phage-type staphylococci that elaborate an epidermolytic exotoxin that produces changes in upper epidermolytic exotoxin that produces changes in upper epidermal layers.

As mentioned in the criteria of SCORTEN (a toxic epidermal necrolysis-specific illness severity score): the ratio of the detached area to the whole body surface was less than 10% for Stevens–Johnson syndrome, more than 30% for toxic epidermal necrolysis, and 10–30% for Stevens–Johnson syndrome/toxic epidermal necrolysis overlap (6). Diverse etiologies have been invoked for Stevens–Johnson syndrome/toxic epidermal necrolysis overlap and toxic epidermal necrolysis. However, the overwhelming majority of occurrences are drug induced. Scores of drugs have been implicated, the most notorious of which are nonsteroidal antiinflammatory drugs, anticonvulsants, and antibiotics such as penicillin and sulfonamides. This patient has developed Stevens–Johnson syndrome/toxic epidermal necrolysis overlap probably caused by semisynthetic penicillin.

Mechanisms leading to toxic epidermal necrolysis and Stevens–Johnson syndrome remain unknown. However, when drugs are incriminated, reactions are immunologically mediated and also related to abdominal drug metabolism. Overlap Stevens–Johnson syndrome/toxic epidermal necrolysis and toxic epidermal necrolysis are characterized by the rapid onset of extensive keratinocyte apoptosis and epidermal detachment accompanied by a high rate of mortality. Paul et al. proposed that keratinocyte apoptosis occurs as a result of enhanced keratinocyte FasL (CD95L) expression, which induces Fas-mediated keratinocyte cell death (9). Other cytokines, such as tumor necrosis factor alpha, which are elaborated by CD8+ and natural killer cells, may also be responsible for apoptosis.

Fas-mediated keratinocyte cell death can be potently inhibited by intravenous immunoglobulin therapy in vitro, and this provided the rationale for investigating the therapeutic potential of intravenous immunoglobulin therapy in the treatment of toxic epidermal necrolysis. Other suggested mechanisms of action of intravenous immunoglobulin therapy include the elimination of circulating immune blockade of antibody Fc receptors and the regulation of cellular immune responses. Intravenous immunoglobulin treatment was used in an open study of ten patients with Stevens–Johnson syndrome or toxic epidermal necrolysis who all survived. The progression of the skin lesions stopped after intravenous immunoglobulin therapy infusion within 24–48 h, and skin healing was rapid and without significant adverse effects. Some investigators have supported the use of intravenous immunoglobulin therapy to treat patients with toxic epidermal necrolysis or Stevens–Johnson syndrome/toxic epidermal necrolysis overlap. Trend et al. reported that based on comparison of their observed mortality rate with SCORTEN prevented mortality rate, treatment with intravenous immunoglobulin therapy significantly decreased mortality in 16 patients with toxic epidermal necrolysis (6). Prins et al. reported that early infusion of high dose intravenous immunoglobulin therapy is safe, well tolerated, and likely to be effective in improving the survival of patients with toxic epidermal necrolysis (total body surface area >10%) in their multicenter retrospective analysis of 48 consecutive cases (9). Tristani-Firouzi et al. reported a series of eight children with toxic epidermal necrolysis who were safely and effectively treated with intravenous immunoglobulin therapy between 1999 and 2001 (10). Despite significant TBSA involvement, all their patients survived. In addition, the treatment with intravenous immunoglobulin therapy resulted of arrest in progression of toxic epidermal necrolysis and rapid reepithelialization, without any toxicity from the drug itself. Bechot et al. reached an opposing conclusion in their study of 34 patients from a single referral center using a comparison of the outcome of these patients with the death rate predicted by the SCORTEN score (11). In that study, SCORTEN predicted a 24% death rate but a death rate of 32% occurred, with the majority of deaths occurring in elderly patients with initial deterioration in renal function.

Early diagnosis and implementation of supportive care and careful monitoring for complication is of vital importance in the management of toxic epidermal necrolysis and Stevens–Johnson syndrome. Although a variety of possible therapeutic modalities have been proposed, not proved and widely accepted treatment regimen exists.

Case 2

A 46-year-old woman was admitted to the hospital with a pruritic, generalized maculopapular eruption (Fig. 6.8). Her medications included fluoxetine hydrochloride, levothyroxine sodium, and nabumetone. Eight days earlier, she had taken two doses of pseudoephedrine hydrochloride for nasal congestion. Two days later, she began taking cefaclor, and the following day, she presented to the emergency department with lip swelling, oral ulcers, and an erythematous, pruritic eruption on her abdomen and thighs. She was treated with diphenhydramine and discharged but was subsequently admitted 2 days later because of a progressive eruption.

On examination, oropharyngeal ulcers and a generalized eruption with occasional target lesions were observed. She was afebrile with stable vital signs. She had no lymphadenopathy. Initial liver, kidney, and thyroid function tests were within normal limits. During the subsequent week, bullae developed over 15% of the patient's body surface. We performed patch testing with nabumetone and pseudoephedrine, with no reactions. Skin biopsy was also performed (Fig. 6.9).

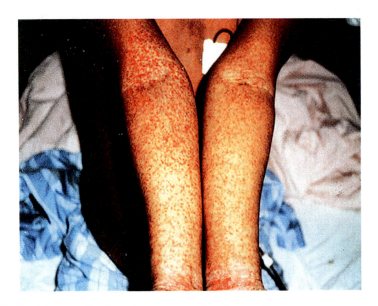

Fig. 6.8 Pruritic, generalized maculopapular eruption of extremities

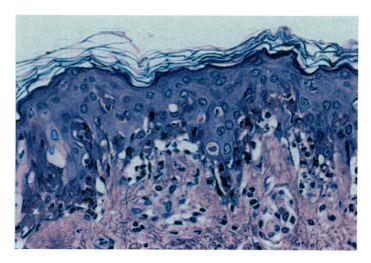

Fig. 6.9 Adepidermal blisters, multiple keratinocyte apoptosis of the epidermis, and lymphocytes infiltration to the upper dermis

3. What medicine is thought to be involved in this patient's progressive eruption?

   (a) Fluoxetine hydrochloride
   (b) Nabumetone
   (c) Pseudoephedrine hydrochloride
   (d) Cefaclor

4. What the skin biopsy demonstrate in this patient? (See Fig. 6.9).

   (a) Epidermal necrolysis
   (b) Vacuolar degeneration of parabasal keratinocytes
   (c) Acantholysis
   (d) Patchy infiltration of lymphocytes

Answers: 3. (b), 4. (a)

Pseudoephedrine is a sympathomimetic agent that is commonly found in over-the-counter cough and cold preparations. In this case, nabumetone was thought to be the most likely culprit for this patient's eruption. Cefaclor was not strongly suspected because the patient had only been taking it for 24 h, and toxic epidermal necrolysis usually takes 1–3 weeks to develop in a patient who has not previously been sensitized to the drug.

Biopsy demonstrated diffuse infiltration of the dermis by lymphocytes and eosinophils. The rash resolved on discontinuation of the use of the dextromethorphan-pseudoephedrine product and treatment with antihistamines, prednisone, and topical corticosteroids. When evaluating a patient with potential adverse drug reactions, clinicians should be aware that culprit drugs might be present in multicompound products. A careful history that includes all drugs exposure can be critical to establishing the underlying cause and preventing recurrence.

Case 3

Three years ago, a 26-month-old boy had developed erythema multiforme after taking amoxicillin-clavulanate and hives after trimethoprim-sulfamethoxazole. Thereafter, he had no history of illness during these 2 years, including no symptoms or signs of infection, or medication use before receiving varicella vaccine. One day after vaccination, he developed a maculopapular exanthema over his face and torso. Three days after vaccination, the rash progressed to target lesions with sporadic bulbous lesions on the arms and vesicular lesions in his conjunctivae and mouth, associated with low-grade fever (Fig. 6.10). On the fifth day after vaccination, he was hospitalized because of mucositis, involving the lips, eyes, anus, and penile meatus (Fig. 6.11). During hospitalization, he developed cholestasis with jaundice and abnormal liver function tests. Ultrasound examination of his abdomen was normal. Blood and urine cultures were sterile, as were lesional cultures for cytomegalovirus, varicella, and herpes simplex virus. Serologic testing for *Mycoplasma pneumonia* was not reported. Skin biopsy of erythematous lesion was performed (Fig. 6.12).

5. What is the possible etiology of progressive rash?

    (a) Adverse effect of varicella vaccine
    (b) Vaccine-related allergic reaction
    (c) Allergic cross-reaction to amoxicillin-clavulanate
    (d) Infection transmitted through contaminated vaccine

6. What pathological findings should NOT be useful for the diagnosis?

    (a) Perivascular infiltration with eosinophils
    (b) Multiple keratinocyte apoptosis of the epidermis

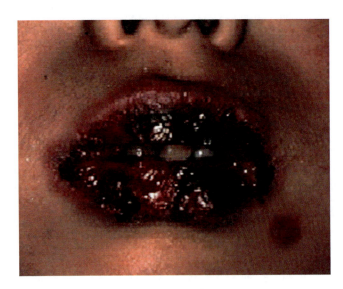

Fig. 6.10 Mouth blisters with crustal and necrotic lesion

6 Stevens–Johnson Syndrome/Toxic Epidermal Necrolysis 107

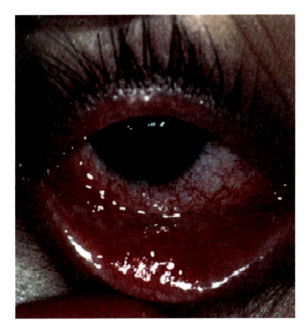

Fig. 6.11 Severe conjunctivitis with microulceration in bulbar conjunctiva or cornea

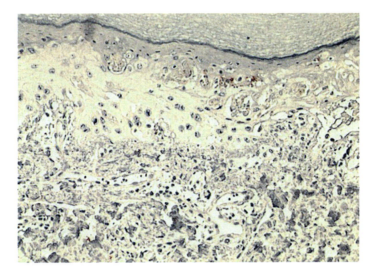

Fig. 6.12 Adepidermal blisters, lymphocytes infiltration to the upper dermis, and dermoepidermal gap

(c) Adepidermal blisters
(d) Lymphocytes infiltration to the upper dermis

Answers: 5. (b), 6. (b, c, d)

A causal link between Stevens–Johnson syndrome/toxic epidermal necrolysis and vaccination has not been established; one reason is that the vaccinated individuals may have inapparent illness or be on mediations at the time of vaccination. In addition, the studies have been limited by the absence of reports demonstrating recurrence of Stevens–Johnson syndrome/toxic epidermal necrolysis with revaccination. Stevens–Johnson syndrome and toxic epidermal necrolysis may also occur ideopathically.

When a case of Stevens–Johnson syndrome or toxic epidermal necrolysis occurs after vaccination, a complete diagnostic evaluation should be undertaken to determine the etiology. The antigen vaccines often contain other components, such as adjuvant and preservative. When evaluating whether a vaccine causes Steven–Johnson syndrome or toxic epidermal necrolysis, the other components can also have important clinical implications. For example, if a person has a previous episode of Stevens–Johnson syndrome or toxic epidermal necrolysis after an antibiotic, the antibiotic content of all vaccines should be reviewed before administration. Varicella vaccine contains the antibiotic neomycin. Neomycin has cross-sensitivity with other aminoglycoside antibiotic; the varicella vaccine might be contraindicated.

Despite the plausibility of a causal relationship between vaccination and Steven–Johnson syndrome/toxic epidermal necrolysis, it happens very rarely and under most circumstances is unlikely to outweigh the benefits of vaccination. Although immunization has not been evaluated as an etiology of Stevens–Johnson syndrome and toxic epidermal necrolysis, the possible role of immunization should be considered in future studies because of the severe morbidity and mortality associated with Stevens–Johnson syndrome and toxic epidermal necrolysis and plausibility of this hypothesis.

In this patient, treatment consisted of intravenous fluids, parenteral nutrition, bacitracin ointment locally on exposed surfaces, hydrogel sheet dressings for open wounds, hydroxyzine hydrochloride for itching, erythromycin ointment and artificial tears in the eyes, and chlorhexidine swabs, magnesium hydroxide, simethicone and viscous lidocaine for dental care.

References

1. Parrillo SJ. Stevens-Johnson syndrome and toxic epidermal necrolysis. Curr Allergy Asthma Rep. 2007;7(4):243–7.
2. Hillebrand-Haverkort ME, Budding AE, bij de Vaate LA, van Agtmael MA. Mycoplasma pneumoniae infection with incomplete Stevens-Johnson syndrome. Lancet Infect Dis. 2008;8(10):586–7.
3. Mockenhaupt M, Messenheimer J, Tennis P, et al. Risk of Stevens-Johnson syndrome and toxic epidermal necrolysis in new users of antiepileptics. Neurology. 2005;64(7):1134–8.
4. Halevy S, Ghislain PD, Mockenhaupt M, Fagot JP, Bouwes Bavinck JN, Sidoroff A, et al. Allopurinol is the most common cause of Stevens-Johnson syndrome and toxic epidermal necrolysis in Europe and Israel. J Am Acad Dermatol. 2008;58(1):25–32.
5. Roujeau JC. The spectrum of Stevens Johnson syndrome and toxic epidermal necrolysis: a clinical classification. J Invest Dermatol. 1994; 102(1): 28S–30S.

6. Bastuji-Garin S, Fouchard N, Bertocchi M, et al. SCORTEN: a severity-of-illness score for toxic epidermal necrolysis. J Invest Dermatol. 2000;115(2):149–53.
7. Gambichler T, Al-Muhammadi R, Boms S. Immunologically mediated photodermatoses: diagnosis and treatment. Am J Clin Dermatol. 2009;10(3):169–80.
8. Redondo P, Vicente J, España A, Subira ML, De Felipe I, Quintanilla E. Photo-induced toxic epidermal necrolysis caused by clobazam. Br J Dermatol. 1996; 135(6):999–1002.
9. Paul C, Wolkenstein P, Adle H, Wechsler J, Garchon HJ, Revuz J, Roujeau JC. Apoptosis as a mechanism of keratinocyte death in toxic epidermal necrolysis. Br J Dermatol. 1996;134(4):710–4.
10. Prins C, Kerdel FA, Padilla RS, Hunziker T, Chimenti S, Viard I, Mauri DN, Flynn K, Trent J, Margolis DJ, Saurat JH, French LE; TEN-IVIG Study Group. Toxic epidermal necrolysis-intravenous immunoglobulin. Treatment of toxic epidermal necrolysis with high-dose intravenous immunoglobulins: multicenter retrospective analysis of 48 consecutive cases. Arch Dermatol. 2003;139(1):26–32.
11. Tristani-Firouzi P, Petersen MJ, Saffle JR, Morris SE, Zone JJ. Treatment of toxic epidermal necrolysis with intravenous immunoglobulin in children. J Am Acad Dermatol. 2002; 47(4):548–52.
12. Bachot N, Revuz J, Roujeau JC. Intravenous immunoglobulin treatment for Stevens-Johnson syndrome and toxic epidermal necrolysis: a prospective noncomparative study showing no benefit on mortality or progression. Arch Dermatol. 2003;139(1):33–6.

Chapter 7
Serum Sickness and Serum Sickness-Like Reaction

Neha Reshamwala and Massoud Mahmoudi

Abstract Serum sickness is an immune complex reaction, hypersensitivity type III, to a protein, serum, or hapten. The manifestations are based on antibody–antigen complexes developing 1–3 weeks postexposure to the antigen, but sooner upon reexposure, with the presentation of a multitude of symptoms (J Microbiol Immunol Infect 34:220–223, 2001). Other similar conditions can mimic or overlap the diagnosis and characteristics of serum sickness. Here, we present two challenging cases of serum sickness and serum sickness-like reaction.

Keywords Serum sickness • Serum sickness-like reaction • Immune complexes • Hypersensitivity reaction

Case 1

The patient is a 6-year-old Caucasian male who was initially seen in the allergy and immunology clinic in 2003 for evaluation. He had a history of prolonged upper respiratory infections followed by numerous sinus infections that were difficult to clear. In February 2005, he received amoxicillin for an unremitting recurrent sinus infection. One to two days into the treatment course, he developed a pinpoint rash. Approximately 4 days into treatment, he had no improvement of his fever, purulent nasal discharge, or upper respiratory symptoms, and was switched to Augmentin (amoxicillin/clavulanic acid). He then developed a progressive and

---

M. Mahmoudi (✉)
El Camino Hospital, Los Gatos, Los Gatos, CA, USA
and
Department of Medicine, University of California, San Francisco,
San Francisco, CA, USA
e-mail: allergycure@sbcglobal.net

diffuse pruritic rash, significant swelling, erythema, and pain of the knee and ankle joints, along with urticaria and bullae. His symptoms continued to be treated and finally resolved.

In February 2009, after being lost to follow-up, the patient presented to the allergy and immunology clinic with hives, throat tightness, knee and ankle joint swelling and pain after starting treatment with Keflex (cephalexin) for group A streptococcus buttock abscess, and throat infection. After the second dose, he developed hives and along with mild throat swelling. Since this episode, he complains of diffuse pruritus, and also knee, ankle, and back pain that is fairly constant but waxes and wanes depending on his activity level. His parents feel that he has intermittent low-grade temperatures and prolonged erythema.

Past medical history. It is significant for mild intermittent asthma since 2 years of age, exercise-induced asthma requiring albuterol, and mild eczema as an infant. Peanut allergy was diagnosed at 3 years, with a history of anaphylactic reaction.

Family history: Mother and father have asthma. Mother has rheumatoid arthritis, hypothyroidism, and type 2 diabetes.

Social and environmental history. The patient lives with his mother and father. There are no other siblings. The mother works as a special education administrator, and the father works as a psychotherapist. There are no pets, no smoke exposure, and no recent travel or sick contacts. His immunizations are up to date. There is no history of reaction to immunizations. He is attending first grade and has normal developmental skills. He is able to participate in sports with the use of mild albuterol for exercise-induced asthma. The family has dust mite protection on the pillow cases and mattress, and has hardwood floors with no carpeting.

Review of systems. He had one episode of vomiting 2½ weeks ago but no recent fevers, diarrhea, or blood in the urine or stool. He has intermittent itchy red and watery eyes and runny nose. Hives now resolved, noted from a week prior.

Physical examination. Vitals: Wt: 23.2 kg, Temp: 36.2°C, Pulse: 83 beats/min, RR: 22 breaths/min, BP: 96/48 mmHg. He is awake, alert, and in no apparent distress. Pupils are equal, round, and reactive to light and accommodation with no conjunctival or scleral injection or discharge. Tympanic membranes are clear bilaterally. Nasal turbinates have a normal hue with some mild bogginess. Oropharynx reveals no erythema or exudates. His neck is supple with now lymphadenopathy. Lungs are clear to auscultation bilaterally with no wheezes, rales, rhonchi, or crackles. Heart has a regular rate and rhythm with normal S1, S2, and no murmurs, rubs, or gallops. Abdomen is soft, nontender, and nondistended with positive bowel sounds. There is no hepatosplenomegaly. Extremities have no clubbing, edema, or cyanosis with less than 2 s capillary refill. There is no significant joint swelling noted on the upper or lower extremities. There is no significant warmth or erythema on the knee joints. Skin shows some mild textured erythematous rash on the upper back and chest.

Diagnostic Testing (Results from 2005)

- 3 View Knee X-ray: soft tissues with considerable swelling, normal bony structures
- CBC: WBC 6.8 μl (6–17.5 μl), neutrophils 51% H (23–45%), lymphocytes 38% (35–65%), rest within normal limits (WNL)
- CRP: 0.70 mg/dl H (<0.9). ESR: 17 mm/h H (0–15)
- Throat culture: negative for Group A Streptococci
- Na 137 mmol/L (135–145), BUN 14 mg/dl (8–22), Cr 0.3 mg/dl (0.4–1.2), Alb 4.5 g/dl (3–5.2)
- ANA negative, HLAB27 not detected, other rheumatologic labs WNL
- C3: 136 mg/dl (90–180), C4: 30 mg/dl (10–40)

With the Presented Data, What Is Your Working Diagnosis?

Impression

1. Diffuse multiforme rash with erythema and pruritus.
2. Arthritis of knees, hands, and feet with overlying erythema/target lesions. The presenting symptoms may be due to infection, exposure to allergen, reaction to medication, or rheumatic disease. Other possibilities include immune reaction or vasculitic process.

Plan

Ibuprofen 200 mg three times a day for 2 weeks, prednisone 20 mg per day for 10 days, hydrocortisone 1% ointment b.i.d. for 3–4 days or until the itching and rash subside, Benadryl (diphenhydramine) 25 mg PO for pruritus, and urinalysis to evaluate for proteinuria or hematuria.

Differential Diagnoses

1. Viral exanthematous infection: can cause fever, rash, malaise, myalgias, and joint pain.
2. Rheumatic juvenile arthritis: due to chronic nature of waxing and waning joint pain and swelling in different joints. Serologic tests seen were consistent with recent streptococcal infection.
3. Henoch–Schonlein Purpura with joint pain, purpura, and possible kidney involvement due to immune complex deposition (1).

4. Immunologic allergic reaction to medication previously taken with or without immune complex deposition.
5. Drug eruption or idiopathic drug reaction: Involves nonspecific exanthems, urticaria, wheezing, shortness of breath, and throat swelling (2).
6. Vasculitis/Cutaneous Vasculitis: Immune complex formation along with hypocomplementemia leading to inflammation, rash, swelling, and arthralgias.
7. Erythema multiforme/Stevens–Johnson syndrome: Hypersensitivity drug reactions with dermatologic manifestations with a prodrome of malaise, fever, arthralgias, and development of erythematous macules or plaques (3).

Workup

- T cell and B cell numbers: Normal
- Lymphocyte mitogen studies: Normal antibody responses
- Lymphocyte antigen studies: Normal T-cell responses
- Immunoglobulin levels IgG: 599 ku/l L (608–1229), IgA: 81 ku/l (33–200) IgM: 77 ku/l (46–197)
- Complement: C3:135 mg/dl (90–180), C4: 45 mg/dl (10–40), CH50 53 mg/dl (>8)
- C1Q binding assay: 1.4 mcgE/ml (0.0–3.9)
- Urinalysis: within normal limits (WNL)
- CRP: 0.2 mg/dl (<0.9), ESR: 7 mm/h (0–15)
- ANA: negative, RF: negative
- AST and ALT: WNL
- Raji Cell immune complex assay: 10 µgE/ml (<63)

What Is Your Diagnosis and Why?

This is a 6-year-old boy who presented with diffuse erythematous rash, fevers, myalgias, arthralgias, and joint swelling after antibiotic treatment, specifically penicillin-based drugs. Initial X-ray showed bilateral knee joint effusion with no evidence of infection.

1. Viral Exanthematous infection: Less likely due to prolonged symptoms over a period of months along with the lack of constitutional symptoms of cough, runny nose, or congestion (1).
2. Rheumatic juvenile arthritis: Less likely due to negative ANA, RF along with normal CRP and ESR levels.
3. Henoch–Schonlein Purpura: Although joint pain is seen in this disease process, the IgA level did not fall, the patient did not develop purpura, and his BUN/Cr level was normal (2).

7 Serum Sickness and Serum Sickness-Like Reaction

4. Vasculitis: Although biopsy of the rash was not performed, vasculitis was considered less likely due to normal complement level, and Raji cell assay.
5. Erythema multiforme: Initial presentation showed target-like lesions, but his rash persisted, and there was no mucosal involvement. Also, the patient had pruritus but no burning sensation (3).

Analysis and review of the clinical presentation of arthritis, hives, low-grade fevers, and joint inflammation and swelling but no significant laboratory changes lead to the diagnosis of serum sickness, or serum sickness-like reaction.

From his initial presentation in 2003 following the course of Augmentin (amoxicillin/clavulanate) antibiotic therapy, his symptoms escalated progressively, resulting in a chronic course lasting approximately 9 months. Because the majority of his symptoms arose within 4–5 days following the treatment with antibiotics, the presentation correlates with the criteria of serum sickness but is complicated by the prolonged course and lack of laboratory findings for immune complexes, leading to an overlapping diagnosis of serum sickness-like reaction.

Case 2

Our patient is a 26-year-old Hispanic male, a construction worker, who was referred to us for the evaluation of recent rash. He reported that while at work, accidentally fired a nail gun to his right knee joint (right femoral medial condyle). As a result, a 3½ in. nail was inserted into the area. He was taken to the emergency room, operated on, and the nail was removed. He was started on cephalexine and acetaminophen with codeine for pain and was discharged the next day. After 7 days, he reported "getting sick," felt feverish (temperature of 103°F), and developed swelling of the legs. Despite his condition, he returned to work but 3 h later he collapsed and was sent home to rest. His condition did not improve, and he was taken to a different hospital for evaluation.

The initial CT of the right knee revealed effusion and no signs of osteomyelitis. An MRI of the right knee revealed the tract in the medial distal femoral condyle with surrounding bone marrow edema. There were also large knee effusion and large soft tissue edema around the knee joint. His right knee was aspirated, and he was placed on intravenous vancomycin and intravenous Rocephin antibiotics. Several days later, he was transferred to the ICU due to elevated temperature; his Rocephin was discontinued, and he was started on ciprofloxacin. Shortly, while still on antibiotic, he developed pruritus and rash on his lower back but got some relief with diphenhydramine. After spending several days in the ICU, his condition stabilized, and he was transferred to the floor. On the hospital day 12, he was discharged with a picc line and intravenous vancomycin and oral ciprofoxacine (to take each twice a day). At home, his hive-like rash spread and developed fever with peaks at noons and midnights. He used diphenhydramine and contacted an allergist for consultation; the allergist instructed him to substitute clindamycin (three times a day) for vancomycin and continue ciprofloxacin. The next day, he developed swelling of hands and feet and made another phone call to the allergist. The allergist on call ordered him to discontinue the ciprofloxacine. The next day, when he contacted his own allergist, he was told to go to an emergency room. He was then admitted to the third hospital for evaluation.

Drug allergies. No known history of drug allergy prior to his recent condition.

Past medical and surgical history. Saw injury to his left fifth digit and subsequent repair, appendectomy.

Social history. He is married and has two daughters. He works as a construction worker. He has a 14-pack-year history of smoking. He was a heavy drinker (6–10 beers a day for 7 years) but quit 2 months ago. He admitted to use of recreational but not intravenous drugs.

Family history. Father has hypertension.

Review of systems. With the exception of need for reading glasses, was unremarkable.

Physical examination. In the initial examination in emergency room, he appeared as an alert Hispanic male in no obvious distress. Vitals included blood pressure of 116/67 mmHg, pulse of 99 beats/min (regular), temperature of 99°F, and respiratory rate of 12 breaths/min. HEENT: except some erythema on the hard and soft palate junction was within normal limits. Heart, lungs, and abdomen were within normal limits. On examination of the inguinal area, moderate bilateral lymphadenopathy noted. Skin: generalized erythematous rash (flat) covering from neck to his waist noted. He also had blanchable raised firm rash covering his abdomen and trunk. The other types of rash were petechial purpuric, nonblanchable from groin down to his medial and lateral aspect of his feet. The arms and hand digits were also covered with papules.

Data

The abnormal results of complete blood counts (CBC) and chemistry are summarized in Table 7.1; EKG: normal; urine analysis (dipstick): except small amount of leukocyte was within normal limits; punch biopsy of a rash (arm): drug eruption.

With the Presented Data, What Is Your Working Diagnosis?

This 26-year-old male had a history of right knee injury due to accidental insertion of 3½ in. nail to the area. This incidence had lead to performing procedures to remove the nail and later on aspiration of the area. His condition required multiple uses of antibiotics and pain medication resulting in generalized rash, swollen joints, and spiking fever. Our initial working diagnosis was drug allergy due to one of the antibiotics.

Table 7.1 Abnormal laboratory findings

Test	Abnormal findings	Range
WBC	18.1 H	4.5–11.0 K/mm^3
RBC	3.9 L	4.6–5.9 M/mm^3
Hgb	12.1 L	14.0–18.0 gm/dl
Hct	35 L	42–52%
Seg	84 H	50–70%
Lymph	7 L	20–40%
Sedimentation rate	16 H	0–15 mm/h
Na	125 L	137–147 mEq/L
Cl	95 L	96–108 mEq/L
Total protein	5.2 L	6.1–8.2 g/dl
Alb	2.2 L	3.2–4.8 g/dl
Ca	7.1 L	8.3–10.3 mg/dl
CRP	16.1 H	0.0–1.0 mg/dl

H denotes higher than normal and L denotes lower than normal values

Differential diagnosis. The differential diagnosis includes viral infection, Stevens–Johnson syndrome, erythema multiforme, vasculitis, serum sickness/serum sickness-like reaction, and other drug eruptions.

Workup

Initial approach consisted of discontinuation of all antibiotics and starting of intravenous solu-medrol 20 mg four times a day. The laboratory workup and the findings included: blood culture (from two sites, negative after 5 days); complements C3 and C4 (within normal limits); urine culture (no growth); stool occult blood (negative); skin biopsy of a rash on the left arm (Fig. 7.1, characteristic of drug eruption); X-ray of hands (soft tissue welling around the fourth digit); and an MRI of the right distal femoral site (findings consistent with trauma).

What Is Your Diagnosis and Why?

Viral infection. Viral exanthematous infection may present with similar symptoms as in our patient. However, our patient did not have involvement of oropharynx and mucosal surfaces that are more common in viral infections.

Stevens–Johnson syndrome. Although several features of our patient resembled those of Steven–Johnson syndrome, we did not notice oral lesions and no involvement of mucus membranes.

Erythema multiforme. This is usually characterized with target-shaped rash and palms and soles are usually involved. Our patient did not have such rash and his palms and soles were spared.

Vasculitis. The biopsy of a rash excluded vasculitis.

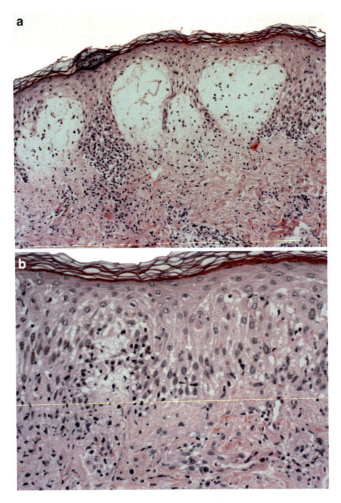

Fig. 7.1 (a) This ×20 view shows skin with spongiotic vesicles and prominent vacuolar change in the basal layers of the epidermis. (b) This high power (×40) demonstrates vacuolar change and a necrotic keratinocyte within the epidermis. The dermis contains a perivascular lymphocytic infiltrate. The features of vasculitis are absent

Serum sickness and serum sickness-like reactions. The reaction due to serum sickness and serum sickness-like reactions consists of arthralgia, fever, rash, and abnormal labs (although not in all patients) such as proteinuria and Complements 3 and 4 (C3, C4) deficiency. Our patient had normal urine analysis, normal C3 and C4, increased C reactive protein (CRP) and hypoalbuminemia.

This patient shared some characteristics of serum sickness, serum sickness-like reactions, Stevens–Johnson syndrome, and general drug eruptions. We believe that his reactions were due to cephalexin, the initial antibiotic. One evidence was the exacerbation of the symptoms after introducing Rocephin; this made sense to us since both antibiotics are members of cephalosporin family. While on corticosteroid and off antibiotics, his rash subsided. He remained afebrile during his hospital stay and was discharged on a course of prednisone.

Discussion

Serum sickness is an allergic disease involving a type III hypersensitivity reaction, which presents with the deposition of immune complexes in small vessels, leading to complement activation and inflammation. Serum sickness was first described by Von Pirquet in 1905 after patients were given antiequine serum to treat diphtheria (4). The most common causes of serum sickness are vaccines, antivenoms and antibiotics, and for serum sickness-like reaction are drug reactions, especially the penicillins and cephalosporins (5) (Table 7.2).

The presentation predominantly includes fever, urticarial exanthems, arthralgias, gastrointestinal problems, myalgias, and lymphadenopathy. Less common signs include dyspnea, carditis, renal, and neurological complications (6). The symptoms are usually self-limiting and last 1–2 weeks before resolving. Primary serum sickness occurs 4–21 days after administering the inciting antigen. The onset may be more rapid with subsequent exposures to the same antigen, with symptoms occurring 1–4 days after repeated exposure (7).

Pathophysiology: Serum sickness is a type III hypersensitivity reaction mediated by the formation of antibody–antigen immune complexes and deposition in tissues leading to an inflammatory response. Importantly, the size of the antigen and antigenic load induces the immune system to produce antibodies against the

Table 7.2 Agents associated with serum sickness and serum sickness-like reaction. Order: most to least common

Serum sickness	Serum sickness-like reaction
Allopurinol	Cefaclor
Antithymocyte globulin	Penicillins (Amoxicillin)
Antivenoms	Trimethoprim–sulfamethoxazole
Cefaclor	Ciprofloxacin
Cephalosporins	Aspirin/salicylates
Cephalexin	Itraconazole
Diphtheria immune globulin	Metronidazole
Metronidazole	Cefuroxime
Griseofulvin	Ceftriaxone
Hymenoptra proteins	Indomethacin
Infliximab	Griseofulvin
Penicillins	Rifampin
Rituximab	Streptomycin
Streptokinase	Minocycline
Vaccines	Fluoxetine

antigen. These antibodies bind the antigens, form complexes, and deposit in the tissues (due to the amount of complexes formed) instead of being cleared; this deposition of complexes causes activation of the complement system which helps to mediate inflammatory responses leading to the physiologic responses seen in serum sickness. Once the complexes are removed from the serum through immune-modulating systems, recovery occurs (1, 2).

Workup. The workup for serum sickness involves a thorough clinical evaluation and laboratory results placed within the context of the timing and appearance of signs and symptoms. The diagnosis should be suspected when manifesting symptoms involve multiple organ systems. It is important to ask about possible exposures preceding the presentation.

The main laboratory evaluation revolves around detecting circulating immune complexes.

Examples of these assays include Raji cell assay, which has receptors that recognize the conserved portions of immune complexes. Commercial assays using monoclonal and polyclonal antibodies directed against complement components of immune complexes are available (2, 7).

Nonspecific markers of inflammation that are also considered in the diagnostic workup include C3, C4, CH50, ESR, and CRP, along with CBC for lymphocytosis and thrombocytosis, chemistry panel for increased liver function tests, albuminemia, and urinalysis for hematuria and proteinuria. While positive test results may support the diagnosis, negative results do not rule out the diagnosis (1, 8).

Management/treatment. The mainstay of treatment is to remove the offending agent from the patient's system. Antiinflammatories help mediate arthralgias, myalgias, and fever. Antihistamines provide symptom relief by inhibiting increased vascular permeability, which can prevent immune complex deposition and inflammation. In chronic or severe cases, corticosteroids are given to suppress the immune response for a short period, such as prednisone 0.5–1.0 mg/kg per day for 5 days (9).

Serum sickness and serum sickness-like reaction have similar clinical presentations. The diagnosis of serum sickness-like reaction is believed to be an abnormal inflammatory response to defective metabolism products of drug byproducts during treatment with a particular agent. It is thought that serum sickness-like reactions are dose-responsive and that higher doses of medication produce a significant amount of metabolites which bind to tissue, thus causing a reaction. The reaction is not associated with immune complex formation or deposition. The result is a similar presentation to classical serum sickness, but usually without high fevers or significant organ involvement. Renal and hepatic involvement is rare and significant decreases in complement level are not seen (10, 11).

The clinical manifestations of serum sickness-like reaction usually present 1–6 days after completing a course of antibiotic treatment. The leading causes of serum sickness-like reactions are the antibiotics Cefaclor and penicillins (7) (Table 7.2). The treatment is similar to that of classical serum sickness with antihistamines, antiinflammatories, and corticosteroids as a therapy but associated with quicker resolution of symptoms than in serum sickness (9) (Table 7.3).

7 Serum Sickness and Serum Sickness-Like Reaction

Table 7.3 Characteristics of serum sickness versus serum sickness-like reaction

Characteristics	Serum sickness	Serum sickness-like reaction
Pathophysiology	Type III immune complex reaction	Nonimmune complex Drug metabolites
Etiology	Antitoxins Vaccines Antibodies	Antibiotics (cefaclor, penicillins)
Onset of symptoms	Within 7 days of receiving inciting agent	Within 1–2 days post completing course of medication
Symptoms	Urticarial rash Fever Malaise Polyarthralgias or polyarthritis	Acute onset of joint pain Lymphadenopathy Urticarial rash With or without fever
Lab findings	Decreased levels C3,C4,CH50 Presence of immune complexes (C1q and Raji cell assays) +CRP, ESR Hypoalbuminemia, proteinuria	BUN/Cr normal Absence of circulating complexes
Treatment	Removal of offending agent Antiinflammatory Antihistamines Corticosteroids	Removal of offending agent Antiinflammatory Antihistamines Corticosteroids
Follow-up	Avoiding the causative drug Further workup if symptoms persist or reoccur	Avoiding the causative drug Further workup if symptoms persist

Summary and conclusion. Serum sickness and serum sickness-like reactions are considered clinical diagnoses. Formation of immune complexes is the key laboratory identifier of serum sickness versus serum sickness-like reactions (noncomplex mediated). While these two conditions are self-limiting, it is important to identify and remove the offending agent and ensure the prevention of future exposure (9).

Questions

1. Which of the following is the time range of symptoms onset in serum sickness reactions?
    (a) 1–2 days
    (b) 7–21 days
    (c) 30–60 days
    (d) 90–180 days

2. Which of the following lab findings is observed in a patient with serum sickness?
    (a) Low levels of IgG and IgM
    (b) Low titers of immune complex

(c) Low levels of serum C3 and C4
(d) Significantly elevated CH50

3. Which of the following skin eruptions is the most common in patients with serum sickness?

   (a) Angioedema
   (b) Exfoliative rash
   (c) Vesiculo-bullous lesions
   (d) Urticaria

4. Immune complexes tend to be large at:

   (a) Equivalence (number of available antigenic sites is equal to the number of available antibody-combining sites)
   (b) Antibody excess
   (c) Antigen excess
   (d) Only when monovalent antigens are present

5. Serum sickness reactions are considered to be mediated by:

   (a) Hypersensitivity type reaction I
   (b) Hypersensitivity type reaction II
   (c) Hypersensitivity type reaction III
   (d) Hypersensitivity type reaction IV
   (e) Cell-mediated reaction

6. Which of the following group of sign and symptoms are typical of serum sickness syndrome?

   (a) Fever, rash, arthralgia, lesions in mucus membranes.
   (b) Fever, rash, arthralgia, angioedema
   (c) Fever, rash, nausea, conjunctivitis
   (d) Oral ulcer, blisters, fever
   (e) Fever, rash, arthralgia, lymphadenopathy

7. Which one of the following is the most common medication causing serum sickness-like reaction in children?

   (a) Penicillin
   (b) Azithromycine
   (c) Cefaclore
   (d) Amoxicillin
   (e) Clindamycin

8. All the followings are management of serum sickness/serum sickness-like reactions except:

   (a) Avoiding the offending agent
   (b) Supportive therapy
   (c) Corticosteroid in some cases

(d) Reintroducing a smaller amount of the offending dose in a month after resolution of symptoms in order to build immunity
(e) Excluding the viral infections

9. Which one of the following feature is not seen in serum sickness-like reaction?

    (a) Formation of immune complexes
    (b) Antibodies as the cause of reaction
    (c) Resolution of symptoms after the removal of the offending agent
    (d) Rash
    (e) Arthralgia

10. Which one of the following is included in differential diagnosis list of serum sickness/serum sickness-like reactions?

    (a) Stevens–Johnson syndrome
    (b) Viral infections with exanthema
    (c) Drug eruptions
    (d) Erythema multiforme
    (e) All of the above

Answers: 1(b), 2(c), 3(d), 4(c), 5(c), 6(e), 7(c), 8(d), 9(a), 10(e).

References

1. Chao, Y.K., et al., Childhood serum sickness: a case report. J Microbiol Immunol Infect, 2001. 34(3): p. 220–3.
2. Schnyder, B., Approach to the patient with drug allergy. Immunol Allergy Clin North Am, 2009. 29(3): p. 405–18.
3. Segal, A.R., et al., Cutaneous reactions to drugs in children. Pediatrics, 2007. 120(4): p. e1082–96.
4. Mener, D.J., C. Negrini, and A. Blatt, Itching like mad. Am J Med, 2009. 122(8): p. 732–4.
5. Tatum, A.J., A.M. Ditto, and R. Patterson, Severe serum sickness-like reaction to oral penicillin drugs: three case reports. Ann Allergy Asthma Immunol, 2001. 86(3): p. 330–4.
6. Baniasadi, S., F. Fahimi, and D. Mansouri, Serum sickness-like reaction associated with cefuroxime and ceftriaxone. Ann Pharmacother, 2007. 41(7): p. 1318–9.
7. Clark, B.M., et al., Severe serum sickness reaction to oral and intramuscular penicillin. Pharmacotherapy, 2006. 26(5): p. 705–8.
8. Mathes, E.F. and A.E. Gilliam, A four-year-old boy with fever, rash, and arthritis. Semin Cutan Med Surg, 2007. 26(3): p. 179–87.
9. Nelson, M., Serum Sickness and Immune Complex Disease. In: Mahmoudi M ed. Allergy and Asthma Practical Diagnosis and Management. New York: Mc Graw-Hill; 2007. p. 195–205.
10. Yerushalmi, J., A. Zvulunov, and S. Halevy, Serum sickness-like reactions. Cutis, 2002. 69(5): p. 395–7.
11. Katta, R. and V. Anusuri, Serum sickness-like reaction to cefuroxime: a case report and review of the literature. J Drugs Dermatol, 2007. 6(7): p. 747–8.

Part III
Allergic Contact Dermatitis

Chapter 8
Preservatives

Sara Flores and Howard Maibach

Abstract Preservatives are common ingredients indicated in allergic contact dermatitis (ACD). Health care practitioners should familiarize themselves with those most frequently used in cosmetics, drugs, and occupational exposure so that they can provide adequate care and education to affected patients. This chapter summarizes the preservatives used in the Standard Series Patch Test, which are also common causes of ACD. We also provide two case examples of ACD resulting from contact with the above additives.

Keywords Preservatives • Quaternium-15 • Parabens • Formaldehyde • Allergic contact dermatitis • Methylchloroisothiazolinone/methylisothiazolinone (MCI/MI) • Methyldibromoglutaronitrile (MDBNG)/phenoxyethanol

Case 1

A 34-year-old African–American woman presented with a chronic rash that had recently exacerbated. The patient reported a history of chronic recurrent dermatitis. Although the cubital fossae were the most common involvement site, at various times she had widespread patchy dermatitis. She was referred for consultation based on an inability to control the dermatitis with topical corticoids and moisturizers.

The patient's past medical history also included asthma and seasonal allergic rhinitis. These were in remission at the time of interview. She was using triamcinolone acetonide 0.10% cream and was experiencing insomnia due to severe pruritis caused by her current condition.

S. Flores (✉)
Department of Dermatology, School of Medicine,
University of California, San Francisco,
San Francisco, CA, USA
e-mail: primaragazzal@yahoo.com

The physical examination showed scaling, induration, and lichenification on the cubital fossae as well as scattered areas on the trunk, arms, and legs.

With the Presented Data, What Is Your Working Diagnosis?

The recent exacerbation, her past medical history, and lack of alleviation through corticosteroids and/or moisturizers suggested that we rule in or out allergic contact dermatitis (ACD) as a secondary factor.

Differential Diagnosis

Seborrheic dermatitis, irritant contact dermatitis (ICD), ACD.

Workup

1. Since the patient was referred on suspicion of dermatitis, a detailed interview and history could have potentially offered further insight as to possible sensitizers. In this patient, the history did not provide clues pointing to the specific allergen.
2. She was patch tested with an extended routine series of the North American Contact Dermatitis Research Group (NACDRG), utilizing Finn Chambers and SCANPOR® (Norgeplaster, Oslo, Norway) tape for 48 h with readings at 49 and 96 h. We used the International Contact Dermatitis Research Group (ICDRG) schema (1). The final reading revealed moderate reaction (2+) to imidazole urea.

What Is Your Diagnosis and Why?

The patient had ACD to imidazole urea. Patch testing was used to find the specific allergen responsible and confirmed/specified our diagnosis.

Management and Follow-Up

The patient returned with her topical products, mainly moisturizers, and two were identified as containing imidazole urea. We requested that she read labels and avoid the use of this preservative. Follow-up at one month and one year revealed that she was now topical corticoid responsive, and the potency and frequency of topical corticoid utilization had decreased rapidly.

Case 2

A 40-year-old Caucasian male visited the dermatology clinic reporting an exacerbation of a chronic dermatitis that had been previously under control. He reported having intermittent hand eczema for about 15 years and was referred due to sudden worsening of the condition. He worked as a machinist. The review of systems was otherwise unremarkable, and the patient was applying 0.10% Betamethasone valerate cream at that time.

On physical examination, his dorsal hands were red, swollen, and scaly. No stigmata of psoriasis were noted.

With the Presented Data, What Is Your Working Diagnosis?

The working diagnosis was possible occupational ACD.

Differential Diagnosis

Differential diagnosis included endogenous dermatitis, not elsewhere classified, atopic dermatitis, irritant dermatitis, and atypical psoriasis.

Workup

1. History often provides clues to the cause and type of dermatitis. In this patient's case, history suggested an occupational dermatitis.
2. He was patch tested to the extended routine series to find specific allergens. In addition, he was tested to his own work chemicals, his gloves, and the oil and coolant series. The positives included fragrance mix, propylene glycol, paraben mix, and 2,5-diazolidinyl urea.
3. Because of the multiple positives, we felt it prudent to rule in or out the likelihood that some results represented false positives due to excited skin syndrome by retesting all the compounds again separately. The only reproducible positive was to 2,5-diazolidinyl urea. The other retests were negative, suggesting that they were false positives due to the excited skin syndrome.

What Is Your Diagnosis and Why?

The diagnosis was ACD to 2,5-diazolidiny This should read "2,5-diazolidinyl urea. In this case, retesting was relevant in that the suspected occupational source was not the one found. Instead, the source was a topical medication. Thus, avoidance of work-related chemicals was unnecessary, and management of the patient's condition was simplified.

Management and Follow-Up

When seen at 1 month and 1 year, he was almost clear. In retrospect, our final diagnosis was endogenous dermatitis (possibly atopic) complicated by ACD to 2,5-diazolidinyl urea contained in several topical medicaments. He found work and home use products with this preservative and discontinued their use.

Discussion

Definition

A preservative is any ingredient added to a product to retard microbial growth and prevent decomposition. Preservatives are widely used since any water-based product needs to withstand the timeframe needed for shipping, distribution, shelf-life, and use by the consumer. Though numerous preservatives exist, the cosmetic market is dominated by a few. A brief description of some common preservatives, including formaldehyde, quaternium-15, imidazolidinyl urea, diazolidinyl urea, Methylchloroisothiazolinone/methylisothiazolinone (MCI/MI), methyldibromoglutaronitrile (MDBNG)/phenoxyethanol, and parabens, is provided below.

Since the above preservatives are consistently encountered, sensitization can occur and result in ACD. It is therefore important for the health care practitioner to have a basic knowledge of the common additives, and so they may aid in the identification of an allergen and educate the patient about preservatives and ACD.

Brief History

Documents recording the use of preservatives in USA date back to the 1800s. However, most early additives were utilized for the conservation of food and drink. In 1938, USA passed the Federal Food, Drug and Cosmetic Act, which was issued by the United States Food and Drug Administration (FDA) and the United States Department of Health and Human Services which required the cosmetic industry to prove product safety before marketing to consumers. The FDA's initial years were marked by new laws intended to protect the consumer against harmful or deadly agents used by manufacturers. Later, during the 1960s and 1970s, microbial contamination of cosmetics led to an increasing awareness of preservatives.

In USA, preservatives used in cosmetics are also evaluated by the Cosmetic Ingredient Review (CIR). The reports include the ingredient's skin sensitization

8 Preservatives 131

potency and the following information: name of ingredient, review conclusion (safe, safe with qualifications, insufficient data to support safety, or unsafe), explanation of the conclusion, and journal citations; all of these findings are then published in the International Journal of Toxicology (2).

Prevalence of AC.D and Types of Preservatives

Most prevalence studies report the results in reference to a specific preservative rather than accounting for all cases of ACD. We present the values for prevalence associated with each of the preservatives in the pages following. However, there are studies that have attempted to assess the prevalence of ACD in the general population regardless of causative allergen. Thyssen et al. and Mirshahpanah and Maibach determined a median prevalence and summarized the main findings from studies on contact allergy in the general population (3, 4). These reviews suggest that the weighted average prevalence was 19.5%, based on the data collected on all age groups and all countries between 1966 and 2007. The median prevalence was 21.8% in women and 12% in men (4). An assessment of the portion of 19.5% due to cosmetic preservatives given the length and scope of this chapter would be impossible. Instead, an introductory presentation of the more common additives serves to familiarize the reader with the occurrence of ACD resulting from these chemicals. Those mentioned below are the most frequently encountered and are included in the Standard Series Patch Test.

Formaldehyde

Formaldehyde is the simplest aldehyde and is a colorless gas that is soluble in polar solvents, most importantly water (5). It is an irritant even in persons not previously sensitized and is also known to cause irritation of the mucous membranes and the conjunctiva. It has been postulated that its small size may allow it to diffuse across the stratum corneum more readily than other compounds (6).

Formaldehyde is used in numerous applications besides cosmetics. Many of these are substances encountered on a daily basis. Some examples include vinyl and rubber gloves, plastic containers, cigarette smoke, and those listed in Table 8.1. Erase possible and the crossed out section. New sentence should be "An allergy to formaldehyde may therefore be difficult for a patient to control since contact with the allergen is harder to avoid.

In the Standard Series Patch Test, formaldehyde is tested at a concentration of 1% in aqueous solution (Table 8.2). In a patch test study done by the North American Contact Dermatitis Group (NACDG) during 2005–2006, 9% of 4,445 patients tested positive to formaldehyde (7). This ranked formaldehyde seventh of the 65 allergens tested. Further, recent studies from Sweden document that the 1% patch test misses clinically relevant patients; Erase the semicolon and add a period at the end of the sentence. Should read: Further, recent studies from Sweden document that the 1%

Table 8.1 Uses of the common preservatives

Formaldehyde	Quaterium-15	Imidazolidinyl urea	Diazolidinyl urea	Parabens
Cosmetics	Cosmetics	Cosmetics	Cosmetics	Cosmetics
Disinfectant	OTC medications	OTC topical drugs	Skin care	Medicines-topical and systemic
Over-the-counter medications	Latex paints		Shampoos and conditioners	Foods-marinated fish, mayonnaise, salad dressings, spiced sauces, mustard, processed vegetables, frozen dairy products, baked goods
Leather tanners	Polishes		Bubble baths	Industrial oils, fats, glues, shoe polish, textiles
Photography	Jointing cements		Baby wipes	
Textiles-permanent press and wrinkle resistant	Metal working fluids		Household detergents	
Paints	Adhesives			
Paper manufacturing	Construction materials			
Fertilizers	Paper or paperboard			
Plastics and resins-particularly urea and phenolic resin				
Metalworking fluids	Inks			
Wood composites-plywood and particle board				
Insulation				

Table 8.2 Preservatives belonging to the Standard Series (modified from Lachapelle and Maibach and Zug et al. (1, 7))

Compound	ECDS and EECDRG[b] (%)	NACDG[c] (%)	JCDS[d] (%)
Formaldehyde	1(aq)	1(aq)	1(aq)
Paraben mix[a]	16	12	15
Quaternium-15	1	2	–
Cl+Me-isothiazolinone	0.01 (aq)	0.01 (aq)	0.01 (aq)
Methyldibromoglutaronitrile	0.5	2 (+phenoxyethanol)	–
Imidazolidinyl urea	–	2	–
2,5-Diazolidinyl urea	2	2	–

[a]The Paraben mix is composed of four constituents: methyl-4-hydroxybenzoate, ethyl-4-hydroxybenzoate, propyl-4-hydroxybenzoate, butyl-4-hydroxybenzoate
[b]The revised 2008 European standard series according to the European Society of Contact Dermatitis and the European Environmental and Contact Dermatitis Research Group. The concentrations quoted refer to petrolatum except where otherwise stated
[c]The revised 2008 North American standard series according to the North American Contact Dermatitis Research Group. The concentrations quoted refer to petrolatum except where otherwise stated
[d]The revised 2008 Japanese standard series according to the Japanese Society for Contact Dermatitis. The concentrations quoted refer to petrolatum except where otherwise stated

patch test misses clinically relevant patients (8). Taking this into account, the prevalence of allergy to formaldehyde is likely greater than the 9.0% reported and is therefore a more frequently encountered cause of sensitization in patients.

Quaternium-15

Quaternium-15 is a water-soluble powder that is compatible with the proteins that are frequently contained in cosmetics. It is effective as a preservative in low concentrations for 2 or more years and has cosmetic, pharmaceutical, and industrial applications, including paper and adhesive production and conservation of over-the-counter medications (Table 8.1). Quaternium-15 belongs to a class of preservatives called formaldehyde-releasing. This means that its chemical structure has one or more formaldehyde groups that are released into the product over time. The amount of formaldehyde released is small and is often insufficient to trigger a reaction in those sensitive to formaldehyde.

Quaterium-15 was ranked fifth in the NACDG study mentioned above and was therefore indicated in cases of ACD more often than formaldehyde. In USA, it is the most frequent preservative causing ACD (5). Of the 4,446 patients in the study, 10.3% had positive reactions to this preservative (7). Health care workers, hair stylists, and machine tool workers may be particularly at risk of sensitization to Q-15 due to frequent exposure to hand cleansers and lotions, hair care products, and cutting fluids containing this compound. In fact, in a study by Park and Taylor, moisturizers were found to be the leading source of Q-15 exposure, occurring in 79% of patients.

Noncoloring hair products accounted for exposure in one-third of the patients, whereas makeup accounted for about 12% (6).

Although the amount of formaldehyde released by quaternium-15 is not usually enough to trigger reactions in those presensitized to formaldehyde, reactions can sometimes occur. Note that patients allergic to quaternium-15 are not always allergic to formaldehyde and vice versa. The allergens must always be confirmed using a patch test with the Standard Series. In this test, a 2% concentration in petrolatum is used.

Imidazolidinyl Urea

Imidazolidinyl urea (IU) is a formaldehyde-releasing biocide found only in cosmetics and over-the-counter topical drugs. It is effective against Gram-negative and Gram-positive bacterial contamination of cosmetics and topical medications and to a lesser degree, fungi. It is therefore usually combined with an antifungal preservative to provide a broader spectrum of protection. Next to the parabens, it is the most commonly used cosmetic preservative.

Its popularity among manufacturers is due to its chemical properties and to its low toxicity. It is a water soluble, odorless, white compound that is compatible with various cosmetic ingredients. In addition, its ability to be combined with other preservatives offering protection against fungi and bacteria offer the final mix a wider spectrum of microbial protection. Finally, imidazolidinyl urea has a relatively low occurrence of irritation or sensitization. The 2005–2006 NADCG study found the prevalence of ACD due to IU to be 2.9% (Table 8.3) (7).

Imidazolidinyl urea is also included in the Standard Series and is tested at 2% (1)

2,5-Diazolidinyl Urea

2,5-Diazolidinyl urea was introduced in 1982 and is the newest of the formaldehyde-releasing preservatives. It is a water-soluble biocide that is, like imidazolidinyl urea, combined with other preservatives for like imidazolidinyl urea, combined with other preservatives for wider antifungal and antimicrobial capacity. The NADCG study

Table 8.3 Prevalence of ACD associated with preservatives (modified from Zug et al. (7))

Preservative	Prevalence (%)
Quaternium-15 2% in petroleum	10.3
Imidazolidinyl urea 2% pet	2.9
Formaldehyde 1% aq	9.0
Diazolidinyl urea 1% pet	3.7
Parabens 12% pet	1.2
MDGN/phenoxyethanol 2.5% pet	5.8
MCI/MI	2.8

revealed the prevalence of positive reactions at 3.7% (7). It is found in skin care products, shampoos and conditioners, cosmetics, baby wipes, and household detergents (5).

Methylchloroisothiazolinone/Methylisothiazolinone

MCI/MI belongs to a group of preservatives called isothiazolinones. The mixture consists of MCI and MI in a 3:1 ratio in water plus 23% magnesium chloride and nitrate to stabilize the combination (5). It is a relatively new additive and has only been used in product over the last 30 years. Europe utilized the compounds first in the 1970s, and USA followed 10 years later. MCI/MI has a wide range of uses and is found in metalworking fluids, soaps, latex paints, detergents, shampoos, hair conditioners, glues, and bubble baths (9).

It is a good preservative in that it is effective in small concentrations against bacteria, yeast, and fungi and thus does not need to be combined with other chemicals (6). In the 2005–2006 study, NACDG found a prevalence of 2.8%, which ranks MCI/MI below formaldehyde but above the parabens (7). Some other names include Kathon CG, Euxyl K100, and Kathon 886. The concentration used in the Standard Series Patch Test is 0.01% in aqueous solution (Table 8.2) (1).

Methyldibromoglutaronitrile (MDBNG)/phenoxyethanol

This mix, commercialized as Euxyl K400, consists of 2-phenoxyethanol and MDBNG in a 4:1 ratio (6). It is the youngest of the preservatives, having been introduced in USA in the 1990s. Though its concentration in cosmetics is restricted, it can be used in higher levels in industrial products such as paints, adhesives, dishwashing fluids, and fabric softeners.

Like MCI/MI, MDBNG/phenoxyethanol is effective against a wide range of pathogenic insult, including bacteria, fungi, and yeasts (9). Prevalence of reaction to the Standard Series Patch Test in a 2005–2006 study by the NACDG was 5.8% to a 2.5% petroleum mix (7). The concentration normally used in the Standard Series is shown in Table 8.2. Most of the ACD caused by this combination can be attributed to the MDBNG rather than to the phenoxyethanol.

Parabens

Parabens are alkyl esters of p-hydroxybenzoic acid and are colorless, odorless, stable- just delete the comma so it reads: "are colorless, odorless, stable and effective over a wide pH, economical, and and effective over a wide pH, economical, and have a broad spectrum of antimicrobial activity with low toxicity. Parabens are the most commonly used preservative in cosmetics and topical medications. Other uses include foods, industrial oils, fats, glues, and textiles. They are mainly effective against yeast and molds and therefore are usually combined with other preservatives that protect against Gram-positive and Gram-negative bacteria, such as quaternium-15 and imidazolidinyl urea. Of all the preservatives listed, the parabens have the lowest percentage of sensitization among consumers and patients. In the 2005–2006 NACDG study, prevalence of reaction to parabens was only 1.2% (7). They are usually patch tested in a paraben mix that exists in petrolatum at a concentration of 16% and that contains 4% each of methyl-, ethyl-, propyl-, and butylparaben (1).

Pathophysiology

There are four types of hypersensitivity reactions. ACD differs from contact urticaria in that it is a type IV hypersensitivity reaction and is therefore mediated by T cells and characterized by the development of immunological memory to the allergen. Upon first exposure to a preservative or fragrance, complexes are formed by binding of these small chemicals to the keratinocytes under the stratum corneum. Langerhans cells recognize this binding and phagocytize the cells and any molecules attached. They then display the engulfed antigen on their surface using a Major Histocompatibility Complex Type II Receptor (MHC II), travel to lymph nodes, and present the antigen to young T cells. The interaction between the Langerhans Cell and the T cell induces the release of cytokines which cause proliferation of memory T cells, capable of recognizing the chemicals on subsequent exposure. This process is called sensitization. Within 48 h after reexposure to an allergen, inflammation is apparent and can last for up to 4 weeks after the allergen has been removed.

Diagnostic Procedures

Following fragrances, preservatives are the most common ingredient indicated in ACD. The specific allergen responsible for a case of dermatitis can often be difficult to diagnose due to the possibility that any ingredient could potentially cause sensitization in a patient. False positives and false negatives also contribute to the difficulty in assessing a particular antigen, particularly when dealing with parabens. The paraben paradox, which describes a reaction in inflamed or diseased skin but not in healthy skin, is just one example of many factors that can lead to difficulty with interpretation. Despite the occurrence of false results, the patch test is still the only sure way to identify the allergens responsible for an ACD.

There exists a variety of patch tests used to assess allergens responsible for hypersensitivity. The TRUE Test (Thin-Layer Rapid Use Epicutaneous Test) is preprepared and consists of 28 allergens and allergen mixes. The North American Contact Dermatitis Standard Screening Series has 65 allergens and is more commonly used by specialists. It must be assembled and is customized to test the allergens indicated by the patient's history and exam (10). The preservatives included in the Standard Series and the concentrations used are outlined in Table 8.1.

As stated above, interpretation of the patch tests is not simple and must result from consideration of changing variables like the type of patch system used, amount of allergen applied, skin area, and variation in responses among patients (1). In addition, the properties of the preservatives influence a physician's understanding of a reaction. Reactions to formaldehyde must be considered cautiously since formaldehyde is an irritant even in those who have not been sensitized. Thus, a slight reaction to formaldehyde during a patch test may not be indicative of an allergic response. Cross sensitization may also muddle interpretation. Cross sensitization occurs when a patient who has previously been sensitized to an allergen reacts to another allergen that is similar in structure. The final diagnosis must be handled carefully by an experienced specialist, who has also weighed the patient's past medical history and physical examination.

Conclusion

Cosmetics contain many ingredients that could potentially act as sensitizers. As stated above, preservatives are the second most common cause of reactions next to fragrances. Patients who develop ACD often experience discomfort and, if the rash is in a conspicuous location, embarrassment. It is therefore important for any health care professional to have some familiarity with common additives so that they can better treat and educate patients.

Questions

1. Which of the following is NOT a formaldehyde-releasing preservative?

    (a) Methylparaben
    (b) Quaternium-15
    (c) Imidazolidinyl urea
    (d) 2,5-Diazolidinyl urea

2. Which preservative has the highest prevalence of sensitization according to the NACDG?

    (a) Formaldehyde
    (b) Quaternium-15
    (c) MDBNG/phenoxyethanol
    (d) Imidazolidinyl urea

3. Which preservative is the most commonly used in cosmetics and topical medications?

    (a) Parabens
    (b) MCI/MI
    (c) Formaldehyde
    (d) 2,5-Diazolidinyl urea

4. If a patient has already been sensitized to formaldehyde, he or she may later have sensitivity to which of the following preservatives?

(a) Propylparaben
(b) MCI/MI
(c) Petrolatum
(d) Quaternium-15

5. Which preservative is most ubiquitous?

    (a) Quaternium-15
    (b) MCI/MI
    (c) Formaldehyde
    (d) Parabens

6. Which preservative is most likely to be tolerated by a patient with a formaldehyde allergy?

    (a) 2,5-Diazolidinyl urea
    (b) MCI/MI
    (c) Quaternium-15
    (d) Imidazolidinyl urea

7. What is the best way to identify an allergen responsible for ACD?

    (a) Patient's past medical history. There is no need for any tests
    (b) A relevant review of systems
    (c) Skin patch test
    (d) Blood test

8. Allergic Contact Dermatitis is characterized by which of the following?

    (a) Type IV hypersensitivity reaction
    (b) Anaphylaxis
    (c) Type I hypersensitivity reaction
    (d) Death

9. Which is the newest preservative?

    (a) Formaldehyde
    (b) Imidazolidinyl urea
    (c) MDBNG/phenoxyethanol
    (d) Methylparaben

10. How can allergic contact dermatitis be differentiated from contact urticaria?

    (a) The reaction persists for a longer amount of time with ACD
    (b) The reaction is more severe in ACD
    (c) The color of the dermatitis is different
    (d) Signs of a reaction occur more quickly in ACD

Answers: 1(a), 2(b), 3(a), 4(d), 5(c), 6(d), 7(c), 8(a), 9(c), 10(a).

References

1. Lachapelle JM, Maibach HI. The Standard Series of Patch Tests. In: *Patch Testing and Prick Testing: A Practical Guide/Official Publication of the ICDRG*. Verlag, Berlin, Heidelberg: Springer; 2009: Chapter 4.
2. Lundov MD, Moesby L, Zachariae C, Johansen JD. Contamination versus preservation of cosmetics: a review on legislation, usage, infections, and contact allergy. *Contact Dermatitis*. 2009; 60: 70–78.
3. Mirshahpanah P, Maibach H. Relationship of patch test positivity in a general versus an eczema population. *Contact Dermatitis*. 2007; 56: 125–130.
4. Thyssen JP, Linneberg A, Menné T, Johansen JD. The epidemiology of contact allergy in the general population-prevalence and main findings. *Contact Dermatitis*. 2007; 57: 287–299.
5. Marks JG, DeLeo VA. *Contact and Occupational Dermatology*. St. Louis (MI): Mosby Year Book; 1992.
6. Rietschel RL, Fowler JF. *Fischer's Contact Dermatitis*. Hamilton (Ontario): BC Decker, Inc; 2008.
7. Zug KA, Warshaw EM, Fowler JF Jr., et al. Patch-test results of the North American Contact Dermatitis Group 2005–2006. *Dermatitis*. 2009; 20: 149–160.
8. Hauksson I, Pontén A, Gruvberger B, Isaksson M, Bruze M. Patch testing with formaldehyde 2.0% (0.60 mg/cm^2) detects substantially more contact allergy to formaldehyde than 1.0%. *Contact Dermatitis*. In press.
9. Sasseville D. Hypersensitivity to preservatives. *Dermatologic Therapy*. 2004; 17: 251–263.
10. Ortiz KJ, Yiannias JA. Contact dermatitis to cosmetics, fragrances, and botanicals. *Dermatologic Therapy*. 2004; 17: 264–271.

Chapter 9
Allergic Contact Dermatitis: Rubber Allergies

Peter Burke and Howard I. Maibach

Abstract Latex (rubber) allergy is a growing health concern among medical and nonmedical fields. Common occupational exposures include, health care and food industry workers using disposable gloves, latex industry employees, and car factory workers assembling rubber details. Additionally, high-risk groups include children with spina bifida or spinal dysraphism. Risk factors for latex allergic contact dermatitis (ACD) include skin damage allowing increased invasion of chemical residues into the skin dermis and atopy inducing an increased prevalence of latex immunologic contact urticaria (ICU). The pathophysiology of latex (rubber) allergy is IgE-mediated (ICU) and type IV ACD related. The IgE-mediated allergy is protein related, while ACD typically results from exposure to chemical accelerators and antioxidants produced during the vulcanization process. The clinical manifestations of latex ACD generally include an erythematous, papular eczema at the site of rubber contact, although distal site involvement is possible. Patch testing is the diagnostic test of choice for type IV latex ACD; however, a thorough history and physical examination are the cornerstone of latex ACD diagnosis. The primary mode of treatment for latex ACD is prevention; however, topical corticosteroids and other medicaments may be used for symptomatic relief.

Keywords Allergic contact dermatitis • Latex • Rubber

Case 1

History of Present Illness

A 28-year-old Caucasian R.N. was referred by occupational medicine clinic to our contact allergy clinic with a chief compliant of recalcitrant hand eczema.

P. Burke (✉)
Philadelphia College of Osteopathic Medicine, Philadelphia, PA 19131, USA
and
University of California San Francisco, San Francisco, CA 94143-0989, USA
e-mail: Peterbu@pcom.edu

Improvement was noted with 0.025 mg triamcinolone acetonide cream and liberal use of lipid rich moisturizers. Lesions extended to the right wrist.

Physical examination

A focused dermatological examination revealed a well-nourished 28-year-old Caucasian woman demonstrating redness, swelling, and scaling on patchy areas of the dorsal hand bilaterally. This included the dorsal right wrist. The remaining skin appeared clear.

Differential diagnosis

Irritant dermatitis, and endogenous eczema such as atopic dermatitis.

Working diagnosis

Allergic contact dermatitis.

Impression and follow-up

Due to the chronicity diagnostic patch testing with routine series of the North American Contact Dermatitis Research Group (NACDRG) utilizing the standard methodology of the International Contact Dermatitis Research Group (ICDRG) was employed (1, 2).

She was patch test positive ++, at 96 h to thiuram mix. The intervention provided to the RN was gloves that are thiuram free. She rapidly healed, returned to work, and was asymptomatic at 1 year follow-up.

Case 2

History of present illness

A 16-year-old Caucasian male was referred from his pediatrician to our Contact Allergy Clinic with a chief compliant of chronic dorsal foot eczema, recalcitrant to topical therapy.

This young man had been seen weekly for 1 year by either his pediatrician or dermatologist. Changing shoes and the use of topical corticosteroids (class I

9 Allergic Contact Dermatitis: Rubber Allergies

clobetasole) produced some improvement, but not clearing. He was referred to rule out ACD from shoes.

Physical examination

A focused dermatological examination revealed a well-nourished 16-year-old Caucasian boy demonstrating marked erythema, edema, and scaling of both dorsal feet. The remaining skin appeared clear.

Differential

ACD to shoes, psoriasis, endogenous dermatitis such atopic dermatitis, and winter eczema.

Working diagnosis

Allergic contact dermatitis.

Impression and follow-up

Due to the chronicity diagnostic patch testing with routine series of the NACDRG utilizing the standard methodology of the ICDRG was employed. She was patch test positive ++ to thiuram mix and to the box of one pair of his sneakers (1, 2).

He was instructed to avoid rubber additive exposure and thiurams in his shoes. This was accomplished by wearing electronically welded plastic shoes – which are typically thiuram free. He was asymptomatic at 1 year follow-up.

Discussion

Historical Background

Latex is obtained by tapping the cultivated rubber tree, *Hevea brasiliensis*. Latex products are produced by placing a porcelain mold into a container of latex and then vulcanizing the complex with chemical accelerators. Thiurams, dithiocarbamates, and mercaptobenzothiazoles (MPT) are added to enhance both the chemical and mechanical properties of the material such as the balance between elongation modulus and tensile strength (3). Vulcanization is a process which utilizes reactive chemicals to alter the chemical structure of the latex in conjunction with the accelerators. After vulcanization, the latex-accelerator complex is washed of excess protein and then dried with an agent such as corn starch.

Latex has an isoprene structure that is classified as a natural rubber polymer. Furthermore, latex is a complex biological molecule of rubber components enveloped by phospholipoprotein matrix complexed with sugars, nucleic acids, lipids, minerals and various associated proteins. Latex sensitivity has two distinct pathways which result in the manifestations of the allergy: (a) IgE mediation with mast cell degranulation and histamine release and (b) ACD with delayed hypersensitivity T-cell mediation (3). The IgE allergy is thought to be protein related, while the ACD results from exposure to chemical accelerators and antioxidants produced during the vulcanization process. It was hypothesized that if additional "leaching" (extraction of epitopes from a liquid medium) steps are undertaken, then several polypeptide epitopes may be removed from the latex polymer minimizing IgE-mediated allergy (3).

Latex exposure is ubiquitous in both medical and nonmedical exposure sources. Allergy to latex and rubber containing products has become increasingly common. Hence, the institution of universal precautions, such as proper glove donning and latex-free medical products, has been adopted to prevent the complications associated with rubber allergy (3).

Prevalence of Rubber-Based Contact Dermatitis

ACD due to rubber latex is a serious occupational health concern among personnel involved in the rubber industry and those who have significant exposure to rubber derivatives. Occupations at risk include, health care workers using disposable gloves, latex industry employees, and car factory workers assembling rubber details (4). Additionally, ACD has been reported in athletes, such as swimmers wearing neoprene suits, bikinis and swimming goggles, football players and cyclists, who had close contact to rubber in their sports equipment (5). Furthermore, several rubber products, including sphygmomanometers, rubber bands, condoms, shoes and bandages have increased the incidence of rubber ACD (6).

There has been a dramatic worldwide increase in type I rubber latex allergy over the past decade. A study involving 1,000 American volunteer blood donors demonstrated a minimal incidence of 0.4% and 6.4% prevalence of detectable antilatex antibodies (7). Latex IgE allergy has been reported in children, particularly in multioperated children with spina bifida or spinal dysraphism. Furthermore, recurrent exposure to latex from urogenital anomalies or ventriculo-peritoneal shunts has also been reported (7). The prevalence of latex sensitization among the pediatric population was reportedly 0.8% among an unselected pediatric population of 1,200 children under 18 years of age (7).

The majority of ACD (type IV) to rubber latex is the result of increased sensitivity to chemical accelerators and antioxidants, such as thiurams, added during the manufacturing of rubber. With the increasing incidence of latex allergy, dithiocarbamates and mercaptobenzothiazole derivatives were added to replace thiurams (3). It was believed that this could potentially decrease latex allergy, nonetheless sensitization incidence has persisted.

Immunology and Pathophysiology of Rubber Allergic Contact Dermatitis

Latex allergy is thought to have two basic mechanisms involved: (1) type I IgE-mediated mast cell degranulation and (2) type IV delayed T-cell hypersensitivity. As previously discussed IgE mediation is related to polypeptide epitopes, while type IV hypersensitivity is related to chemical accelerators during the manufacturing process (3, 7). Clinically, IgE mediation manifests as either atopy or life-threatening anaphylaxis, while type IV results in ACD. The focus of this work is on ACD; however, it has been demonstrated that chronic exposures to rubber ACD can increase the likelihood of IgE-mediated anaphylaxis. For instance, a study among 1,800 children were investigated for contact dermatitis with standard diagnostic patch testing, as well as immunological blood tests to detect IgE-mediated allergy (7). Thirty-two of the 1,800 children had positive patch tests while the immunoassays for IgE mediation were negative at the time of diagnosis. However, only after 2 years this same patient population depicted that 10 of 27 patients had positive immunoassays, indicating sufficient IgE levels for the subsequent development of atopy or anaphylaxis. This demonstrates the ever increasing predilection of type I allergy resultant from ACD latex exposure (7).

ACD is a type IV hypersensitivity reaction. It manifests clinically as the contact hypersensitivity after presensitization with antigenic haptens. The reaction is a mixed TH1/TH2 cell response eliciting both the inflammatory cascade and atopy–anaphylaxis axis (8). ACD from rubber results from chemical residues added during the vulcanization process during manufacturing. Initial hypothesis was that this allergenic profile was thought to be directly attributed to thiuram, hence other additives, such as dithiocarbamates and MPT, were used as alternative accelerators aimed at reducing the allergenic response thought to be elicited solely from thiuram. However, these actions did not significantly decrease latex allergy. Bergendorff et al. used high performance liquid chromatography (HPLC) to determine the exact chemical composition of rubber gloves thought to cause rubber ACD (9). Thiurams and MPT were readily isolated and analyzed using a diode spectrometric detector after separation using HPLC; however, dithiocarbamates were more difficult to isolate. Dithiocarbamates have an increased propensity to chelate metal ions from the solvent or contact surfaces (9). This demonstrates that the rubber additives are quite reactive prior to manufacturing (vulcanization).

Hence, the determination of allergenicity prior to vulcanization may not be accurate given the known reactivity.

One study focused on analyzing the chemical composition of the rubber before, during, and after the vulcanization process. Given the reactivity of the chemicals, it was postulated that the end products after vulcanization would be different from the initial additives. Major chemical changes occur during the vulcanization process. Thiuram disulfides rarely are detected in the end product of vulcanized rubber (4). Thiurams are converted to dithiocarbamates or the derivatives of MPT (Fig. 9.1). Therefore, from a theoretical chemical perspective, the dialkyl thiocarbamoyl structure may be responsible for the allergic rubber reactions rather than the thiuram structure (4). Examination of the chemical structure may explain why the reduced thiuram use in rubber products has not decreased latex ACD. Therefore, the positive patch reactions to patients with suspected latex ACD may be explained by cross-reactivity among thiurams and dithiocarbamates (4). This shows that chemical analysis must be taken into consideration because the allergens may be chemically converted or replaced during the vulcanization process. The determination of specific allergens for latex allergy may then be very difficult to determine due to the chemical processing as well as differences in manufacturers practices. Thus, latex manufacturers may need to reduce dithiocarbamate additives to latex rubber and physicians may need to expand their traditional patch test series to include dithiocarbamates.

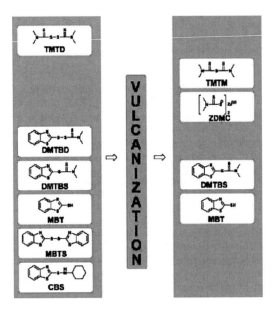

Fig. 9.1 An overview indicating the rubber chemicals present at different stages in the process. TMTM, tetramethylthiuram monosulfide; ZDMC, zinc dimethyldithiocarbamate; DMTBD, *N,N*-dimethylthiocarbamylbenzothiazole disulfide; DMTBS, *N,N*-dimethylthiocarbamylbenzothiazole sulfide; MBT, 2-mercaptobenzothiazol (Courtesy of Bergendorff et al. (4))

Clinical Manifestations of Rubber Allergic Contact Dermatitis

The general clinical manifestations of latex allergy vary from mild (contact urticaria, rhinoconjunctivitis, mucosal swelling) to severe (generalized urticaria, asthma, anaphylaxis). Type I reactions generally occur within minutes, while type IV reactions typically respond 96 h after cutaneous contact (3). The most common presentation of rubber contact dermatitis is an erythematous, papular eczema at the site of rubber contact. In general, the lesions are a patchy eczema; however, a systemic papulo-vesiculous reaction can take place if there is enough cutaneous latex deposition (Figs. 9.2 and 9.3) (10).

There are certain risk factors which place patients at increased risk for the development of latex allergy. Hence, knowledge of these risk factors will better enable physicians to screen and diagnose latex allergy.

In general, there is a greater degree of exposure in females. This may be attributed to a larger number of women involved in medical fields experiencing an

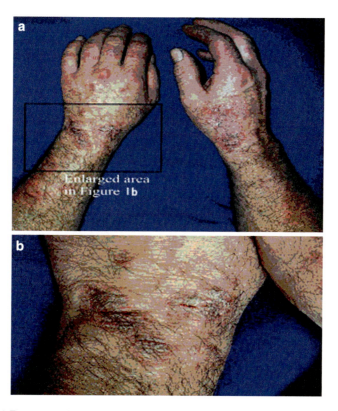

Fig. 9.2 (**a**) Forearms and hands of a patient demonstrating well-defined, erythematous, hyperkeratotic, fissured plaques limited to areas covered by cuffed, 14-in gloves. (**b**) Close-up view of plaques on the back of wrist and hand. (Courtesy of Kwon et al. (13))

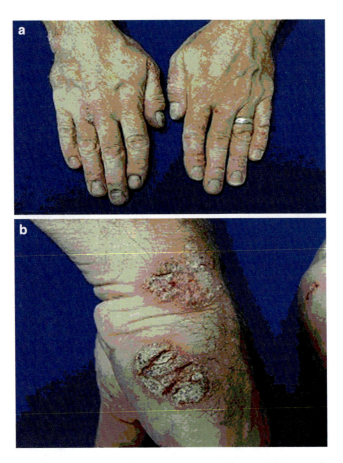

Fig. 9.3 (**a**) Back of hands of a patient demonstrating well-defined, erythematous, hyperkeratotic, fissured plaques. (**b**) Close-up view of plaques on side of right hand (Courtesy of Kwon et al. (13))

increased exposure to rubber containing products such as gloves. Additionally, latex allergy appears to have increased frequency among young people since they tend to be employed as workers in industries requiring greater exposure to latex products such as gloves used in food preparation. A major risk factor for latex allergy are predisposing skin injuries. Any trauma or break in the skin disrupts the skin barrier and leads to increased invasion of chemical residues into the skin dermis hypothesized to cause ACD (13). Interestingly, a risk factor for ICU is atopy. Among patients with atopy, a prevalence of 3–9.4% ICU has been reported (10). It must be mentioned that children with spina bifida or spinal dysraphism have an increased predilection for IgE-mediated latex allergy making this disease an additional risk factor for latex sensitization (4). Thus, the major risk factors for developing latex allergy appear to be female sex, young age, skin injuries, and atopy.

Diagnosis and Treatment

To diagnose either type I latex allergy or latex ACD, the most important measure is the history taking and physical examination by a physician. The dermatologist must ascertain whether the patient has an occupation or risk factors which could potentially predispose the patient to latex allergy. Additionally, inspection of the dermal quality, distribution, and morphology can direct the dermatologist toward the correct diagnosis. Nonetheless, there are diagnostic tests of choice for both type I latex allergy and latex ACD. The type I rubber allergy diagnostic test of choice is the immunological prick test (11). The epicutaneous prick test is a quick and inexpensive test that detects latex-specific IgE on skin mast cells. Additionally, in vitro immunoassay can be performed to detect the specificity with which IgE binds latex. However, the sensitivity and specificity between a simple prick test versus immunoassay ranges from 50% to 100% and 63% to 100%, respectively (10, 11). This leads to a very broad range of false positive and negatives making it a rather unreliable diagnostic marker.

The diagnostic test of choice for latex ACD is patch testing. As with other diagnostic patch testing, the chemical moiety, namely, either thiuram (25 $\mu g/cm^2$) or mercaptobenzothiazole (75 $\mu g/cm^2$) obtained from NACDRG standard series for latex allergy, is applied to a patch in 1% petrolatum (12). However, given recent research it may be prudent for physicians to add dithiocarbamate mixtures to the standard series. The patch is then applied directly to the skin. The patch is read at 48 h and 96 h, respectively. A positive reaction involves erythema, induration, and papules, strong reactions result in a bullous reaction. The patch test uses a simple three point grading system as follows: +, ++ & +++ in order of increasing severity (12).

The primary means of treatment for type I allergy is prevention of exposure by presensitized individuals. Given the ubiquitous nature of latex containing products, this is virtually impossible. It is of particular concern for high-risk groups such as health care workers or spina bifida patients. In order to avoid IgE-mediated latex allergy, there are number of precautions that can be taken to avoid sensitization. To avoid occupational exposure, all operating rooms should be latex free, and the use of low protein nonpowdered gloves should be adopted (3, 10). All hospital patients with known latex allergy should be required to wear hospital bracelets indicating the sensitization. Additionally, the use of nitrile or neoprene gloves have been adopted by most institutions to prevent cutaneous exposure to latex; however, one study has shown that permeation times for nitrile gloves are 10 min for toluene, 30 min for xylene, and 60 min for acetone (10, 13). This demonstrates that frequent glove redonning must be adopted.

Medical therapy may be employed for symptomatic relief. Pruritus may be treated with oral antihistamines or other antipruritus medications. Topical corticosteroids remain the most effective treatment of latex ACD. Short-term use of topical corticosteroid preparations, such as fluticasone propionate or clobetasole butyrate, is well tolerated. However, long-term use may result in local and systemic side effects. For severe recalcitrant disease states, systemic corticosteroids may be appropriate (12).

Questions

1. A 27-year-old laboratory technician presents with a pruritic, erythematous rash on the dorsal aspect of her right hand. She is known to have similar reactions to rubber in the past. She uses proper hygiene and wears latex-free gloves. Some of the materials which she is known to handle are acetone and toluene. What risk factor directly predisposed her for recurrent latex ACD?

    (a) Improper glove donning
    (b) Skin damage
    (c) Female sex
    (d) Latex-free gloves

2. What is the typical reaction time for a latex ACD?

    (a) 15 min
    (b) 1–2 min
    (c) 1 week
    (d) 24–96 h

3. A 45-year-old man with a known type I latex allergy is scheduled for a routine laparoscopic cholecystectomy. The unit clerk unknowingly forgot to create a bracelet making the house staff aware of the allergy. What complication of latex allergy is she at greatest risk for?

    (a) Contact urticaria
    (b) Rhinoconjunctivitis
    (c) Anaphylaxis
    (d) Generalized erythema

4. What is the diagnostic test of choice for type I latex allergy?

    (a) Patch testing
    (b) IgE immunoassay
    (c) Prick testing
    (d) CBC

5. What is the most effective way to diagnose a latex allergy due to either type I or type IV?

    (a) Patch Testing
    (b) Prick Testing
    (c) Good history and physical examination
    (d) Liver function studies

6. At the end of the vulcanization process the thiuram additive remains unchanged?

    (a) True
    (b) False

9 Allergic Contact Dermatitis: Rubber Allergies

7. What are the primary constituents of latex type IV ACD?

   (a) Latex protein
   (b) Chemical accelerators
   (c) Dithiocarbamates
   (d) All of the above

8. A 15-year old-football player develops a pruritic, erythematous dermatitis in a preauricular and postauricular distribution. Two years later the patient had a period of severe wheezing and atopy with no known associated infectious etiology. What is the associated pathophysiology?

   (a) IgE-mediated atopy and anaphylaxis
   (b) Type IV delayed T-cell hypersensitivity
   (c) Type IV delayed T-cell presensitization with subsequent type I atopy and anaphylaxis
   (d) Type I presensitization with subsequent type IV atopy and anaphylaxis

9. What is the treatment of choice for latex ACD?

   (a) Prevention
   (b) Topical Corticosteroids
   (c) Systemic Corticosteroids
   (d) Oral antihistamines

10. Which of the following is a common product with latex exposure?

    (a) Condoms
    (b) Erasers
    (c) Bandages
    (d) All of the above

Answers: 1(b), 2(d), 3(a), 4(c), 5(c), 6(b), 7(d), 8(c), 9(a), 10(d).

References

1. Lachapelle JM, Maibach HI. Patch Testing and Prick Testing. A Practical Guide. Berlin: Springer-Verlag Berlin Heidelberg: 2003, 2009, pp. 46–50.
2. Warshaw Erin M, Furda Laura M, et al. Angiogenital dermatitis in patients referred for patch testing. Retrospective analysis of cross-sectional data from the North American Contact Dermatitis Group, 1994–2004. Archives of Dermatology. 2008: 144(6): 749–755.
3. Boguniewicz M, Covar R, Fleischer D. Allergic Disorders. In: Hay WW, Jr., Levin MJ, Sondheimer JM, Deterding RR: Current Diagnosis and Treatment: Pediatrics, 19th Ed. Denver, CO: The McGraw-Hill Companies, Inc; 2008: http://www.accessmedicine.com/content.aspx?aID=3409411.
4. Bergendorff O, Persson C, Ludtke A, Hansson C. Chemical changes in rubber allergens during vulcanization. Contact Dermatitis. 2007: 57: 152–157.
5. Moritz K, Sesztak-Greinecker G et al. Allergic contact dermatitis due to rubber in sports equipment. Contact Dermatitis. 2007: 57: 131–132.

6. Hann S, Hughes M, Stone N. Self-adherent wrap bandages – a hidden source of natural rubber latex. Contact Dermatitis. 2006: 55: 194–195.
7. Gilbert G, Gilbert MH, Dagregorio G. Allergic contact dermatitis from natural rubber latex in atopic dermatitis and the risk of later type I allergy. Contact Dermatitis. 2005: 53: 46–51.
8. Xu H, DiIulio NA, Fairchild RL. T cell populations primed by hapten sensitization in contact sensitivity are distinguished by polarized patterns of cytokine production: interferon gamma-producing (Tc1) effector CD81 T cells and interleukin(Il) 4/Il-10-producing (Th2) negative regulatory CD41 T cells. The Journal of Experimental Medicine. 1996: 183: 1001–1012.
9. Bergendorff O, Persson C, Hansson C. High performance liquid chromatography analysis of rubber allergens in protective gloves used in health care. Contact Dermatitis 2006: 55: 210–215.
10. Nettis E, Colanardi MC, Ferrannini A, Tursi A. Latex hypersensitivity: personal data and review of the literature. Immunopharmacology and Immunotoxicology. 2002: 24: 315–324.
11. Nitti JT, Nitti GJ. Anesthestic Complications. In: Morgan GE, Jr., Mikhail MS, Murray MJ: Clinical Anesthesiology, 4th Ed. New York, NY: The McGraw-Hill Companies, Inc; 2006: http://www.accessmedicine.com/content.aspx?aID=895440.
12. Cohen David E, Jacob Sharon E. Allergic Contact Dermatitis. In: Wolff K, Goldsmith LA, Katz SI, Gilchrest B, Paller AS, Leffell DJ: Fitzpatrick's Dermatology in General Medicine, 7th Ed. New York, NY: The McGraw-Hill Companies, Inc; 2008: http://www.accessmedicine.com/content.aspx?aID=2966976.
13. Kwon S, Campbell L, Zirwas MJ. Role of protective gloves in the causation and treatment of occupational irritant contact dermatitis. Journal of the American Academy of Dermatology. 2006: 55: 891–896.

Chapter 10
Jewelry: Nickel and Metal-Based Allergic Contact Dermatitis

Peter Burke and Howard I. Maibach

Abstract Metal allergic contact dermatitis (ACD) is a type IV delayed hypersensitivity reaction. Nickel allergy is the most prevalent of ACD and is the most common positive reaction from diagnostic patch testing. Recently, there has been a growing prevalence of patch test reactivity among other metals such as gold, cobalt, and palladium. Classically, the allergy is associated with pre-sensitization and resultant erythema, edema, and lichenification in the distribution of metal contact. The diagnostic standard is patch testing using the standard NACDRG (North American Contact Dermatitis Research Group) series, or the allergen suspended in petrolatum. The primary method of treatment consists of prevention of metal contact; however, medical therapy may be employed for symptomatic relief. Therapy consists of the use of topical corticosteroids in mild–moderate cases and the use of systemic corticosteroids in moderate–severe cases, while other symptoms such as pruritus may be controlled with antipruritics or oral sedating antihistamines.

Keywords Allergic contact dermatitis • Metal • Nickel • Gold • Cobalt • Palladium

Case 1

History of Present Illness

An 8-year-old Caucasian boy was referred by his pediatrician to our contact dermatitis clinic with a chief complaint of a gradually extending peri-umbilical dermatitis (eczema). The history of present illness revealed that the eruption had been present for approximately 6 months and exacerbated and remitted, but without an obvious explanation to the parents or referring physician. Treatment consisted of

---

P. Burke (✉)
Philadelphia College of Osteopathic Medicine, Philadelphia, PA 19131, USA
and
University of California San Francisco, San Francisco, CA 94143-0989, USA
e-mail: Peterbu@pcom.edu

over-the-counter 1% hydrocortisone cream and proprietary topical medicaments. Past medical and surgical history was otherwise unremarkable.

Physical Examination

A focused dermatological examination revealed a well-nourished 8-year-old Caucasian boy demonstrating redness, scaling, edema, and lichenification in a periumbilical area, measuring 7 cm in diameter. The remaining skin appeared clear.

Differential Diagnosis

Differential diagnosis includes endogenous dermatitis, such as atopic dermatitis and nummular eczema, and exogenous dermatitis, such as allergic contact dermatitis (ACD).

Working Diagnosis

ACD.

Impression and Follow-Up

On further questioning, our clinical suspicion was blue jean button dermatitis in a boy who frequently did not wear underpants. We suggested to the parents the possibility of blue jean (nickel) ACD and demonstrated that the buttons on his blue jeans were dimethylglyoxime (DMG) positive, revealing a clinically relevant nickel release.

We elected to not perform confirmatory patch testing with 5% nickel sulfate in petrolatum, as we believed that the history, morphology, and DMG-positive button strongly suggested nickel ACD.

His parents removed the nickel-containing blue jean buttons and replaced them with DMG negatives. Complete healing occurred in 3 weeks and he has been asymptomatic at follow-up 1 year later.

Case 2

History of Present Illness

An 18-year-old woman was self-referred to our contact dermatitis clinic with a 1-year history of dermatitis that started on the ears and gradually progressed to involve several anatomic sites.

A general physician made a diagnosis of atopic dermatitis and treated with topical corticosteroids, moisturizers, and oral antihistamines. The extent of the lesions and severity went through periods of exacerbation and remission without a clear explanation to the patient.

Physical Examination

A focused dermatological examination revealed a well-nourished 18-year-old woman demonstrating erythema, edema, and lichenification of cubital and popliteal fossae, and scattered eczematous rashes on the trunk and buttocks. The remaining skin appeared clear.

Differential Diagnosis

Differential diagnosis includes atopic dermatitis, nonspecific dermatitis, eczematous psoriasis, exogenous dermatitis, such as ACD, and systemic contact dermatitis.

Working Diagnosis

ACD.

Impression and Follow-Up

As the patient had been carefully followed by her personal physician and failed to clear, diagnostic patch testing with the NACDRG extended series was performed, revealing a 3+ reaction with intense erythema with infiltration and coalescing vesicles to 2.5% nickel sulfate in petrolatum. The scale utilized was that of the International Contact Dermatitis Research Group (ICDRG).

On retrospective historical review, she revealed that the dermatitis started on her ears and may have been related to the use of costume jewelry, explaining the possible diagnosis of ACD to nickel with distal spread. She agreed to discontinue the use of costume jewelry. Several earrings were DMG positive. Complete clearing occurred in 3 weeks, with no exacerbation at 1 year.

The presumed pathology at distal sites with minimal contact, such as the cubital and popliteal fossae suggests that the nickel has been percutaneously absorbed and deposited in the distal sites (systemic contact dermatitis).

Discussion

Historical Background

Nickel, a ubiquitous metal found worldwide, occurs in the earth's core as well as in soil, water, and air. The Swedish chemist Baron Axel Fredrik Cronstedt discovered nickel in 1751 (1). Nickel is used extensively worldwide because of its reproducibility, strength, and oxidation resistance. Metals such as nickel and molybdenum are utilized as additives to stainless steel to prevent staining, rusting, and corrosion. However, other transitional metals may be combined with steel to form other alloys, including elements such as cobalt, palladium, iron, titanium, vanadium, and magnesium. Nickel-containing alloys are abundant in most industrialized nations due to its ability to enhance the metallurgical properties. It may be found in everyday items such as jewelry, eyeglass frames, watchbands, belt buckles, snaps, and coins (2). Nickel is the most prevalent positive patch test in the general population; however, other metals such as gold, cobalt, and, to a lesser extent, palladium may also evoke such sensitivities.

Prevalence of Metal-Based Contact Dermatitis

Positive patch test results for nickel sensitivity have been reported in up to 5.8% of US adults (9% women and 0.9% men). Additionally, another study ($n=399$) depicted that 7.6–12.9% of US infants and children were affected. The NACDG conducted a patch test frequency study from January 1, 2001, to December 31, 2002, on 4,193 patients using 65 allergens (2). The top ten allergens from this period were repeated in the 2001–2002 case report with the following allergic patch test reaction rates: nickel sulfate (16.7%), neomycin (11.6%), Myroxilon pereirae (balsam of Peru) (11.6%), fragrance mix (10.4%), thimerosal (10.2%), sodium gold thiosulfate (10.2%), quaternium-15 (9.3%), formaldehyde (8.4%), bacitracin (7.9%), and cobalt chloride (7.4%) (2). This study indicated that two of the three common metal antigens (nickel and cobalt) were among the top ten reactants.

The ubiquitous presence of nickel and nickel-containing alloys makes frequent contact with this metal practically unavoidable. The frequency of nickel sensitization has been increasing, especially among women and children. The NACDG reported an increase in positive patch tests to nickel from 10.5% between 1985 and 1990 to 18.8% between 2003 and 2004 (2). The alarming frequency of sensitization to nickel led to nickel being named the 2008 "Allergen of the Year" by the American Contact Dermatitis Society. In 1992, the Danish government enacted legislation requiring that elemental nickel released from products that are in prolonged contact with the skin, such as earrings, buttons, and spectacle frames, should be less than

0.5 µg/cm² per week. In response to the legislation, rates of nickel sensitization in the Danish population decreased. In Danish children from 0.5 to 18 years of age, the prevalence of nickel allergy decreased from 24.8 to 9.2% between 1985 and 1998 (3). The European Union (EU) passed a similar legislation in 1994, issuing "The Nickel Directive," which mandated that the limit be less than 0.5 µg/cm² per week in objects containing nickel that come into direct and prolonged contact with the skin (4).

Despite the increasing frequency of nickel exposure and the success observed in Europe, USA has failed to enact a directive against excessive nickel exposure. These positive test results coupled with as many as 20–33% of children from recent studies having positive patch tests show the imminent need for a US legislation relative to nickel release due to chronic exposure potential.

Impact of Patient Factors on Contact Allergy with Nickel and other Metals

The prevalence for nickel and other metals is well known. We believe that the US legislation should be enacted to combat the increasing frequency of metal allergy; however, it is appropriate to study patient factors in an effort to avoid and reduce metal exposure in high-risk groups. Ruff et al. demonstrated that of 208 patients tested, 5.8% had a positive metal allergy to either cobalt, nickel, or chromate with additional concurrent co-metal sensitivities, and the prevalence of isolated metal allergy was consistent with the literature (5). For instance, nickel and cobalt allergies are more prominent in women, while chromate allergy is more prominent in men (occupational exposure from cement). Note that nickel sensitization has been theorized as being a prerequisite for cobalt allergy.

Overall, the high-risk groups for developing metal allergy appear to be females and young children. The relative risk in women is 3.7 more prevalent when compared with that in men and 3.2 for those aged 30 years or less (2). However, it must be mentioned that 13% of children were found to be nickel sensitive in a Denver study of 85 children. As can be expected, an important risk factor for metal exposure is ear piercing. A study of 567 Danish citizens determined that nickel sensitization was higher among patients with pierced ears (14.8%) compared to that in a like population without ear piercing (1.8%) (6). The higher rates of ear piercing in women compared with that in men can explain the predilection of metal allergy for women. However, as the popularity of body piercing increases in both genders, the rate of metal allergy will probably also increase concomitantly in both. Occupations at high risk for metal exposure and sensitization include metal workers, retail clerks, hairdressers, domestic cleaners, and caterers. Tasks performed by metal workers include welding, nickel electroplating, metal wires and alloys operating machine bending, lining of steel furnaces, metal cutting, and sheets metal pattern designs (2).

Immunology and Pathophysiology of Metal ACD

ACD is a type IV delayed hypersensitivity reaction. ACD manifests clinically as contact hypersensitivity after sensitization with low molecular weight haptens (Figs. 10.1 and 10.2) (7). The reaction requires uptake of allergen by antigen-presenting cells (APCs) in the skin (Langerhan's cells, APCs) and activation of allergen-specific T cells. The mechanism can be attributed to the activation of CD8+ cytotoxic T-cells and the IL-4, IL-5, and IL-10 producing CD4+ TH2 cells, eliciting a mixed TH1/TH2 cytokine response (7). For instance, after nickel contacts the skin, it forms an antigenic complex with a specific self-peptide and major histocompatability complex on Langerhan's cells in the skin (7). This APC then migrates to the regional lymph nodes to activate immature T-cells (Figs. 10.1 and 10.2).

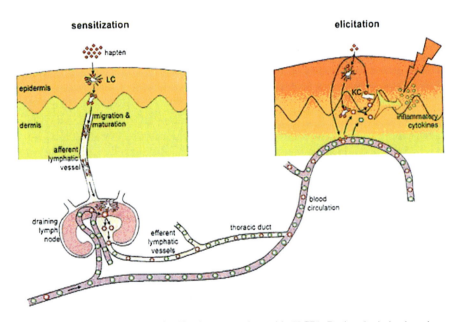

Fig. 10.1 Immunological events in allergic contact dermatitis (ACD). During the induction phase (*left*), skin contact with a hapten triggers migration of epidermal Langerhan cell (LC) via the afferent lymphatic vessels to the skin-draining lymph nodes. Haptenized LC home into the T-cell rich paracortical area. Here, conditions are optimal for encountering naïve T cells that specifically recognize allergen-MHC molecule complexes. Hapten-specific T cells now expand abundantly and generate effector and memory cells, which are released via efferent lymphatics into the circulation. With their newly acquired homing receptors, these cells can easily extravasate peripheral tissues. Renewed allergen contact sparks off the effector phase (*right*). Due to their lowered activation threshold, hapten-specific effector T cells are triggered by various haptenized cells, including LC and keratinocytes (KC), to produce proinflammatory cytokines and chemokines. Thereby, more inflammatory cells are recruited, further amplifying local inflammatory mediator release. This leads to a gradually developing eczematous reaction, reaching a maximum within 18–48 h, after which the reactivity successively declines (courtesy of Ref. [8])

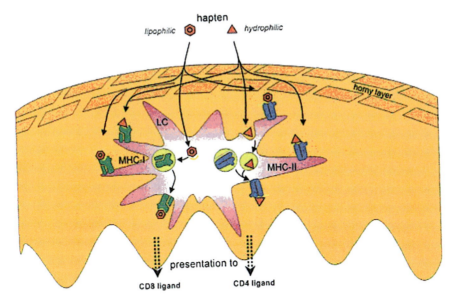

Fig. 10.2 Hapten presentation by epidermal Langerhans cells (LCs). Allergen penetrating the epidermis readily associates with all kinds of skin components, including major histocompatibility complex (MHC) proteins, abundantly present on epidermal LC. Both MHC class I and class II molecules may be altered directly or via intracellular hapten processing and, subsequently, be recognized by allergen-specific CD8$^+$ and CD4$^+$ T cells (courtesy of Ref. [8])

The MHC–nickel–peptide complex is eventually presented to a series of T-cell receptors, which consequently results in a cytokine inflammatory cascade (7). Since, the activation of the reaction requires specific dermal peptide–antigenic interaction only pre-sensitized individuals will express an allergic reaction.

Larsen et al. proposed an additional mechanistic explanation of ACD in IL-23 and TH17-mediated inflammation in human ACD (9). A novel IL-17 producing CD4+ T-cell has been described that preferentially targets epithelial cells, endothelial cells, and macrophages to express proinflammatory cytokines to activate and recruit neutrophils to the sensitized tissue (9). Pre-sensitized keratinocytes express IL-23 in response to allergen exposure, which activates IL-17 producing TH-17 cells (9). The role of IL-17 in the inflammatory cascade has been demonstrated by impaired cellular and humoral immunity in IL-17 knockout mice. Additionally, allergen-specific IL-17 producing CD4+ and CD8+ T cells develop in sensitized mice. Furthermore, in vitro treatment with IL-17 neutralizing antibodies inhibits the immune response mobilization of monocytes, macrophages, and granulocytes in sensitized tissue (9). The clinical importance of the mechanism may be realized as a novel approach for the treatment of contact dermatitis.

Allergenicity of Gold, Cobalt, and Palladium

Gold

Prior to the early 1990s, gold allergy was thought to be rare. Gold is a ubiquitous metal that has been valued for thousands of years without obvious complaints of skin problems (10). Gold as a metal is inert. Therefore, in order to be sensitized to gold, the metal must be ionized. Chemically, gold salts are very reactive, and thus have been used as a therapeutic modality for rheumatic and dermatologic diseases such as rheumatoid arthritis and pemphigus vulgaris, respectively (10). It was surprising when patch testing for gold allergy consistently showed 10% positive patch tests of patients presenting with dermatitis. In 1998–2000, the NACDG ranked gold as the sixth most frequent cause of positive patch tests (2).

One must speculate whether gold allergy is a novel ACD or the result of co-sensitivity/cross-reactivity to other metals such as nickel. Irritant dermatitis is similar to contact dermatitis from visual patch test analysis; however, serial dilutions of gold sodium thiosulfate have conclusively proved the allergenicity of gold (10). The co-sensitivity/cross-reactivity can be appreciated by understanding the dermatopathological mechanistic aspects of ACD. Gold ACD is also a type IV hypersensitivity reaction involving both CD4+ and CD8+ T cells. The production of IFN-γ is a typical sign of TH-1 response. Christiansen et al. showed the up-regulation IFN-γ in gold-sensitive patients independent of nickel allergy (11). It has been postulated that gold directly binds the MHC-II molecule independent of APC presentation. This mechanism varies from the traditional APC presentation that is observed in traditional type IV hypersensitivities such as that observed with nickel.

Gold allergy normally presents as a dermatitis at the site of contact; however, solitary eyelid and oral gold allergy has been reported. It has been postulated that the allergen is transferred from the hands to the eyelids without causing any hand dermatitis. This might be resultant from the more delicate epidermal skin structure of the eyelids. A strong correlation has also been drawn between gold allergy and gold dental restorations. Although reports are rare, symptoms have manifested in patients with a lichenoid mucositis similar in nature to lichenoid planus. This has prompted some physicians to add gold to the regular tray of allergy patch testing.

Cobalt

Cobalt is an abundant metal found in the environment that is essential since it is a major component of vitamin B12, cyanocobalamin. Cobalt can form many alloys with metals such as iron, nickel, chromium, and molybdenum, which are heavily used in industry. Numerous occupations have increased exposure to cobalt, including cement workers and bricklayers. Cobalt is reported as the tenth most common sensitizer in USA with a patch test reaction rate of approximately 7.6% (2).

Many patients with cobalt sensitivity have a concurrent nickel sensitivity as well, leading to the assumption of a cross-reactivity between cobalt and nickel. This suggests an enhanced development of allergy to either metal if a sensitivity already exists (12). Hence, some may speculate the efficacy of concurrent cobalt and nickel in patch testing.

A recent study has demonstrated that different cobalt-containing alloy discs allow the release of significant amounts of cobalt when suspended in human sweat. The cobalt released from one of the alloys was reportedly 2–3 times greater than that in a serial dilution (93 $\mu g/cm^2$) patch test in the same study (12). This reflects the potential importance of biological fluids in this reaction. This shows that the metal release from an alloy is not directly correlative with the cobalt concentration of the alloy. Furthermore, cross-reactivity was studied in guinea pigs induced with cobalt and then challenged with chromate or nickel (13). No cross-reactivity was observed. The excessive release of cobalt coupled with the lack of cross-reactivity in guinea pigs suggests that cobalt allergy is induced by multiple exposure and co-sensitization with nickel rather than by cross-reactivity (12). This warrants the concurrent patch testing of both cobalt and nickel.

Palladium

Palladium is used in the telecommunications industry, high temperature solders, dentistry, and jewelry. Palladium chloride suspended in 1% petrolatum is found in dental and metal patch test series, and the prevalence of allergy has been increasing. Since 1990, there have been numerous reports of palladium allergy with almost every patient having a reaction to another metal, usually nickel. In a population of 2,300 patients, 171 were patch test positive to palladium (7.4%) (14). Of those 171 patients, cross-sensitivity was detected in 169 patients. Since both metals belong to group VIII of the periodic table, there is a strong likelihood of cross-reactivity/co-sensitivity between nickel and palladium due to the chemical properties (14).

Clinical Presentation of Metal Allergy

The most common presentation of metal contact dermatitis is a well-demarcated, erythematous, popular eczematous plaque at the site of metal contact (15). Common locations for dermatitis include earlobes from earrings, neck from necklaces, periumbilically from belt buckles or snaps, and periorbitally from glasses. In general, once sensitization has been established, the acute phase of the reaction progresses from erythema to edema to papulo-vesiculation, while chronically lichenification and scaling are common (15). One exception may be the areas of thin skin that has higher absorption coefficients, such as the eyelids, mucosal surfaces, and genitalia.

While metal contact dermatitis may result in different areas, including the face, neck, and earlobes, hand dermatitis tends to be the most prevalent.

Systemic metal contact dermatitis has been described two-fold, by either oral ingestion or long-lasting immunologic memory in previously sensitized areas of skin. Systemic contact dermatitis is a relatively uncommon and poorly understood aspect of ACD. With oral ingestion a mere 0.22–0.35 mg of nickel, the most sensitive patients may respond with a fulminant systemic dermatitis (15). Foods with high metal content include whole wheat, oatmeal, chocolate, beans, nuts, and dried foods (1). High metal content may also be found in vitamins, fruits, and vegetables. Thus, in rare individuals with high sensitivity to metal, it is recommended to minimize the intake of these food products containing high metal content.

It may be possible for metal contact dermatitis to manifest systemically from simple contact without ingestion. This is possible, because Langerhan's and T cells circulate throughout the body; hence, areas not exposed to the metal may become involved. This is referred to as auto-eczematization. This phenomenon occurs primarily in individuals who are initially sensitized to the metal and then subsequently have systemic exposure, resulting in extensive dermatitis and erythroderma (15).

Of paramount concern is the increasing use of stainless steel medical devices in patients with metal allergy. There have been some reports of metal orthopedic implants that have caused generalized eczematous rashes provoking the removal of the implant (16). Patients may react to dental prosthesis, orthodontic wiring, and peripheral intravenous catheters. Yet, the most concerning is allergy of endovascular stents causing a re-stenosis effect (16). Such events are extremely rare; however, patch testing prior to implantation of the device in a patient with either known allergy or general allergic physiology is warranted.

Diagnosis and Treatment

Metal ACD should be suspected in anybody with an eczematous dermatitis present in locations in the skin with prolonged metal exposure. Classically, the standard diagnostic technique for metal ACD is patch testing. Patch testing for metal ACD involves suspending metals such as nickel sulfate (2.5 or 5%) or gold sodium thiosulfate (0.5%) in petrolatum. The patch is applied directly to the patient's skin for 48 h and then examined at 72 h and 96 h respectively. A positive reaction involves erythema, induration, and papules; strong reactions result in a bullous reaction (Fig. 10.3). Often the NACDRG test is used, which is a commercially available patch test containing two standard trays (Table 10.1) (15).

Recently, there has been controversy concerning delayed patch test reading in metal alloys known to cause contact dermatitis. It was determined that the standard patch test reading is still appropriate; however, patient's with suspected metal allergy should have the standard patch reading with an additional reading after day 5 (17). For instance, it was demonstrated that of the 353 patch tests to gold sodium thiosulfate 0.5%, 22 (6.2%) were negative at day 5, but positive between days 7 and 21. Additionally, cobalt, nickel, mercury, and palladium had similar results on delayed reading at days 7–21 (17).

10 Jewelry: Nickel and Metal-Based Allergic Contact Dermatitis

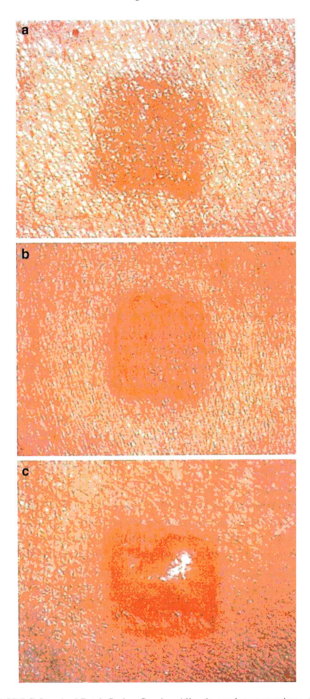

Fig. 10.3 NACDRG Standard Patch Series. Scoring Allergic patch test reactions. (**a**) + reaction; (**b**) ++ reaction (**c**) +++reaction (courtesy of Ref. [18])

Table 10.1 The NACDRG standard series (courtesy of Ref. [18])

Allergens	µg cm^{-1}
Panel 1	
1. Nickel sulfate	200
2. Wool alcohols	1,000
3. Neomycin sulfate	230
4. Potassium dichromate	23
5. Caine mix	630
6. Fragrance mix	430
7. Colophony	850
8. Epoxy resin	50
9. Quinoline mix	190
10. Balsams of Peru	800
11. Ethylenediamine dihydrochloride	50
12. Cobalt chloride	20
Panel 2	
13. *p-tert*-Butylphenol formaldehyde resin	50
14. Paraben mix	1,000
15. Carba mix	250
16. Black rubber mix	75
17. Cl + Me-isothiazolinone (Kathon CG)	4
18. Quaternium 15	100
19. Mercaptobenzothiazole	75
20. *p*-Phenylenediamine	90
21. Formaldehyde (*N*-hydroxymethyl succinimide)	180
22. Mercapto mix	75
23. Thiomerosal (thiomersal)	8
24. Thiuram mix	25

Patch testing remains the clinical diagnostic standard for metal contact dermatitis; however, a rapid and simple to use DMG test could be used for patients to identify nickel-containing metal alloys such as gold or palladium alloys (17). DMG may be applied to a cotton swab and exposed to the metal object such as earrings. If the alloy has greater than 5 ppm nickel, the DMG reacts as an indicator of metal alloys by turning into a pink color. This rapid assay will quickly alert the patient to the presence of nickel and avoid the purchase without damaging the merchandise (19). In all, 69% of local artists, 42.9% of tourist stores, and 24.1% of chain stores targeting younger women in San Francisco had positive DMG reactions (19). Considering the increasing prevalence of nickel sensitization, and unavoidability of nickel exposure, this rapid assay should be mandated to be made available to patient's with known allergy.

The primary mode of treatment for metal ACD is aimed at minimizing exposure. Physical or chemical barriers may be employed to prevent the release of metal ions. For example, physical barriers may be used by placing adhesives such as duct tape to the inside of buckles or snaps. Additionally, nail polish has shown to be effective in preventing metal ion release as evidenced by negative DMG tests.

Finally, chemical means using non-chelating barrier creams (9% glycerin and 4% primose oil) may be used. The effect of the cream is to provide protection against foreign particles, such as metal, against excessive trans-dermal water loss. Nonetheless, avoidance is the most successful preventative measure.

Medical therapy may be employed for symptomatic relief. Vesicular eruptions are best treated with drying agents such as aluminum sulfate/calcium acetate, while chronic lichenified skin may be treated with moisturizers or emollients (15). Pruritus may be controlled with topical antipruritics or oral antihistamines. Nonetheless, corticosteroids remain the most effective treatment of ACD. Topical corticosteroid preparations such as fluticasone proprionate or clobetasole butyrate are well tolerated with short-term use (15). However, long-term use may result in cutaneous atrophy, hirsutism, hypopigmentation, folliculitis, acne, and systemic absorption. Systemic corticosteroid administration is indicated only in moderate to severe cases.

Recently, calcineurin inhibitors have been used in the treatment of ACD. Tacrolimus inhibits the up-regulation of TH-2 cell production of IL-4, IL-5, and IL-10 resulting in allergy. Tacrolimus has shown to reduce signs and symptoms of nickel ACD, including erythema, pruritus, induration, and vesiculation, without the associated negative symptoms and medical complications with long-term steroid administration (15).

Questions

1. A 35-year-old Caucasian female presents with a well-demaracated erythematous lesion over the lower neck extending to the upper trunk. She was known to wear a nickel-containing necklace in the distribution of the dermatitis. She was referred to her local dermatologist and the diagnosis of nickel contact dermatitis was determined. She has been treated with oral antihistamines, moisturizers, and topical corticosteroids for 6 months duration without improvement. What is the treatment of choice?

    (a) Oral prednisone
    (b) Zieulton
    (c) Tacrolimus
    (d) Topical fluticasone

2. A 12-year-old girl is found to have edematous earlobes with papulo-vesiculation after exposure to nickel-containing earrings. What is the mechanism of the dermatitis?

    (a) Type 4 delayed hypersensitivity with mixed TH-1/TH-2 reaction
    (b) Type 1 IgE-mediated mast cell degranulation
    (c) Type 3 immune complex deposition
    (d) Type 2 delayed hypersensitivity with mixed TH-1/TH-2 reaction

3. What is the percentage of US adults who manifest a clinically relevant nickel contact dermatitis?

   (a) 7%
   (b) 5.8%
   (c) 9.0%
   (d) 4.6%

4. A 35-year-old Caucasian female presents with an erythematous lichenified circular lesion over the left fourth digit that has persisted for 3 months duration. She was known to wear her wedding band in the distribution of the dermatitis. Serial patch testing was conducted to determine the etiology of the dermatitis. When should the patch test be read?

   (a) 72 and 96 h
   (b) 48 and 96 h
   (c) 24 and 96 h
   (d) 72 h, 96 h, days 7–21 post-patch placement

5. A 10-year-old boy presents with an erythematous lichenified circular lesion measuring 8 cm in diameter in the peri-umbilical area that has persisted for 6 months duration. Subsequently, 3 months later, lichenifications appear in the popliteal fossae bilaterally. What is the most likely diagnosis?

   (a) Nickel contact dermatitis with atopic dermatitis
   (b) Systemic contact dermatitis (nickel)
   (c) Atopic dermatitis
   (d) Nickel contact dermatitis

6. What is the morbid complication of stent placement in patients with known contact allergy?

   (a) Anaphylaxis
   (b) TEN (toxic epidermal necrolysis)
   (c) Steven–Johnson's Syndrome
   (d) Re-stenosis event

7. A 20-year-old woman presents with an erythematous, lichenified lesion on her lower neck and upper trunk. She was known to previously wear a cobalt/nickel-containing metal alloy. What is the pathophysiology of the ACD?

   (a) Cross-reactivity between nickel and cobalt creating a delayed type IV hypersensitivity reaction.
   (b) Co-sensitivity between nickel and cobalt creating a delayed type IV hypersensitivity reaction.
   (c) Type III immune complex deposition
   (d) Type I IgE-mediated mast cell degranulation

8. In the early 1990s the governments of Denmark and the EU sanctioned the "Nickel Directive", which subsequently decreased nickel exposure in Denmark and Europe, respectively. What is the amount of µg/cm^2/week release allowed from nickel-containing products?

    (a) 5 µg/cm^2/week
    (b) 15 µg/cm^2/week
    (c) 0.5 µg/cm^2/week
    (d) 0.05 µg/cm^2/week

9. A 35-year-old male construction worker developed an erythematous and papulo-vesiculous dermatitis status post-diagnostic patch testing for a suspected chromate allergy. What is the likely source of exposure?

    (a) Earrings
    (b) Cement
    (c) Bowling ball
    (d) Rubber bands

10. What is the most prevalent metal ACD on diagnostic patch testing?

    (a) Cobalt
    (b) Gold
    (c) Nickel
    (d) Palladium

Answers: 1. (a), 2. (a), 3. (b), 4. (d), 5. (b), 6. (d), 7. (b), 8. (c), 9. (b), 10. (c).

References

1. Sharma AD. Relationship between nickel allergy and diet. Indian J Dermatol 2007;73(5):307–12.
2. Pratt MD, Belsito DV, DeLeo VA, et al. North America contact dermatitis group patch test results, 2001–2002 study period. Dermatitis 2004;15(4):176–83.
3. Johansen J, Menne T, Christophersen J, Kaaber K, Veien N. Changes in the pattern of sensitization to common contact allergens in Denmark between 1985–86 and 1997–98, with a special view to the effect of preventive strategies. Br J Dermatol 2000;142:490–5.
4. Commission Directive 2004/96/EC of September 2004 amending Council Directive 76/769/EEC as regards restriction on the marketing and use of nickel for piercing post assemblies for the purpose of adapting its Annex I to technical progress.
5. Ruff C, Belsito D. The impact of various patient factors on contact allergy to nickel, cobalt and chromate. J Am Dermatol 2006;55:32–9.
6. Neilsen NH, Menne T. Nickel sensitisation and earpiercing in an unselected Danish population. Glostrup allergy study. Contact Derm 1993;29:16–21.
7. Xu H, DiIulio NA, Fairchild RL. T cell populations primed by hapten sensitization in contact sensitivity are distinguished by polarized patterns of cytokine production: Interferon gamma-producing (Tc1) effector CD81 T cells and interleukin(Il) 4/Il-10-producing (Th2) negative regulatory CD41 T cells. J Exp Med 1996;183:1001–12.

8. Frosch, P, Menne, T. et. al. Contact Dermatitis, 4th Edition. 2006. Berlin: Springer Berlin Heidelberg New York, pp. 12–14.
9. Larsen, J, Bonefeld C, Poulsen S. IL-23 and TH17-mediated inflammation in human allergic contact dermatitis. J Allergy Clin Immunol 2009;123:486–92.
10. Bjorkner B, Bruze M, Moller H. High frequency of contact allergy to gold sodium thiosulfate, an indication of gold allergy? Contact Derm 1994;30:144–51.
11. Christiansen J, Farm G, Eid-Forest R. Interferon-γ secreted from peripheral blood mononuclear cells as a possible diagnostic marker for allergic contact dermatitis to gold. Contact Derm 2006;55:98–109.
12. Juliander A, Hindes M, Skare L. Cobalt-containing alloys and their ability to release cobalt and cause dermatitis. Contact Derm 2009;60:165–70.
13. Liden C, Wahlberg JE. Cross-reactivity to metal compounds studied in Guinea pigs induced withchromate or cobalt. Acta Derm Venereal (Norway) 1994;74(5):341–3.
14. Vincenzi C, Tosti A, Guerra L, et al. Contact dermatitis to palladium: A study of 2300 patients. Am J Contact Derm 1995;6:110–2.
15. Cohen DE, Jacob SE. Allergic Contact Dermatitis. In: Wolff K, Goldsmith LA, Katz SI, Gilchrest B, Paller AS, Leffell DJ: Fitzpatrick's Dermatology in General Medicine, 7th Ed. New York, NY: The McGraw-Hill Companies, Inc; 2008: http://www.accessmedicine.com/content.aspx?aID=2966976.
16. Kanerva L, Forstrom L. Allergic nickel and chromate hand dermatitis induced by orthopaedic metal implant. Contact Derm 2001;44:103–4.
17. Thyssen J, Maibach H. Nickel release from earrings purchased in the United States: The San Francisco earring study. J Am Acad Dermatol 2008;58:1000–5.
18. Lachapelle JM, Maibach HI. Patch Testing and Prick Testing. A Practical Guide, 2nd Edition. Berlin: Springer-Verlag Berlin Heidelberg 2003, pp. 46–50.
19. Davis M, Bhate K, Rohlinger A. Delayed patch reading after 5 days: The Mayo Clinic experience. J Am Acad Dermatol 2008;59:225–33.

Chapter 11
Allergic Contact Dermatitis to Fragrances

Sarah J. Gilpin and Howard I. Maibach

Abstract Allergic contact dermatitis (ACD) is a specific type of contact dermatitis that develops after more than one skin contact with an allergenic chemical. Such contact results in an inflammatory skin response that manifests as a redness, edema, and sometimes skin lesions (Zhai and Maibach, Dermatotoxicology, 2004). ACD to fragrances is alleged to be a common cause of contact allergy to cosmetic products. It has been estimated that approximately 1% of the unselected population is allergic to fragrance materials (Frosch et al., Contact Derm 33:333–342, 1995). Since fragrance are no longer used only in fine perfumes and colognes, but also in popular, daily use products such as skin and hair care products, deodorants, and household products, identifying the causative agent can be problematic. Here we present three interesting clinical cases of contact allergy to fragrances and/or fragranced products, which demonstrate the complexity and breadth of the syndrome.

Keywords Allergic contact dermatitis • Fragrance allergy • Contact allergy

Case 1

Chief Complaint. A 40-year-old female reported to our clinic with a chief complaint of "rash in armpit."

History of Present Illness. The patient has been essentially rash free life long until a fortnight earlier when dermatitis began in the axilla and gradually became more progressive. The patient had used the same brand of deodorant for approximately 5 years.

Past Medical History. Her past medical history revealed no medical or surgical events relevant to the exhibited dermatitis.

Family History. Unremarkable in relationship to current event.

S.J. Gilpin (✉)
University of Minnesota, 4000 Pheasant Ridge Dr, Blaine,
MN 55449, USA
e-mail: gilp0004@tc.umn.edu

Review of Systems. Unremarkable in relationship to current event.
Social History. Unremarkable in relationship to current event.
Physical Examination. Both axillae were red and swollen; however, the vault was largely spared.

With the Presented Data, What Is Your Working Diagnosis?

The rapid onset of axillary dermatitis, bilateral and symmetrical, with sparing of the vault led to an impression of allergic contact dermatitis (ACD) to the deodorant. Irritant dermatitis and inverse psoriasis were also considered.

Differential Diagnosis

ACD to the fragrance in a deodorant product.

Work-Up

Diagnostic patch testing utilizing the International Contact Dermatitis Research Group (ICDRG) classification was performed (3). This included the routine series of the North American Contact Dermatitis Group (NACDG) (3), the extended fragrance series (4), and the patient's deodorant.

At 48 and 96 h post-application, the deodorant as is revealed a 1+ and geraniol (2% pet) a 2++.

What Is Your Diagnosis and Why?

The patient had ACD to the fragrance that included geraniol in her deodorant product. Patch testing identified the causative allergens and confirmed our working diagnosis.

Management and Follow-Up

The patient substituted a fragrance-free formula for the previously utilized fragranced deodorant. She cleared within a fortnight and has remained asymptomatic for 1 year. Although we were able to identify the probable cause and effect relationship of fragrance dermatitis in our patient, such causative relationships are often challenging to determine definitively.

Case 2

Chief Complaint. A 55-year-old female arrived at our clinic with a red, splotchy rash.
History of Present Illness. The rash has been intermittent for approximately 3 months and was a diffuse, scattered rash over parts of her neck, breasts, and wrists. It was worse on the right side compared to the left.
Family History. Unremarkable in relationship to current event.
Review of Systems. Unremarkable in relationship to current event.
Social History. Unremarkable in relationship to current event.
Physical examination. This revealed a barely visible macular erythema on the neck, above the breasts, and wrists.

With the Presented Data, What Is Your Working Diagnosis?

The history suggested a dermatitis that was either endogenous and/or exogenous. As this had been intermittent for 3 months, we felt that exogenous factors might be considered.

Differential Diagnosis

Exogenous or endogenous atopic dermatitis.

Work-Up

Diagnostic patch testing utilizing the standard ICDRG classification and methods was performed (2). This included the extended routine series of the NACDG (2) and the patient's own consumer products.

She was patch test positive to her fine fragrance and from the routine fragrance series, eugenol (2% pet).

What Is Your Diagnosis and Why?

We suspected but did not prove that the dermatitis might have been due to intermittent use of fine fragrance. The patient declined serial dilution and provocative use testing (PUT); therefore, the diagnosis remained suggestive but was not proven as ACD due to intermittent use of a fine fragrance. Causation was assumed but required clinic follow-up as the splotchy lesions and the patch test positivity might have been coincidental. Her declining serial dilution and use testing made for a less certain causation.

Management and Follow-Up

The patient discontinued the use of her fine fragrance and has remained clear at 6 months.

Case 3

Chief Complaint. A 35-year-old woman reported to our clinic with a chief complaint of a chronic rash that was intermittent and of 1 year duration.

History of Present Illness. She had been on intermittent courses of topical corticoids from hydrocortisone to clobetasol, and three courses of prednisone taper. The rash was corticoid responsive, but her condition flared when prednisone and/or higher potency corticoid was removed.

Family History. Unremarkable in relationship to current event.
Review of Systems. Unremarkable in relationship to current event.
Social History. Unremarkable in relationship to current event.
Physical Examination. This revealed patchy erythema and edema of the arms, forearms, anterior trunk, and thighs.

With the Presented Data, What Is Your Working Diagnosis?

Our working diagnosis was ACD to tixicortal pivilate and hydrocortisone.

Differential Diagnosis

Recalcitrant atopic dermatitis, dermatitis not elsewhere classified (NEC) and/or occult ACD.

Work-Up

Diagnostic patch testing utilizing the ICDRG classification and standard methods was performed (2). This included the extended routine series of the NACDG (2).

She was patch test positive at 48 and 96 h to tixicortal pivilate and geraniol (2% pet).

Repeat patch tests were done with both positives to rule out excited skin syndrome (ESS). Results were reproducible.

The patient declined serial dilution and PUT.

A review of the patient's full regimen of skin care products failed to show a fragranced product that contained geraniol.

What Is Your Diagnosis and Why?

We believe that she had a reliable positive diagnostic patch to geraniol but did not find clinical significance.

Management and Follow-Up

We discontinued the use of hydrocortisone product, for which tixicortal is a surrogate marker. We did not interdict fragrances as we had no direct proof that the geraniol positive patch test result was clinically relevant.

She remained well on the above regimen, suggesting clinical relevance of the corticoid patch. Additional relevance could have been obtained with a provocative use test of hydrocortisone.

Discussion

Definition

Contact dermatitis is a general classification of inflammatory skin conditions resulting from exposure to environmental agents (1). It is one of the most common skin diseases affecting over 30% of the population at some time during life (5). Contact dermatitis consists of two different subtypes: irritant and allergic. Irritant contact dermatitis results from single or multiple exposures to non-protein chemicals called haptens that induce an inflammatory skin response through activation of innate skin immunity. ACD is due to more than one contact with an offending chemical that results in activation of acquired specific immunity (6).

History and Prevalence

Skin reactions to manmade and natural products have been occurring since time immemorial. The first systematic study of allergic response goes back to 1895 by a

Polish dermatologist, Jozef Jadassohn. Since then, patch testing methodology to describe and characterize such types of response has steadily evolved to become a complex science unto itself (7).

Surprisingly, there is little reliable data on the prevalence of ACD. Most studies do not show a causative effect, only positive or negative results which may or may not be relevant to the symptoms.

Pathophysiology

ACD is classified as a type IV delayed-type hypersensitivity reaction mediated by hapten-specific T cells. It manifests as varying degrees of erythema, edema, and vesiculation (1). ACD requires two phases of activation; an induction phase in which sensitization develops, and a second stage of exposure which elicits the inflammatory skin reaction and corresponding disease characteristics (1). ACD results from exposure to common allergens, including poison ivy/oak/sumac, nickel and other metals, medications, rubber, adhesives, detergents, fragrances, and many others. These materials invoke a series of events that lead to inflammation. These events are characterized by specific molecular and immunologic phenomena that govern the resultant disease pattern.

The skin plays a huge role in ACD as it allows the low molecular weight allergens, called haptens, to enter the suprabasilar layer of the epidermis. This layer is where the Langerhans cells (LCs), the antigen presenting cells (APCs), and the keratinocytes are located. These cell types play key roles in triggering the inflammation response that leads to sensitization (8). Activated keratinocytes then express many types of cytokines which in turn activate more T cells, creating an up-regulation cycle that leads to activation of mast cells and macrophages, resulting in histamine generation and infiltration of leukocytes and pro-inflammatory soluble factors and cells. All of this leads to the characteristic signs of ACD; redness, edema, and vesiculation (8).

Clinical Presentation, Testing, and Diagnosis

Diagnostic testing requires care when interpreting the results and linking them to a clear diagnosis of ACD (1, 9). Positive patch results must be consistent with the history of exposure to the compound in question. The connection must further be verified by looking at the location of exposure as well as at the patch test concentration. The expertise of the dermatologist is paramount to ensure that patching serves as a key method in the evaluation of contact allergy (9). An operational step-wise protocol for clinicians has been suggested to make the most effective use of diagnostic patch testing. It involves a seven-point investigation that evaluates the following patch conditions and the resulting ACD diagnosis (Table 11.1). These

11 Allergic Contact Dermatitis to Fragrances 175

Table 11.1 Steps for investigation of diagnostic patch test results (1)

History of exposure

Appropriate methodology

Positive patch test to a non-irritating concentration of the offending allergen

Repeat patch test if excited skin syndrome is exhibited

Serial dilution patch testing is used to distinguish an allergen from an irritant

Home in-use testing or open patch tests are used to corroborate ACD findings

Resolution of dermatitis after removal of offending material

Table 11.2 Patch test scoring using the ICDRG scale (2)

Score indicator	Determination and visual characteristics
+?	Doubtful reaction: mild redness only
+	Weak positive reaction: red and slightly thickened skin
++	Strong positive reaction: red, swollen skin with individual small blisters
+++	Extreme positive reaction: intense redness and swelling with coalesced large blisters or spreading reaction
IR	Irritant reaction: red skin improves once patch is removed
NT	Not tested

seven steps should be followed to make a more definitive link between the material and ACD in those with dermatitis to help prevent misdiagnosis (1). For fragrance ACD, this link between causation and allergic response depends on the ability to link relevant exposure, such as the presence of the fragrance in the consumer product that is the cause of the patient's allergy, to the response. For fragrances in particular, the assumption of ACD due to presumed intrinsic allergenic nature is not enough to show clinic relevance (10).

The distinction between allergic and irritant reactions is of major importance when patch testing. An irritant reaction is most prominent immediately after the patch is removed and often fades over the next day. An allergic reaction takes a few days to develop, so is more prominent on day five than when the patch is removed.

Any reaction seen is scored according to the ICDRG (Table 11.2). The scores are then evaluated to determine a causative agent and to rule out irritation and ESS. Further testing using serial dilution or PUT may be needed to strengthen validity of results.

The testing of fragrance materials for their link to ACD is increasingly important due to their widespread use and the elicitation of positive patch results by specific fragrance compounds. These led to the adoption of two diagnostic test series for fragrance components called Fragrance Mix I and Fragrance Mix II (Table 11.3) by

Table 11.3 Fragrance components of Fragrance Mix I and Fragrance Mix II (11)

Fragrance material	Fragrance Mix I (%)	Fragrance Mix II (%)
Oak moss extract	1	
Isoeugenol	1	
Eugenol	1	
Cinnamal	1	
Hydroxycitronellal	1	
Geraniol	1	
Cinnamyl alcohol	1	
Amyl cinnamal	1	
Citronellol		0.5
Hydroxyisohexyl 3-cyclohexene caboxaldehyde (Lyral)		2.5
Hexyl cinnamal		5.0
Citral		1.0
Coumarin		2.5
Farnesol		2.5

Table 11.4 Fragrance allergen series(12)

Compound	Concentration/vehicle % (w/w)
Cinnamic aldehyde	1.0 pet[a]
Cinnamic alcohol	2.0 pet
Amylcinnamaldehyde	2.0 pet
Eugenol	2.0 pet
Isoeugenol	2.0 pet
Geraniol	2.0 pet
Oakmoss absolute	2.0 pet
Hydroxycitronellal	2.0 pet
Narcissus absolute	2.0 pet
Musk xylene	1.0 pet
Methyl anthranilate	5.0 pet
Musk moskene	1.0 pet
Musk ketone	1.0 pet
Jasmine synthetic	2.0 pet
Benzyl salicylate	10.0 pet
Benzyl alcohol	10.0 softisan[b]
Vanillin	10.0 pet
Lavender absolute	2.0 pet
Cananga oil	2.0 pet
Rose oil Bulgarian	2.0 pet
Ylang-Ylang oil	2.0 pet
Geranium oil Bourbon	2.0 pet
Jasmine absolute, Egyptian	2.0 pet
Sandalwood oil	2.0 pet
Lyral	5.0 pet
Citral	2.0 pet
Farnesol	5.0 pet

(continued)

11 Allergic Contact Dermatitis to Fragrances

Table 11.4 (continued)

Compound	Concentration/vehicle % (w/w)
Citronellol	1.0 pet
Hexyl cinnamic aldehyde	10.0 pet
Coumarin	5.0 pet
Fragrance Mix II	14.0 pet
Amyl cinnamyl alcohol	5.0 pet
Anise alcohol	10.0 softisan
Benzyl benzoate	10.0 pet
Benzyl cinnamate	10.0 pet
Butylphenyl methylpropional	10.0 pet
Evernia furfuracea	1.0 pet
a-Isomethyl ionone	10.0 pet
d-Limonene	10.0 pet
Linalool	10.0 pet
Methyl-2-octynoate	0.2 pet

[a] Pet = petrolatum vehicle used for lipid and water soluble fragrance compounds
[b] Softisan = vegetable fatty acid derivative preferred as a vehicle for some fragrance compounds

dermatologists across the globe. These series are now used extensively for testing patients with suspected fragrance sensitivity.

Conclusion

Fragrances are an important part of everyday life and are enjoyed by many people. However, as our case studies demonstrate, they can also be an important contributor to ACD in the clinic. Such importance is exemplified by the creation of specific fragrance series (Table 11.4) and defined diagnostic patch test methods to aid the dermatologist in identifying and alleviating symptoms. For fragrance materials in particular, the link between positive patch results and causation must be thoroughly evaluated to prevent return visits from patients.

Questions

1. What two conditions are included in the grouping of contact dermatitis?

    (a) Delayed and chronic dermatitis
    (b) Acute sub-irritant and irritant dermatitis
    (c) Eczema and psoriasis
    (d) Allergic and irritant contact dermatitis
    (e) Hyper-immune and immune dermatitis

2. When experiencing a presumed allergy to a deodorant, which allergen patch series should be administered?

(a) The North American Standard Series
(b) The Japanese Standard Series and the North American Series
(c) The Fragrance Series
(d) All of the above
(e) Selection of patch series depends on a subject's history of use and etiology

3. Which one of the following is not a reason for addition of fragrance to a deodorant?

   (a) Scent and odor-masking
   (b) Consumer acceptance
   (c) Product stability
   (d) FDA requirement
   (e) Anti-oxidation

4. Which of the following materials is NOT a component of the fragrance mix as used in the standard series?

   (a) Geraniol
   (b) Isoeugenol
   (c) Hydroxycitronellal
   (d) Citronellol
   (e) Eugenol

5. Which one is the main difference between irritant and ACD?

   (a) Involvement of an immune response in irritant but not ACD
   (b) Irritant contact dermatitis requires one exposure but ACD requires a second exposure.
   (c) Itching, redness and skin lesions are signs of irritant but not ACD.
   (d) Irritant contact dermatitis lasts for 24 h whereas ACD lasts for much longer.
   (e) ACD requires a greater dose to elicit response than does ACD

6. Which of the following is NOT a characteristic of eugenol?

   (a) Found in oil of cloves and cinnamon leaf
   (b) Used as a flavoring for toothpaste and foods
   (c) Has anti-septic properties
   (d) Non-sensitizing
   (e) An ingredient in Fragrance Mix I

7. Principle forms of endogenous eczema include all of the following except:

   (a) Follicular eczema
   (b) Atopic eczema
   (c) Seborrhoeic dermatitis
   (d) Discoid eczema
   (e) Statis dermatitis

8. Principle forms of exogenous dermatitis include all of the following except:

   (a) Irritant contact dermatitis

11 Allergic Contact Dermatitis to Fragrances   179

  (b) Irritant fibrosis
  (c) ACD
  (d) Photoallergic contact dermatitis
  (e) Occupational dermatitis

9. ACD, such as that seen to this patient's fragrance, is classified as what type?

  (a) Type I IgE mediated
  (b) Type II IgM mediated
  (c) Type III immune complex
  (d) Type IV cell-mediated
  (e) Unknown non-mediated

10. Which of the following is NOT true about PUT?

  (a) Reflects real-life exposure of an allergen
  (b) Adds causative weight to positive patch test results
  (c) Helps minimize false-positive reactions
  (d) Are done using occlusion only
  (e) Helps deter-mine clinical relevance of patch test results

11. Which of the following is NOT true of ESS?

  (a) Also referred to as "angry back"
  (b) Can lead to false-positive patch reactions
  (c) Indicates that a patient can no longer be patch tested to determine allergy
  (d) Involves a generalized state of skin hyperactivity
  (e) Is ruled out by testing one suspected allergen at a time

12. Which of the following is not a characteristic of geraniol?

  (a) Is used in approximately 70% of perfumes and as a flavor ingredient
  (b) Is a component of Fragrance Mix II
  (c) Upon oxidation becomes geranial or citral
  (d) Is commonly found in the following essential oils: bergamot, carrot, coriander,lavender, lemon, lime, orange, and rose
  (e) Is cited as a moderately frequent cause of ACD

13. Which of the following determines the clinical relevance to patch test result?

  (a) Ruling out ESS
  (b) Performing serial dilution testing
  (c) Performing PUT
  (d) Patch testing to standard series as well as patient's consumer products and occupational exposures
  (e) All of the above

14. Tixocortal pivilate is described by which of the following statements?

  (a) No longer used to treat contact dermatitis
  (b) Not included in the standard patching series
  (c) A marker for topical corticosteroid allergy

(d) A corticosteroid body creme
(e) Only a sensitizer in Europe and Japan

15. Which of the following is NOT true about topical steroid usage?

    (a) Most common treatment for irritant and ACD
    (b) Can be used in many vehicle types from creams to ointments to aerosols
    (c) Are classified into seven groups depending on potency
    (d) Can inhibit patch test reactions
    (e) Can be used without concern for adverse effects

Answer key: 1(d), 2(e), 3(d), 4(d), 5(b), 6(d), 7(a), 8(b), 9(d), 10(d), 11(c), 12(b), 13(e), 14(c), 15(e).

References

1. Zhai H, Maibach HI (eds) Dermatotoxicology. 6th ed. Boca Raton: CRC Press, 2004.
2. Frosch PJ, Pilz B, Andersen KR et al. (1995) Patch testing with fragrances: results of a multicenter study of the European Environmental and Contact Dermatitis Research Group with 48 frequently used constituents of perfumes. Contact Derm 33, 333–342.
3. Lachapelle JM. The Standard Series of Patch Tests. In: Patch Testing and Prick Testing: A Practical Guide Official Publication of the ICDRG. Lachapelle JM, Maibach HI (eds). Berlin, Heidelberg: Springer Berlin Heidelberg, 2009: Chapter 4.
4. Trattner A, David M (2004) Patch testing with fine fragrances: comparison with fragrance mix, balsam of Peru and a fragrance series. Contact Derm 49, 287–289.
5. Fyhrquist-Vanni N, Alenius H, Laurerma A (2007) Contact dermatitis. Dermatol Clin 25, 613–623.
6. Saint-Mezard P, Rosieres A, Krasteva M et al. (2004). Allergic contact dermatitis. Eur J Dermatol 14, 284–295.
7. Lachapelle JM, Maibach HI. Patch Testing Methodology. In: Patch Testing and Prick Testing: A Practical Guide Official Publication of the ICDRG. Lachapelle JM, Maibach HI (eds). Berlin, Heidelberg: Springer Berlin Heidelberg, 2009: Chapter 3.
8. Marks JG, Elsner P, DeLeo V. Contact and Occupational Dermatology. 3rd ed. St. Louis: Mosby, 2002.
9. Storrs FJ, Fowler JF (1994) Patch testing technique-reading patch tests: some pitfalls of patch testing. Am J Cont Derm 5, 170–172.
10. Hostynek JJ, Maibach HI (2003) Operational definition of a causative contact allergen – a study with six fragrance allergens. Exog Derm 2, 279–285.
11. Storrs FJ (2007) Fragrance – Contact allergy of the year. Dermatitis 18, 3–7.
12. Allergen Series. 2009. Chemotechnique Diagnostics. 07 Nov 2009. <http://www.chemotechnique.se/index2.htm>.

Part IV
Other Allergies Affecting Skin and Mucous Membranes

Chapter 12
Atopic Dermatitis

Albert E. Rivera and Lloyd J. Cleaver

Abstract Atopic dermatitis is both a chronic and relapsing skin condition frequently seen by all of those in healthcare. The condition leads to multiple stresses for patients: physically, emotionally, professionally, and financially. Knowledge and understanding of the pathophysiology and available treatments may help lessen the burden of a disease and improve the patients' quality of life.

Keywords Atopic dermatitis · Atopy · Pruritus · Lichenification · Filaggrin

Case 1

History of present illness. The patient is a 4-year-old female presenting with a "rash" that has been present for several months but never formally diagnosed. The family reports that it is the worst on her antecubital areas, wrists, and the popliteal regions. The patient has difficulty sleeping due to the severity of the itching. Antihistamines have not helped and a previous prescription for pimecrolimus (Elidel) possibly made it worse. Occasional use of over the counter moisturizers did not seem to be of benefit either.

Past medical and surgical histories are unremarkable at this time. Though the "rash" has been present for some time, it has not received a prior diagnosis. Relevant *social and family histories* are denied by patient's mother.

Medications currently include only a children's multivitamin and infrequent use of various over the counter moisturizers. *Medication allergies* are denied.

Review of systems is unremarkable other than the itching, skin findings, and difficulty sleeping.

A.E. Rivera (✉)
Northeast Regional Medical Center, 700 West Jefferson Street, Kirksville 63501, MO, USA
e-mail: bo_rivera@yahoo.com

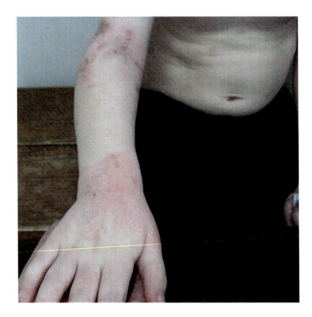

Fig. 12.1 Erosions and lichenification of the right dorsal arm of a 4-year-old female

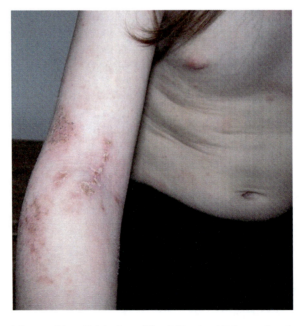

Fig. 12.2 Excoriations and impetiginization of the right antecubital space in a 4-year-old female

Physical examination was notable for fairly diffuse xerosis, erythema, fissuring, excoriation, lichenification, and mild exudate primarily in the antecubital area as well as lateral elbow, extensor aspects of the wrists, upper chest, and popliteal fossae (Figs. 12.1–12.3). Dennie–Morgan lines were noted on examination of the face. White dermatographism was demonstrated on the back. The remainder of the examination was normal.

With the Presented Data, What is Your Working Diagnosis?

Impression. Eczema with secondary excoriations and impetiginization.

Differential diagnoses considered for this case included atopic dermatitis, atypical seborrheic dermatitis, contact dermatitis, psoriasis, asteatosis, lichen simplex chronicus, arthropod insult, infectious etiology (viral, fungal, bacterial), cutaneous malignancies (T-cell lymphoma, langerhans cell histiocytosis), numerous nutritional abnormalities, metabolic disorders, immunodeficiency (Wiskott–Aldrich, hyperimmunoglobulin-E syndrome, severe combined immunodeficiency, DiGeorge syndrome), and autoimmune conditions (dermatomyositis, lupus erythematosus). Of course, specific patient's age and history will serve as a guide in creating the optimal, individualized differential for each patient.

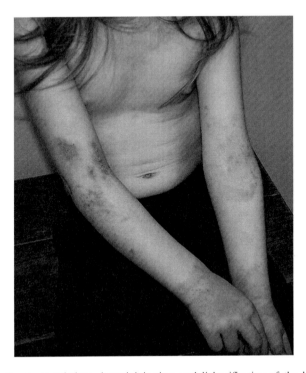

Fig. 12.3 Erythema, excoriations, impetiginization, and lichenification of the bilateral upper extremities and chest in a 4-year-old female

Workup

The workup of a patient presenting with these clinical findings will vary. Often clinical examination and patient history are sufficient for the diagnosis. Obtaining a thorough family history may, as in this patient, alleviate concerns for specific conditions. However, oftentimes, a more elaborate search may be required. In this case, a basic complete blood count (CBC) and comprehensive metabolic panel (CMP) were utilized to eliminate several concerns from the differential. Other serologic testing for antibodies was obtained to eliminate an autoimmune disease from consideration. Often, in infants or children, genetic testing is required for persistent cases to rule out potentially severe diseases. However, genetic tests were not felt to be necessary initially. Microscopic search for fungal or arthropod etiology was deemed valuable to perform. A biopsy was discussed with the mother but was deferred unless necessary at a future visit.

Data

The patient's CBC, CMP, and antinuclear antibodies (ANA) were returned without significant findings. Cultures of the impetiginized lesions revealed only *Staphylococcus epidermidis* at this time. A potassium hydroxide scraping for fungal organisms revealed no hyphae. Three separate mineral oil scrapings of slightly linear lesions for *Sarcoptes scabiei* did not reveal any organisms. The mother reported that the patient's diet is sufficient and that she rarely misses taking her multivitamin. Specifically, revisiting the physical examination, no nail pitting or oil spots were noted on the nails. As noted, the patient's mother deferred a biopsy at this time, opting instead for a gradual, conservative approach to management.

What is Your Diagnosis and Why?

This 4-year-old female patient demonstrates acute childhood atopic dermatitis due to the age range, history, laboratory data, and physical findings. The history of present illness and physical examination confidently allowed exclusion of several conditions within the differential. Further evaluation with the microscopic and laboratory data led to greater specificity of the diagnosis.

Management and Follow-Up

The patient was instructed to use gentle skin care, including fragrance and dye free soap, and moisturize after baths as well as frequently during the day. Class V (and later Class III) topical steroids, antihistamines, and empiric antibiotics were

12   Atopic Dermatitis

also prescribed. Extensive education was provided regarding the use of the medications prescribed in addition to optimal skin care practices.

Upon follow-up, the patient had significant improvement in her skin lesions and symptoms. Maintenance was achieved with continued meticulous skin care and moisturization. Topical steroids were then used only on an as-needed basis for flares. Should the lesions recur or inadequate control develops, then a biopsy for confirmation would be recommended.

Case 2

History of present illness. The patient is a 23-year-old female presenting with a prolonged history of uncontrolled "eczema" treated by her primary care physician with mid-potency topical steroids and antihistamines. She reports that the itching is severe enough to interfere with daily activities and sleep. The associated fissuring and pain limit her physically and are emotionally stressful. Currently the outbreak is extensive and "covering the whole body." She has itching in her scalp that is not currently being treated.

Past medical history includes asthma, seborrheic dermatitis, and seizures which recently presented. *Past surgical history* includes a plate in her right arm to repair a fracture post motor vehicle accident, tubal ligation, and cesarean section.

Social history is significant for one pack per day tobacco use. Concerning *family history*, the patient does not know her father's medical history, and she denies any maternal health problems.

Medications only include the recent topical steroids, antihistamines, and newly started phenytoin (Dilantin). *Allergies* are to pimecrolimus (Elidel) which causes a "rash."

Review of systems is significant for itching, skin findings, difficulty sleeping, cutaneous pain, and mildly depressed mood.

Physical examination was notable for diffuse erythema, fissuring, excoriation, and lichenification with several foci of serous exudates and crusting (Figs. 12.4–12.7). There are mild scale and erythema within the scalp. Surgical scars are present consistent with the patient's medical history.

With the Presented Data, What is Your Working Diagnosis?

Impression. Diffuse xerosis with secondary excoriations and focal areas of crusting and exudate.

Differential diagnoses considered for this patient included atopic dermatitis, severe seborrheic dermatitis, contact dermatitis, psoriasis, asteatosis, lichen simplex chronicus, arthropod insult, infectious etiology (viral, fungal, bacterial), cutaneous malignancies (primarily cutaneous T-cell lymphoma), numerous nutritional abnormalities, metabolic disorders, drug eruption, and immunologic conditions (dermatomyositis,

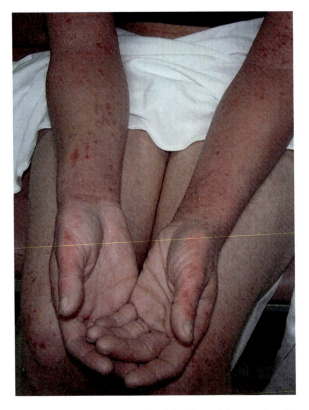

Fig. 12.4 Excoriations, lichenification, and scale of the bilateral forearms in a 23-year-old female

lupus erythematosus, dermatitis herpetiformis, pemphigus foliaceus). Again, each patient's history and examination will serve as a guide in creating the optimal, individualized differential.

Workup

Often clinical examination and patient's (plus family) history are sufficient for the diagnosis of some conditions. Since the patient has had the condition for several years without adequate control under prior therapy and no specific diagnosis has been reached, the workup of this patient requires a more aggressive initial plan. As usual, a basic CBC and CMP were utilized to eliminate several concerns from the differential. Scrapings to exclude fungi or arthropods helped in establishing a diagnosis. Cultures of the impetiginized lesions were taken to verify antibiotic necessity and selection. In this patient, systemic, immunologic, and malignant conditions are imperative to exclude. Therefore, a full autoimmune panel was ordered as well

12 Atopic Dermatitis

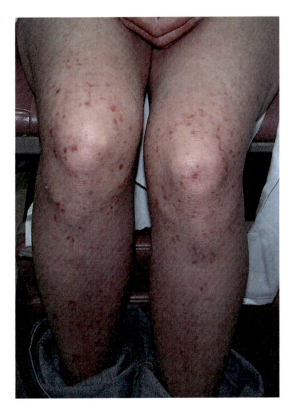

Fig. 12.5 Excoriations and lichenification of the bilateral anterior lower extremities in a 23-year-old female

as taking a punch biopsy of two separate representative lesions to assist in the final diagnosis. In general, adults are more concerning for cutaneous malignancies and, therefore, the threshold for biopsy should be lower. She was additionally provided information and a referral for allergy testing.

Data

Lab work, including CBC, CMP, thyroid stimulating hormone (TSH), and autoimmune testing (ANA, Sm, Ro, La, Scl-70, and Jo-1 antibodies), was normal other than slightly elevated cholesterol, LDL, and triglycerides. Potassium hydroxide scrapings for fungal organisms were without finding on the trunk but did reveal yeast on the scalp. Three separate mineral oil scrapings for scabies mites were negative. Cultures of the impetiginized areas were notable for *Staphylococcus aureus*. The organisms were susceptible to all antibiotics except the tetracycline family. Histopathology of both specimens demonstrated subacute spongiotic dermatitis with no other significant findings. The patient has not yet been able to undergo allergy testing.

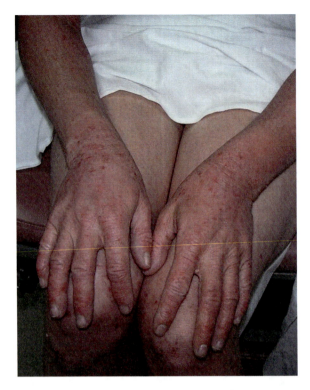

Fig. 12.6 Excoriation, fissuring, impetiginization, and lichenification of the bilateral hands and wrists in a 23-year-old female

What is Your Diagnosis and Why?

This 23-year-old female typifies a chronic, refractory adult atopic dermatitis with secondary impetiginization due to the age, history, physical examination, lab work, cultures, and histopathology. Also, seborrheic dermatitis was secondarily confirmed. Combining the patient's history and complete physical examination sufficiently allowed exclusion of several conditions within the differential. The addition of microscopic and laboratory data also narrowed the diagnostic possibilities. The histologic exclusion of other pathologies and confirmation of the suspected diagnosis were the final keys to diagnosis.

Management and Follow-Up

The patient was instructed to use gentle skin care, including fragrance and dye free soap, and moisturize after baths as well as frequently during the day. High and mid-potency topical steroids, antihistamines (H1 and H2), and empiric

12 Atopic Dermatitis

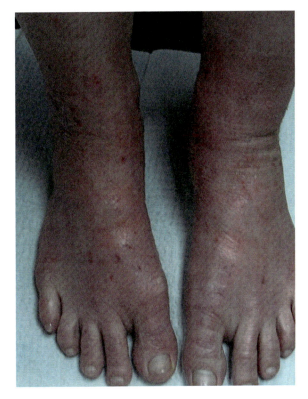

Fig. 12.7 Fissuring, impetiginization, and lichenification of the bilateral dorsal feet in a 23-year-old female

antibiotics were also prescribed. She was given an anti-yeast shampoo and topical steroid solution for use on her scalp. Extensive education was provided regarding the use of the medications prescribed in addition to optimal skin care practices. Compliance was stressed with the patient multiple times. She was encouraged to schedule testing with an allergist as soon as possible. Smoking cessation was encouraged. Upon questioning, the patient did not meet the criteria for depression but her emotional health will be monitored closely and referred if necessary.

Upon follow-up, the impetiginized lesions had resolved and her scalp complaints had improved. Otherwise, treatment of the remaining skin lesions over several months has been frustrating with slow, gradual improvement. In this patient, multiple gentle skin care emollients, products and soaps, Classes V, III, II and I topical steroids, one course of oral steroids, topical and oral antibiotics, various antihistamines, and, most recently, cyclosporine have been utilized with only modest success.

Discussion

Atopic dermatitis is both a chronic and relapsing skin condition frequently seen by numerous medical professionals. It places multiple stresses not only on the patient but also on those associated with the patient. Physically it can be painful, leading to shunning of certain activities. The inconvenience of avoiding certain irritants or products may be troublesome at times as well. Along with the difficulty in daily life, duties at work may also be affected causing loss of productivity or time. This directly or indirectly leads to financial strains through loss of time on a job or through the purchase of multiple, different adjuncts or medicines for preventative skin care; maintenance of skin barrier; or improvement of a deteriorated condition. The time and effort used in the management of atopic dermatitis may be psychologically and socially detrimental also.

Prevalence

The prevalence of atopic dermatitis has been quoted by various sources and determined by multiple methodologies. General agreement is seen at approximately 10–25% of adolescent or pediatric age populations, with the numbers increasing. One study notes an overall prevalence of atopy in 20% of children less than 15 years of age, specifically reporting 11.5% for those 0–3 years old, 21.4% in those 4–6 years old, and 27.2% of 7–14 year olds (1). Usually atopic dermatitis is first noted in childhood. Often there is subsequent development of allergies, asthma, rhinitis (the "atopic march") or other symptoms.

Typical Presentation

The infantile form of atopic dermatitis is seen in those aged 2 months to 2 years. Up to 60% of cases present within the first year. Often the cheeks demonstrate the first manifestation of the disease. Primary lesions may include papules, pustules, or plaques. Secondarily there may be excoriation, crusts, exudates, or lichenification. Typically, the condition will be worse during winter months. The risk factors for persistence of atopic dermatitis beyond infancy and into childhood are egg, peanut, and dust mite allergies as well as possibly even peripheral eosinophilia contributing to the increased risk (2).

Childhood atopic dermatitis includes those patients who are roughly 2–12 years of age. Common anatomic locations include the antecubital area, popliteal region, flexures, and also the face. Frequently seen presentations are those of erythema, scale, papules, and plaques. Again, excoriation, lichenification, exudate, or other secondary findings may coexist. Pruritus is a very prominent finding associated with almost every case. Growth retardation may be seen in patients with more than half of their body surface involved. Social development may also be delayed. It has been found that dust mite allergy (odds ratio 3.68) and peanut allergy (odds ratio 2.63) are significant risk factors for the persistence of atopic dermatitis beyond childhood and that the rate is approximately 40% (2, 3).

In general, presentation beyond 10–12 years of age is considered to be included within the adult presentation of atopic dermatitis. An estimated 1–3% of adults are affected by atopic dermatitis. Often many of the same symptoms such as xerosis, skin sensitivity, and especially pruritus persist in adults. As before, the physical findings in adults may include papules, plaques, erythema, scale, exudate, lichenification, or other presentations. Common locations include the antecubital and popliteal fossae, neck, facial areas, and hands. Frequently, the most persistent problem encountered is intermittent or chronic dermatitis of the hands. Often there is coexistent bacterial colonization. Heat, contactants, and emotional or physical stress are some of the involved triggers.

Histology

The histologic presentation of atopic dermatitis is due to increased transepidermal water loss secondary to barrier dysfunction. There is subsequent decrease in sebum production along with altered fatty acid composition of the sebum produced. As a whole, the histology is fairly nonspecific. There is often localized parakeratosis with possible crust; if impetiginization is present, there may be neutrophils within the stratum corneum. If the lesion is acute, there may be spongiosis, occasionally with vesicles or bullae, presence of superficial dermal (or occasionally also epidermal) perivascular lymphocytes, possible histiocytes, or eosinophils. If chronic, there could be hyperkeratosis (which correlates with lichenification) and acanthosis. Inflammatory cells or spongiosis may be present as well but often to a lesser extent. Frequently, a clinical-histologic correlation allows more precise diagnosis of the condition.

Genetics

The genetic findings associated with atopic dermatitis can be attributed to multiple factors. There is a significant increase in atopic dermatitis if both parents are atopic, but there has been shown to be an even stronger link between siblings. In addition, there seems to be more of an influence attributed to maternal inheritance rather than paternal. Overall, however, the condition is multifactorial in its etiology. Even with a strong genetic component, there is an environmental contribution involved. Atopic dermatitis is found more commonly now than in the past and also more frequently in developed countries. This supports the environmental contribution to the genetic predisposition.

Genetic research has uncovered numerous causative or associated factors involved in this predisposition. In more than half of the atopic dermatitis patients, there is a defective region of chromosome 1q21 leading to faulty Filaggrin (FLG) gene expression. The inactive, phosphorylated precursor profilaggrin is the primary component of the keratohyalin F granules within the epidermal granular layer. Normally, this peptide is dephosphorylated as part of the production of normal Filaggrin (4). Other possible, associated genes are interleukin 4 receptor α chain (IL4RA), toll-like receptor 2 (TLR2), kallikrein-related peptidase 7 (KLK7), epidermal collagen 29 (COL29), and serine protease inhibitor, Kazal-type 5 (SPINK5). Further potential genes of interest and research are located on chromosomes 3q21, 5q31, 11q13, and 14q11 (5).

Immunology

The immunology associated with atopic dermatitis is an extremely complex interaction and expression of immunological markers and mechanisms. Differences have been found in multiple factors within lesional compared to nonlesional skin of atopic patients. There are increased corneocyte tryptic enzymes, which lead to poor connections between the corneocytes as well as thinning of the cornified layer as a whole. Skin injury (whether self-induced or by exogenous chemicals or organisms) causes keratinocytes to emit cytokines and chemokines promoting inflammatory cell invasion. Though not wholly supported yet, even possible vitamin levels, specifically vitamin D3, and viruses have been questioned (6).

Within *acute* atopic dermatitis there are increased numbers of CD4+ cells and T-helper 2 cells. T-helper 2 cells express cutaneous lymphocyte-associated antigen (CLA), which guides them to the skin. There is activation of the T-helper 2 immune response along with production of cytokines IL-3, IL-4, IL-5, IL-6, IL-10, and IL-13. IL-4 and IL-5 lead to increased levels of IgE as well as elevated levels of eosinophils. IL-4 also leads to decreased production of interferon-gamma (IFN-γ). IL-10 leads to inhibition of the delayed-type hypersensitivity response. There is inhibition of the T-helper 1 immune response leading to impaired acute, but not necessarily chronic, antigen exposure sensitivity (7, 8).

Langerhans cells have increased expression of high affinity IgE receptors (FcεRI), leading to stimulation and activation of helper T cells. Also, IL-16 production by Langerhans cells is an attractant for additional T cells. Monocytes produce elevated levels of prostaglandin E2, which reduces IFN-γ production and also increases levels of IgE. Mast cells become activated, releasing multiple chemical mediators including plasma and tissue histamine, cAMP (cyclic adenosine monophosphate) specific phosphodiesterase, leukotriene B4, and histamine releasing factor. The chemokines CCL5 (RANTES; regulation on activation, normal

T-cell expressed and secreted), CCL11 (eotaxin), CCL13 (monocyte chemoattractant protein 4), CCL18 (pulmonary and activation-regulated chemokine), CCL27 (CTACK; cutaneous T cell-attracting chemokine), and MCP4 (monocyte chemotactic protein-4) lead to increased numbers of inflammatory cell types in the skin of atopics (9). However, even with the entire storm of inflammatory cells, there is a decreased antiviral, antifungal, and antibacterial response due to decreased levels of IL-8, human β-defensin 2, human β-defensin 3, nitric oxide synthetase, and cathelicidins.

In contrast, the *chronic* form of atopic dermatitis transitions to a T-helper 1 immune response rather than T-helper 2 response. There is less production of IL-4 and IL-13 with an increase in IL-5, IL-11, IL-12, IFN-γ, and granulocyte-macrophage colony-stimulating factor (GM-CSF). Also noted are cytokines stimulating fibrosis such as IL-11, IL-17, and transforming growth factor beta (TGF-β1).

Diagnosis

The diagnosis of atopic dermatitis using Hanifin and Rajka method must have three "Major Criteria" including: (1) pruritus, (2) typical flexural lichenification in adults or facial and extensor lesions in childhood or infants, (3) chronic or chronically relapsing dermatitis, or (4) personal or family history of atopic disease (asthma, allergic rhinitis, or atopic dermatitis); *PLUS* three of the "Minor Criteria" which include: (1) xerosis, (2) ichthyosis, hyperlinear palms, or keratosis pilaris, (3) IgE reactivity (immediate/Type 1 skin test reactivity, positive radioallergosorbent test (RAST)), (4) elevated serum IgE, (5) early age of onset, (6) tendency for cutaneous infections (especially *S. aureus* or herpes simplex) or impaired cell-mediated immunity, (7) tendency to nonspecific hand or foot dermatitis, (8) nipple eczema, (9) cheilitis, (10) recurrent conjunctivitis, (11) Dennie–Morgan infraorbital lines, (12) keratoconus, (13) anterior subcapsular cataracts, (14) orbital darkening, (15) facial pallor or erythema, (16) pityriasis alba, (17) anterior neck folds, (18) pruritus associated with sweating, (19) wool or lipid solvent intolerance, (20) perifollicular accentuation, (21) food hypersensitivity, (22) symptoms influenced by environmental or emotional factors, or (23) white dermatographism or delayed blanch to cholinergic agents (10).

Treatment

Treatment of atopic dermatitis should be individualized and factors to consider include the severity, location, prior management, psychological effect, age of the patient, self-treatment capacity (vs. required assistance), current medications, allergies, and medical history. There are numerous treatment variables to contemplate and medications that are available. The following paragraphs will briefly cover several of the most commonly encountered therapies but is not exhaustive. Other appropriate texts may be referenced for further detail regarding any of the topics below.

Patient preference of a quality emollient is often recommended to enhance compliance. Many patients may request to use a "favorite" moisturizer and this may be permitted, but they should avoid fragrance or other sensitizers. If the product does not seem to be benefitting the patient, or actually making them worse, a more appropriate product should be suggested early in the course. Quality moisturization should be applied often, and one frequently made recommendation is to utilize the products shortly after bathing.

Though many chemicals, foods, antigens, products, etc., are cited as potential causes, every patient is different and should be managed as such. Potential dietary intake, chemical exposure, soaps or surfactants, fabrics, dust, animals, and mites are commonly reported causes or associated factors. Some physicians recommend high-efficiency particulate air (HEPA) filters to aid in allergen filtration. Avoidance of specific allergens known or suspected to lead to symptomatic exacerbation for each individual patient should be stressed (11). Single element elimination trails can potentially identify the factor(s) if desired. Usually, allergy testing is not recommended unless the patient experiences prolonged disease, has persistent asthma, or is refractory to most treatment strategies. The current recommendations by the American Academy of Pediatrics' Committee on Nutrition and Section on Allergy and Immunology note that delayed food exposure is not beneficial and that breastfeeding for at least 4 months does reduce the incidence of atopic dermatitis within the first 2 years (12). However, if elimination diets are considered, they should be done with care and under appropriate supervision as the effect of poor nutrition could possibly be more troublesome than the original condition.

Bacteria may also be part of the pathogenesis of atopic dermatitis. Up to 90% of atopic patients become colonized with *S. aureus* though cultures may not always confirm this. These bacteria secrete superantigen toxins that may stimulate the inflammatory cell cascade, thus, continuing the cycle. If bacterial colonization is suspected, sodium hypochlorite baths may be utilized. One quarter to one half of a cup of bleach may be combined with a tub full of water and mixed adequately. The patient is then instructed to cleanse for several minutes before washing off with regular water. When taking showers or baths, the water should not be scalding or extremely hot, rather it should be tepid or even cool if tolerated. Harsh scrubbing with bathing adjuncts such as loofas or wash cloths should be avoided. Mild fragrance-free, dye-free soaps are optimal for cleansing. The skin should be gently patted dry after bathing is complete, and a quality hypoallergenic emollient should be generously applied over the entire body. When dressing, bland fabrics, most commonly cotton, washed in fragrance-free, dye-free detergents are frequently better tolerated than those washed in harsh chemicals.

Topical corticosteroids are generally agreed upon as first line therapy for medical management. The treatment protocols are quite varied, and there is no one correct method. If high potency corticosteroids are chosen, the body surface area and duration of use should be limited. The risks include atrophy of the skin and, rarely, inhibition of the hypothalamic-pituitary axis. If lower potency corticosteroids are utilized, then a longer treatment period is attainable. However, that is often at a loss of maximal results. Prolonged use of any steroid class may eventually lead to tachyphylaxis and decreased control. Therefore, other adjuncts or treatment regimens are necessary. Certainly, regular barrier protection and barrier repair are to be utilized along with the steroids.

The use of systemic corticosteroids for atopic dermatitis may lead to dramatic improvements for some patients. Often, this will lead to the frequent request by patients and the overuse by some physicians. The side effects associated with long-term use of systemic corticosteroids should be respected. Loss of bone density, elevated blood sugar, elevated blood pressure, inhibition of the hypothalamic-pituitary axis and post-treatment flares are all associated. If used for an acute episode, the plan for future management and transition to other therapies should start being formulated at that time.

The calcineurin inhibitors are a second line, alternative or complimentary treatment to topical corticosteroids. Tacrolimus (Protopic) and pimecrolimus (Elidel) are included in this group. Those patients who would require continuous, high potency steroids or those requiring care in sensitive, intertriginous or thin skinned regions are good candidates for use. This limits the potential for any untoward side effects. Generally, these products are not for use in patients younger than 2 years old. The most common side effect is stinging or burning at the site of use. No other studies conclusively support human, systemic complications from use of this medication class in the strength and use indicated.

Systemic antihistamines may also be considered as part of a management strategy. The primary benefit of first generation antihistamines is obtained through sedation, allowing the patient to rest and decrease manipulation. Second generation antihistamines may be beneficial if the patient has associated allergic symptoms in addition to atopic dermatitis. Doxepin hydrochloride has both H1 and H2 antagonist properties. Topical antihistamines are generally not used in treatment protocols. Typically, only more bothersome or severe cases are treated with this medication class early in their course.

Antibiotics are often used for cases with secondary excoriations or impetiginization. They may also be used if a patient is suspected to be colonized with bacteria that lead to flares of their disease. Use of antibiotics must be as directed for short periods of time to minimize the potential for antibacterial resistance. Some cases may require prolonged treatment with an antibiotic, however. If the patient has significant fungal lesions of the skin or scalp, appropriate antifungals should be begun. Should the patient develop eczema herpeticum, then antiviral therapy should be instituted promptly.

Phototherapy is a valid treatment modality in certain patients. Ultraviolet A-1 (UVA-1), broadband ultraviolet A (UVA), psoralens plus ultraviolet A (PUVA), narrowband ultraviolet B (UVB), broadband ultraviolet B (UVB), and natural sunlight are all potential considerations for treatment. For this strategy also, the side effect profile and ease of use must be considered as well. There must be both physician and patient access to the phototherapy, which is not always common. The effects to the skin, both cosmetically and medically, are concerns with long-term use. Rhytides, lentigines, and various skin carcinomas are all potential unwanted results.

Systemic immunosuppressants are a valuable alternative for refractory cases of atopic dermatitis. Methotrexate, an analog of folic acid, inhibits dihydrofolate reductase leading to interference of DNA synthesis. The greatest concerns with this medication are hepatotoxicity and anemia, so liver associated enzymes and blood counts should be monitored. Mycophenolate mofetil inhibits inosine monophosphate, which is involved in purine synthesis. Leukopenia and anemia may be associated, so lab work should be monitored. Also, dosage adjustment and close monitoring in patients who have renal insufficiency is indicated. Cyclosporin, a systemic calcineurin inhibitor, inhibits T-cell activation and decreases cytokine transcription. It is recommended that treatment be limited to less than 1 year since renal toxicity, hypertension, and malignancy are potential side effects. Interferon-gamma limits IgE response and inhibits Th2 cell proliferation and function. Azathioprine is an analog of 6-mercaptopurine that effectively inhibits purine synthesis. Before starting this medication, thiopurine methyltransferase levels should be checked and dosing based accordingly. Regular monitoring should be performed should marrow suppression or hepatotoxicity develop. The biologics as a medication class have also been used with varying success. Additional, larger studies are needed regarding the effectiveness of these agents.

Questions

1. Which is not considered to be a "major" criterion in the diagnosis of atopic dermatitis?

    (a) Xerosis
    (b) Pruritus
    (c) Chronic dermatitis
    (d) Family history of atopic disease

2. Within what age range is a patient considered to have "childhood" atopic dermatitis?

    (a) 0–5 years
    (b) 1–7 years
    (c) 2–12 years
    (d) 10–18 years

3. What is frequently the most persistent cutaneous problem for adults with a history of atopic dermatitis?

    (a) Bullae
    (b) Ecchymoses
    (c) Nail dystrophy
    (d) Hand dermatitis

4. What is the pathognomonic finding on histopathology to diagnose atopic dermatitis?

    (a) Hyperkeratosis
    (b) Eosinophils

(c) Acanthosis
(d) Findings are nonspecific

5. What is the most commonly found genetic defect in patients with atopic dermatitis?

   (a) PTCH
   (b) FLG
   (c) EBP
   (d) p53

6. Which type of atopic dermatitis is considered to be a T-helper type 2 (Th-2) associated condition?

   (a) Acute atopic dermatitis
   (b) Chronic atopic dermatitis
   (c) Both acute and chronic atopic dermatitis
   (d) Neither acute nor chronic atopic dermatitis

7. Which type of atopic dermatitis is considered to be a T-helper type 1 (Th-1) associated condition?

   (a) Acute atopic dermatitis
   (b) Chronic atopic dermatitis
   (c) Both acute and chronic atopic dermatitis
   (d) Neither acute nor chronic atopic dermatitis

8. What bacteria commonly colonize the skin of atopic individuals?

   (a) *Streptococcus viridans*
   (b) *Staphylococcus aureus*
   (c) *Pseudomonas aeruginosa*
   (d) *Escherichia coli*

9. What management is required for all patients with atopic dermatitis to ensure improvement?

   (a) Management is individualized
   (b) High efficiency particulate air (HEPA) filter
   (c) Allergy testing
   (d) Delayed food exposure

10. What is the most common first line therapeutic class chosen for treatment of atopic dermatitis?

    (a) Systemic antibiotics
    (b) Topical calcineurin inhibitors
    (c) Topical corticosteroids
    (d) Phototherapy

Answers: 1(a), 2(c), 3(d), 4(d), 5(b), 6(a), 7(b), 8(b), 9(a), 10(c).

References

1. Garde J, Hervas D, Marco N, Milan JM, Martos MD. Calculating the prevalence of atopy in children. Allergol Immunopathol (Madr). 2009;37(3):129–134.
2. Horowitz AA, Hossain J, Yousef E. Correlates of outcome for atopic dermatitis. Ann Allergy Asthma Immunol. 2009;103:146–151.
3. Wasserbauer N, Ballow M. Atopic dermatitis. Am J Med. 2009;122(2):121–125.
4. O'Reagan GM, Sandilands A, McLean WH, Irvine AD. Filaggrin in atopic dermatitis. J Allergy Clin Immunol. 2008;122:689–693.
5. Bieber T, Novak N. Pathogenesis of atopic dermatitis: New developments. Curr Allergy Asthma Rep. 2009;9:291–294.
6. Kumar A, Grayson MH. The role of viruses in the development and exacerbation of atopic disease. Ann Allergy Asthma Immunol. 2009;103:181–187.
7. Spergel JM. Atopic dermatitis. Internet J Asthma Allergy Immunol. 1999;1(1).
8. Fiset P-O, Leung DYM, Hamid Q. Immunopathology of atopic dermatitis. J Allergy Clin Immunology. 2006;118:287–290.
9. Spergel JM. Immunology and treatment of atopic dermatitis. Am J Clin Dermatol. 2008; 9(4):233–244.
10. Bolognia JL, Jorizzo JL, Rapini RP, et al. Dermatology. Second Edition. Mosby, Spain 2008.
11. Ricci G, Dondi A, Patizi A. Useful tools for the management of atopic dermatitis. Am J Clin Dermatol. 2009;10(5):287–300.
12. Greer FR, Sicherer SH, Burks AW; the Committee on Nutrition and Section on Allergy and Immunology. Effects of early nutritional interventions on the development of atopic disease in infants and children: the role of maternal dietary restriction, breastfeeding, timing of introduction of complementary foods, and hydrolyzed formulas. Pediatrics. 2008;121(1): 183–191.

Chapter 13
Allergic Reactions Affecting Mucosal Surfaces

J. Wesley Sublett and Jonathan A. Bernstein

Abstract Local vaginal IgE immune responses have been underappreciated by allergists. Seminal plasma (SP) hypersensitivity and chronic vulvovaginal *Candida* hypersensitivity are two examples or such reactions that respond to desensitization to relevant seminal plasma proteins and *Candida albicans*, respectively. Both disorders probably occur more frequently in the general population than realized and therefore clinicians should be familiar with the evaluation, diagnosis, and treatment options available for these disorders.

Keywords Human seminal plasma • Vulvovaginal candidiasis • Immunotherapy

Case 1

A 27-year-old woman presented with a 3-year history of postcoital vulvovaginal burning, pruritus, and pain. The pain, which occurred approximately 10 min postcoitally, was described as "a thousand needles being injected into the vagina," and persisted for up to 7 days postcoitus. She denied urticaria, angioedema, difficulty breathing, or syncope, but did develop an erythematous skin rash after contact with seminal fluid. The subject reported that her symptoms occurred after the first intravaginal contact with seminal fluid and became progressively worse with each episode of sexual intercourse. There was slight vaginal and labial swelling but no evidence of blisters or ulcerations. Due to pain, she initially abstained from unprotected sexual intercourse for periods up to 6 months, during which she was symptom free. However, despite this period of abstinence, symptoms immediately returned after

J.A. Bernstein (✉)
Division of Immunology/Allergy Section, Department of Internal Medicine,
University of Cincinnati College of Medicine, 231 Albert Sabin Way, ML#563,
Cincinnati, OH 45267-0563, USA
e-mail: jonathan.bernstein@uc.edu

unprotected sexual intercourse. She subsequently noted that the use of condoms completely prevented symptoms during sexual intercourse. The patient had no prior sexual partners and was currently monogamous. She denied a history of sexually transmitted diseases and or recurrent vulvovaginal *Candida* yeast infections. She denied the use of vaginal douches, spermatocidal gels, vaginal lubricants, sanitary napkins, and scented or colored toilet paper. She had never seen an allergist in the past and had no documented history of symptoms consistent with allergic rhinitis, asthma, eczema, or food or drug allergy. She had no pets or other environmental exposures at home or work that she could attribute to her symptoms.

Laboratory Data

After consultation with our group and her gynecologist, the patient had testing to exclude underlying causes, including a pap smear, *Candida* culture, KOH prep, and vaginal cultures for bacteria and viruses, including herpes simplex virus (HSV) culture and a human papilloma virus (HPV) DNA probe. The Pap smear was negative for intraepithelial lesions or malignancy. The KOH prep was negative for *Gardnerella* and *Trichomonas*. Vaginal cultures were negative for *Chlamydia*, *Mycoplasma*, *Gonorrhea*, HSV I and II, and cytomegalovirus (CMV). Both low-risk and high-risk HPV DNA probes were negative. She was also HIV negative. All other laboratory tests, including a CBC with differential, renal panel, liver panel, thyroid stimulating hormone, Complement 3 and 4, and antinuclear antibody, were normal. The subject also received skin pricks to several seasonal and perennial aeroallergens which indicated that she was sensitized to dust mite, dog, and cat.

Initial Impression

Probable localized SP hypersensitivity. Diagnosis based on immediate pain/burning after intravaginal contact with seminal fluid and alleviation of symptoms with the use of a condom.

Differential Diagnosis

Conditions that should be considered in the differential diagnosis of localized SP hypersensitivity include (a) sexually transmitted diseases (viral and/or bacterial) (b) seasonal allergic vulvovaginitis, (c) latex sensitivity, (d) contact dermatitis, (e) exercise or vibratory associated urticaria, (f) transmission of food or drug protein and metabolites, respectively through body fluids to a sexual partner sensitized to these proteins or metabolites, and (f) physical factors such as small introitus which could cause dyspareunia.

Clinical Evaluation

Initially, a fresh ejaculate was obtained from the women's sexual partner, allowed to liquefy at room temperature for 30 min, and then centrifuged at 10,000 rpm for 10 min to separate out precipitant (spermatozoa) from the supernatant (seminal fluid). The supernatant was then used to perform a skin prick test (SPT) on the volar surface of the patient's forearm in conjunction with positive histamine (10 mg/ml) and negative saline controls. The subject's sexual partner was also tested in a similar manner as a negative control. The patient had a positive SPT (defined as a 3 mm wheal with erythema greater than the negative saline control) which was measured as a wheal of 5 mm and erythema of 10 mm. Her sexual partner's SPT test was negative. Intracutaneous testing to whole seminal fluid was not done to the high incidence of irritant-induced responses.

Identification and Confirmation of Relevant Seminal Plasma Sensitizing Proteins

Gel Filtration Chromatography

SP samples to isolate relevant seminal plasma proteins (SPP) are fractionated by fast protein liquid chromatography (FPLC) as described elsewhere (1, 2). Figure 13.1 illustrates the fractional peaks of SPP. Fraction 1 containing large molecular weight proteins are routinely excluded for use in desensitization because of prior experience, where the treatment with whole seminal fluid was often ineffective. This observation is supported by previous studies demonstrating that these

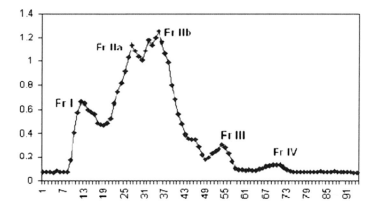

Fig. 13.1 WSP can be resolved into 4–6 fractions using Sephacryl S200 Gel Filtration Chromatography. These fractions are usually used for skin testing and desensitization excluding fraction 1. Prostate-specific antigen (PSA) resolves usually in Fraction IIb and Fraction III

large molecular weight proteins in fraction 1 can inhibit lymphocyte cell-mediated responses in vitro (3).

IgE-Specific Enzyme-Linked Immunosorbent Assay and ELISA Inhibition

To confirm SPT test responses to whole seminal fluid, direct enzyme-linked immunosorbent assay (ELISA) and ELISA inhibition is performed to identify specific IgE levels against whole seminal plasma (WSP) and the fractionated SPP (2, 4). Figure 13.2 illustrates the results of an ELISA inhibition experiment.

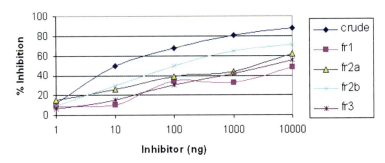

Fig. 13.2 ELISA inhibition using seminal plasma protein fractions: Of the four fractions used, the highest inhibition was exhibited by Fr 2b (50% inhibition exhibited at about 100 ng protein content), followed by Fr3 and Fr2a

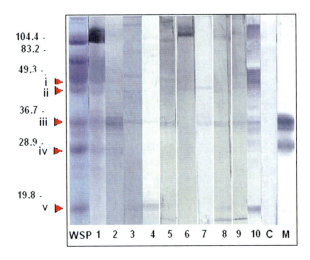

Fig. 13.3 IgE-specific immunoblot to whole seminal plasma (WSP) proteins (*Lanes 1–10* are IgE binding to WSP using ten individual patients' sera, *M* marker for Monoclonal anti-PSA detecting PSA bands)

Sodium dodecyl sulfate – polyacrylamide gel electrophoresis and Western Immunoblotting of SP

We performed Sodium dodecyl sulfate – polyacrylamide gel electrophoresis (SDS-PAGE) of WSP followed by Western Immunoblotting to identify specific IgE antibody responses to specific protein fractions. Figure 13.3 illustrates IgE-specific immunoblots using sera from ten patients with localized SP hypersensitivity. Note the heterogeneous responses between individuals, but all have specific IgE antibodies to fraction 3 which corresponds to prostate-specific antigen (PSA), previously identified as one of the relevant proteins in SP hypersensitivity (5, 6).

With the Presented Data, What Is Your Diagnosis?

Human localized SP hypersensitivity.

Discussion

Human seminal plasma (HSP) hypersensitivity was first reported by a Dutch gynecologist, J.L.H. Specken, in 1958 (7). Since that time, numerous cases of HSP hypersensitivity have appeared in the literature (1, 7, 8), HSP hypersensitivity is defined as a spectrum of systemic and/or localized symptoms after exposure to specific protein components in SP. Women with systemic HSP hypersensitivity present with symptoms of diffuse urticaria, facial, tongue, lip, and throat angioedema with or without stridor, wheezing with severe dyspnea, pelvic and vulvovaginal pain, nausea, vomiting, diarrhea, general malaise and in the most extreme circumstance, life-threatening hypotension, loss of consciousness, and complete circulatory failure that occur within 30 min after exposure to seminal fluid. Symptoms usually resolve over a 24-h period, although urticaria, vaginal pain, and malaise may persist for several days to weeks (8). A previous review of HSP found that 32 cases had been reported between 1958 and 1989 (7). Of reported cases, most were between 20 and 30 years of age and reported localized vaginal pain associated with systemic symptoms of urticaria and pruritus. Forty percent of cases reported symptoms the first time they had intercourse (7). Although the true prevalence of SPH in the general population is unknown, a questionnaire study conducted on a group of women with suspected SPH revealed that 88 out of 1,073 women (8%) surveyed had probable SPH based on their symptoms and resolution of symptoms with the use of a condom. If one were to extrapolate this figure to the normal population, then approximately 20–40,000 women in the United States could potentially have this condition (8). Although avoidance of semen is an effective solution to this problem, it is not usually acceptable by women desiring to have a normal sexual relationship and/or who want to conceive (9). Therefore, SPH not only causes a serious clinical dilemma for affected women, but also leads to significant emotional strain on the interpersonal relationship with their sexual partner (2, 8, 9).

For localized SP hypersensitivity, the most common age of onset is between the ages 20 and 30 year-old. Up to 30–40% of patients experience symptoms with first intercourse and a common feature of both localized and systemic SPH is that the use of condoms prevents symptoms in all cases (2, 8). In our experience, localized SPH reactions are more common than systemic reactions. In general, whereas atopy appears to be a risk factor for systemic SPH, it does not appear to be a risk factor for localized SPH. Women with SPH are not promiscuous as the average number of sexual partners reported is 1.5 (8). Symptom onset is rapid for both systemic and localized SPH occurring within seconds to minutes and can last several hours and for localized reactions vaginal discomfort can persist for several days (8).

There is controversy regarding the most relevant sensitizing allergen(s) for patients with SPH. Investigators have reported that PSA, a 33–34 kD glycoprotein, is the sole allergen in SP causing SPH. However, we have found that other proteins may be involved as well (Fig. 13.3) (5, 6). Because of the high incidence of reactions after first time intercourse, many have proposed a cross-reacting common protein may be involved. Recent studies have reported that dog epithelial extract is cross-reactive to SP, and is likely due to the significant homogeneous structure of dog PSA to human PSA (5).

The diagnosis of HSP hypersensitivity is made mainly by clinical history and complete prevention of symptoms with condom utilization during intercourse. The use of skin prick testing to the subject's sexual partner human seminal fluid and confirmation by serologic testing as described above (1, 2, 8). Various treatments for women with HSP hypersensitivity have been described. The use of prophylactic antihistamines, 30–60 min before sexual intercourse, has been reported to control localized and systemic symptoms in some cases (8). In some cases, the use of a nonsteroidal antiinflammatory agent 30 min before intercourse has alleviated symptoms in the female. This suggests that prostanoids might be involved in some of these cases. Several cases of successful desensitization by intravaginal graded challenge using whole seminal fluid have been reported (10). However, in our experience, the most effective treatment approach for women with IgE-mediated HSP hypersensitivity has been immunotherapy using relevant SPP isolated by fractionation of WSP (1, 2, 4, 11). After skin testing the patient and her sexual partner to the fractionated SPP to determine the ones that elicit a specific IgE-mediated response, a rapid immunotherapy protocol using the relevant SPP is initiated over approximately 3 h. This requires administering a series of subcutaneous injections in the upper arm, similar to traditional allergy injections, of each SP protein beginning at low concentrations and building up until a total of 60–100 µg of each protein is delivered (1, 2, 4, 11). Following immunotherapy with HSP fractions, women must maintain their tolerance to seminal fluid proteins by having frequent and regular sexual intercourse with their partner two to three times a week. This treatment has been very successful in significantly attenuating or completely alleviating symptoms. In our experience, in properly selected patient, SPP desensitization is over 95% successful in resolving symptoms over time. Furthermore, women successfully treated have been able to become pregnant by natural unprotected sexual intercourse. SP hypersensitivity has not been associated with infertility; women unable to get pregnant after desensitization are advised to see a fertility specialist to investigate other causes other than SPH (9).

In summary, this case depicts a patient with localized SP hypersensitivity confirmed by SPT and serologic testing who was successfully treated with rapid immunotherapy to fractionated SPP. The observation that a significant percentage of women experience symptoms without prior exposure to semen illustrates the possibility of developing a localized mucosal immune response as a result of cross-reactivity to proteins structurally similar to human PSA.

Questions

1. Seminal plasma protein hypersensitivity (SPH) occurs after first time intercourse:

    (a) Never
    (b) 30–40% of cases
    (c) 50% of the time
    (d) 75% of the time

2. The most common cross-sensitizing protein associated with localized SPH originates from:

    (a) Cat
    (b) Dust mite
    (c) Dog
    (d) Mold
    (e) None of the above

3. All of the following statement are true except:

    (a) Patients with SPH are more likely to have infertility
    (b) Prostate-specific antigen is believed to be the major allergen causing SPH
    (c) Atopy is a risk factor for systemic SPH
    (d) Large molecular weight seminal plasma proteins can inhibit T-cell-mediated immunity

4. The most effective treatment of SPH is:

    (a) Graded intravaginal challenge with whole seminal fluid
    (b) Intravaginal instillation of cromolyn sodium
    (c) Pre-treatment with antihistamines
    (d) Rapid subcutaneous desensitization using relevant seminal plasma proteins

5. All of the following are true statements except:

    (a) The use of a condom should alleviate all symptoms in women with SPH
    (b) After rapid desensitization, booster injections should be administered initially weekly followed by monthly injections

(c) After rapid desensitization, women should have unprotected sexual intercourse with their sexual partner two to three times a week
(d) Atopy is not a risk factor for localized seminal plasma hypersensitivity

Answers: 1. (b), 2. (c), 3. (a), 4. (d), 5. (b).

Case 2

A 35-year-old woman presented with an 8-year history of recurrent vaginal candidiasis. In the past year, she reported 12 episodes of profuse white curd-like vaginal discharge that was confirmed to be vaginal candidiasis by her gynecologist by KOH prep and a positive culture for *Candida albicans*. She had previously been treated with multiple local antifungal creams and vaginal suppositories as well as repeated treatments with systemic antifungal agents that included ketoconazole, itraconazole, and fluconazole. Use of systemic antifungal agents, such as ketoconazole, resulted in short-term resolution of symptoms from 7 to 14 days before reoccurrence. The subject denied exacerbation of symptoms with antibiotic use, sexual intercourse, or the use of latex condoms. She denied any other contributing conditions such as sexual transmitted diseases, HIV, or diabetes mellitus. There was not reported use of vaginal douches, spermatocidal gels, vaginal lubricants, sanitary napkins, and scented or colored toilet paper. She denied concurrent use of oral contraceptive pills. She had no documented history of allergic rhinitis, asthma, or eczema. The reactions occurred regardless of whether or not her husband used a condom during intercourse.

Laboratory Data

The subject had documented *C. albicans* vulvovaginitis confirmed by positive KOH preps and vaginal fungal cultures demonstrating *C. albican* isolates. Testing was performed by her gynecologist at a recent annual examination. Her Pap smear was normal, the KOH prep was negative for *Gardnerella* and *Trichomonas,* and vaginal cultures were negative for *Chlamydia, Mycoplasma, Gonorrhea,* HSV I and II, and CMV. Both low-risk and high-risk HPV DNA probes were negative. The patient was skin tested to common seasonal and perennial aeroallergens to assess her atopic status.

Initial Impression

Probable vulvovaginal *Candida* hypersensitivity.

Differential Diagnosis

Conditions that should be considered in the differential diagnosis include (a) sexually transmitted diseases, (b) localized seminal plasma hypersensitivity, (c) seasonal allergic vulvovaginitis, (d) latex sensitivity, and (e) contact dermatitis.

Clinical Evaluation

Skin prick testing to *C. albicans* was performed using commercially available *C. albicans* extract. Histamine hydrochloride 10 mg/ml was used as the positive control and saline as the negative control. SPT to the *C. albicans* extract was negative. A positive SPT was defined as 3 mm wheal with erythema greater than the negative saline control. However, the patient exhibited a positive intracutaneous test response to *C. albicans* at a 1:1,000 dilution measured as a wheal of 6 mm and erythema of 12 mm. The subject also experienced a late phase cutaneous response (>3 mm) after 8 h.

IgE Measurement and C. albicans *Immunocap Testing*

Serum obtained from the subject was sent for measurement of total IgE and specific IgE to *C. albicans*. Her total IgE level was 64 IU/ml (normal < 18 IU/ml), while serum-specific IgE to *C. albicans* was <0.4 IU/ml. No prior laboratory test results for total serum IgE or anti-*Candida* IgE were available for comparison.

With the Presented Data, What Is Your Diagnosis?

Vulvovaginal *Candida* hypersensitivity; her diagnosis was based on her history and skin test results.

Discussion

An estimated 75% of the female population will have a *Candida* vulvovaginal infection occur at least once during their lifetime (12, 13). Risk factors commonly associated with vulvovaginal candidiasis include diabetes mellitus, HIV, oral contraceptive use, and antibiotic administration. However, the majority of women will have no recognizable risk factors (12, 13). Topical antifungal agents and/or systemic antifungal agents, such as ketoconazole, are usually effective in treating vulvovaginal candidiasis. Despite effective treatment in most women, 5% will subsequently experience recurrent *Candida* infections (12, 13). These recurrent vulvovaginal *Candida* infections pose a frustrating problem to gynecologists and other primary care providers as no completely effective treatment, including topical or systemic antifungal agents such as ketoconazole and diflucan, has been found (12, 13).

Evidence suggests that women with recurrent vulvovaginal *Candida* infections have developed localized hypersensitivity reactions to *C. albicans* (13, 14). It has been postulated that allergic *Candida* vaginitis is a consequence of either transient inhibition of cell-mediated immunity or mast cell-mediated mediator release, or a combination of both (15, 16). Reduced in vitro lymphocyte proliferation in response to *C. albicans* has been demonstrated in women with recurrent *Candida* vulvovaginitis. This response may be the result of a macrophage-driven increase in the production of prostaglandin E2 (PGE_2) which directly inhibits IL-2 production and subsequent T-cell proliferation. Vaginal washings from some of these women contain elevated PGE_2 levels, supporting a role for PGE_2-induced inhibition of cell-mediated immunity and subsequent occurrence resulting in the development of localized vaginal allergic responses to *Candida* (15, 16). Vaginal washings analyzed for specific IgE antibodies by radioallergosorbent testing in recurrent *Candida* vulvovaginitis cases during episodes of vaginitis revealed anti-*Candida* IgE in 17.2% of cases. Only 6.2% of cases demonstrated serum-specific IgE antibodies to *Candida* and 1.6% of cases had both vaginal fluid and serum anti-*Candida* IgE (17). In some cases, women grow other yeast species such as *Torulopsis globrata* in their vaginal cultures with is cross-reactive *C. albicans* (18).

Several reports claiming success in desensitizing women with recurrent *Candida* vulvovaginitis to *C. albicans* have been published (19, 20). In a prospective study, women with recurrent *Candida* vulvovaginitis confirmed by a positive prick or intracutaneous skin test to *C. albicans* who subsequently were treated with conventional immunotherapy to *C. albicans* over 1 year, demonstrated a reduction in vaginitis episodes from a mean of 17.2 ± 1.98 to 4.3 ± 1.8 (19). Similarly, in another study of women with recurrent *Candida* vulvovaginitis with a positive immediate SPT to *C. albicans* subsequently treated with *C. albicans* allergen immunotherapy for a period of 24 months, there was a decrease in the mean incidence of vaginitis episodes per year from 8.5 ± 2.6 to 3.6 ± 4.3 (20).

In our case, *C. albicans* allergen immunotherapy was initiated after the demonstration of a positive SPT to *C. albicans* and confirmation of a positive vaginal culture for *C. albicans* yeast. Similar to conventional immunotherapy for allergic rhinitis, a series of subcutaneous injections using commercial *C. albicans* extract was administered initially twice a week a lower dilution of 1:100,000 w/v and gradually increasing by one log concentration until a dilution of 1:100 w/v was achieved at which point the frequency of injections was decreased to every 2–4 weeks. In our experience, which is similar to others, increasing the allergen concentration above a 1:100 or 1:1,000 dilution actually makes the vaginitis episodes in many women (19, 20). After 3 months of treatment, the patient noticed a significant reduction in her *Candida* vulvovaginitis episodes. After 1 year of immunotherapy, she had only experienced three episodes of vaginitis which were rapidly responsive to a topical antifungal agent and she was able to resume normal sexual relations with her husband. Table 13.1 summarizes the demographic characteristics of 12 women

Table 13.1 Demographics of 12 patients with chronic vulvovaginal *Candida* hypersensitivity treated with *C. albicans* immunotherapy

Age	Race	OCP	DM	Caused by ABX	ST	Atopic	LPR	Total IgE (IU/ml)	Specific IgE (IU/ml)	Culture for Candida	Maximum [IT]	Duration of IT (months)
40	C	N	N	N	ID	Y	+	ND	ND	+	1:1,000	66[a]
15	C	Y	N	Y	ID	N	+	<18	<18	+	1:1,000	33[a]
62	C	N	N	N	ID	N	+	ND	ND	+	1:1,000	30[a]
26	C	N	N	Y	ID	Y	+	ND	ND	+	1:1,000	86
34	C	N	N	Y	ID	N	+	ND	<18	+	1:1,000	16[b]
29	C	N	N	Y	ID	Y	+	64	ND	+	1:500	12[b]
48	C	N	N	Y	ID	N	+	55	<18	+	1:5,000	21[b]
41	C	N	N	Y	SPT	N	+	47	ND	+	1:10,000	2[c]
30	C	N	N	Y	ID	N	+	ND	ND	+	1:1,000	17
40	C	N	N	Y	ID	N	+	ND	ND	+	1:1,000	9
64	C	N	N	N	ID	N	+	ND	ND	+	1:50,000	39
40	C	N	N	N	ID	N	+	<28	ND	+	1:1,000	91

Abbreviations: *C* Caucasian, *ND* not done, *ABX* antibiotics, *IT* immunotherapy, *OCP* oral contraceptive, *DM* diabetes mellitus, *ID* intradermal, *ST* skin test, *SPT* skin prick test, *LPR* late phase response, [ ] concentration

[a]Denotes patient currently still on immunotherapy
[b]Denotes patient lost to follow-up
[c]Denotes patient cessation due to reaction

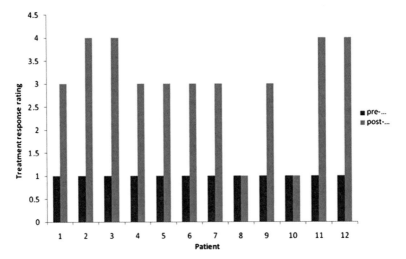

Fig. 13.4 Treatment response rating by 12 patients chronic vulvovaginal *Candida* hypersensitivity treated with *C. albicans* immunotherapy. Rating scores based on a 5 point likert scale; 1 = no response, 2 = minimal barely noticeable response; 3 = partial but noticeable response; 4 = noticeable response as episodes are significantly fewer; 5 complete response – no longer experiencing episodes

with chronic vulvovaginal hypersensitivity treated with *C. albicans* immunotherapy. Figure 13.4 illustrates their treatment response. Only two patients did not exhibit a therapeutic response, one of which was lost to follow-up.

In summary, this case is an example of vulvovaginal *Candida* hypersensitivity confirmed by skin prick testing and immunocap testing to *C. albicans*. This case illustrates the potential for localized IgE reactions to occur intravaginally which may be due to a combination of a defective localized mucosal barrier and increased PGE_2 levels in vaginal fluids which can inhibit cell-mediated immunity. The potential benefit of *C. albicans* immunotherapy in reducing the occurrence of recurrent vaginitis in patients with vulvovaginal *Candida* hypersensitivity is highlighted by this case.

Questions

1. Which of the following statements regarding Recurrent Vulvovaginal *Candida* Hypersensitivity is incorrect?

    (a) These women experience improvement in symptoms in response to condoms
    (b) Chronic treatment with antifungal agents is ineffective
    (c) Use of oral contraceptives can contribute to recurrent yeast infections
    (d) Up to 75% of females in the United States will have at least one yeast infection in their lifetime

13 Allergic Reactions Affecting Mucosal Surfaces

2. Treatment of women with chronic *Candida* vulvovaginal hypersensitivity using immunotherapy:
   (a) Results in a significant reduction in recurrent vaginal yeast infections within 24 months
   (b) Can be performed in women with positive cultures to *Torulopsis globrata*
   (c) Neither a or b
   (d) Both a and b

3. All of the following are true statement except;
   (a) Recurrent use of antibiotics predisposes women to recurrent vaginal yeast infections
   (b) PGE_2 is believed to decrease cell-mediated immune responses
   (c) IgE-mediated mast cell activation is believed to play a role in vulvovaginal *Candida hypersensitivity* reactions
   (d) High dose immunotherapy using *C. albicans* is necessary to achieve maximal tolerance

4. Which of the following statements are true?
   (a) Localized specific IgE *candida* antibodies have been isolated in the majority of women with recurrent vulvovaginal *Candida hypersensitivity*
   (b) Being atopic is not a risk factor for chronic vulvovaginal *Candida* hypersensitivity
   (c) Recurrent vulvovaginal yeast infections are a risk factor for cervical cancer
   (d) Chronic vulvovaginal *Candida* hypersensitivity typically goes into spontaneous remission

5. Diagnosis of recurrent vulvovaginal *Candida* hypersensitivity requires all of the following except:
   (a) A positive skin test to *Candida albicans*
   (b) A positive vaginal culture for yeast
   (c) A history of recurrent yeast infections
   (d) A family history of recurrent yeast infections

Answer: 1. (a), 2. (d), 3. (d), 4. (b), 5. (d).

References

1. Bernstein, I.L., et al., *Localized and systemic hypersensitivity reactions to human seminal fluid.* Ann Intern Med, 1981. **94**(4 Pt 1): p. 459–65.
2. Bernstein, J.A., et al., *Evaluation and treatment of localized vaginal immunoglobulin E-mediated hypersensitivity to human seminal plasma.* Obstet Gynecol, 1993. **82**(4 Pt 2 Suppl): p. 667–73.
3. Marcus, Z.H., et al., *In vitro studies in reproductive immunology. 1. Suppression of cell-mediated immune response by human spermatozoa and fractions isolated from human seminal plasma.* Clin Immunol Immunopathol, 1978. **9**(3): p. 318–26.

4. Bernstein, J.A., et al., *Is burning semen syndrome a variant form of seminal plasma hypersensitivity?* Obstet Gynecol, 2003. **101**(1): p. 93–102.
5. Basagana, M., et al., *Allergy to human seminal fluid: cross-reactivity with dog dander.* J Allergy Clin Immunol, 2008. **121**(1): p. 233–9.
6. Weidinger, S., et al., *Prostate-specific antigen as allergen in human seminal plasma allergy.* J Allergy Clin Immunol, 2006. **117**(1): p. 213–5.
7. Presti, M.E. and H.M. Druce, *Hypersensitivity reactions to human seminal plasma.* Ann Allergy, 1989. **63**(6 Pt 1): p. 477–81.
8. Bernstein, J.A., et al., *Prevalence of human seminal plasma hypersensitivity among symptomatic women.* Ann Allergy Asthma Immunol, 1997. **78**(1):p.42–8.
9. Resnick, D.J., et al., *The approach to conception for women with seminal plasma protein hypersensitivity.* Am J Reprod Immunol, 2004. **52**(1): p. 42–4.
10. Lee, J., et al., *Anaphylaxis to husband's seminal plasma and treatment by local desensitization.* Clin Mol Allergy, 2008. **6**: p. 13.
11. Mittman, R.J., et al., *Selective desensitization to seminal plasma protein fractions after immunotherapy for postcoital anaphylaxis.* J Allergy Clin Immunol, 1990. **86**(6 Pt 1): p. 954–60.
12. Sobel, J.D., *Recurrent vulvovaginal candidiasis. A prospective study of the efficacy of maintenance ketoconazole therapy.* N Engl J Med, 1986. **315**(23): p. 1455–8.
13. Rosedale, N. and K. Browne, *Hyposensitisation in the management of recurring vaginal candidiasis.* Ann Allergy, 1979. **43**(4): p. 250–3.
14. Witkin, S.S., *Immunology of recurrent vaginitis.* Am J Reprod Immunol Microbiol, 1987. **15**(1): p. 34–7.
15. Witkin, S.S., J. Hirsch, and W.J. Ledger, *A macrophage defect in women with recurrent Candida vaginitis and its reversal in vitro by prostaglandin inhibitors.* Am J Obstet Gynecol, 1986. **155**(4): p. 790–5.
16. Meech, R.J., J.M. Smith, and T. Chew, *Pathogenic mechanisms in recurrent genital candidosis in women.* N Z Med J, 1985. **98**(771): p. 1–5.
17. Witkin, S.S., J. Jeremias, and W.J. Ledger, *A localized vaginal allergic response in women with recurrent vaginitis.* J Allergy Clin Immunol, 1988. **81**(2): p. 412–6.
18. Koivikko, A., et al., *Allergenic cross-reactivity of yeasts.* Allergy, 1988. **43**(3): p. 192–200.
19. Rigg, D., M.M. Miller, and W.J. Metzger, *Recurrent allergic vulvovaginitis: treatment with Candida albicans allergen immunotherapy.* Am J Obstet Gynecol, 1990. **162**(2): p. 332–6.
20. Moraes, P.S., S. de LimaGoiaba, and E.A. Taketomi, *Candida albicans allergen immunotherapy in recurrent vaginal candidiasis.* J Investig Allergol Clin Immunol, 2000. **10**(5): p. 305–9.

Part V
Immunologic Diseases of the Skin

Chapter 14
Vasculitis

Satoshi Yoshida

Abstract The vasculitides span a wide range of disease severity, extending from illnesses that rarely produce death to those almost universally fatal before the introduction of effective therapy. Clinical manifestations of specific vasculitic disorders are diverse and depend on the size of the involved vessels and the organs affected by ischemia. Most damage results when inflammation narrows vessels and causes tissue necrosis.

Immunosuppressive and cytotoxic agents are used to treat many vasculitic diseases. Although such approaches can be effective, long-term treatment may be complicated by chronic sequelae from organ damage, disease relapses, and medication side effects. Recent investigations have focused on understanding the pathophysiology of these diseases, which may lead to more efficacious and less toxic therapeutic options.

Two cases related to the presentation and management of vasculitis are discussed.

Keywords Vasculitis • Wegener's granulomatosis • Necrotizing sialometaplasia • Churg-Strauss syndrome • Antineutrophil cytoplasmic antibodies

Case 1

A 23-year-old man presented with a 5-day history of vomiting and passing dark urine. He gave an approximately 6-month history of arthralgias and joint swelling particularly affecting larger joints. He had recurrent epistaxis and recent episcleritis. He was noted to be thin and pale with conjunctival suffusion and deformity of his nasal bridge. His vitals included blood pressure of 126/70 mmHg and temperature of 36.2°C. Clinical examination revealed no focal neurologic deficits. Renal indices were abnormal (blood urea nitrogen 29.5 mmol/L, creatinine 802 μmol/L, and potassium 5.4 mmol/L).

S. Yoshida (✉)
Department of Allergy and Immunology,
Johns Hopkins Medicine International,Tokyo Midtown
Medical Center, Tokyo, Japan
e-mail: syoshida-fjt@umin.ac.jp

Cytoplasmic antineutrophil cytoplasmic antibodies (cANCAs) was strongly positive (titer: 1280) Enzyme-Linked ImmunoSorbent Assay was positive (ELISA PR3+). He was diagnosed with Wegener's granulomatosis. He started hemodialysis, corticosteroids, and oral cyclophosphamide and subsequently was discharged home.

He presented 2 months later with recurrent partial seizures and severe throbbing headaches characteristic of migraine with aura. He described episodes of body image distortion (macrosomatognosia) with his hand "balooning," colored visual spectra phenomena characterized as a "kaleidoscope" effect, a light moving diagonally across his visual field from left to right, and an impaired sense of passage of time (a perceived increased speech velocity). These episodes heralded the onset of headache, seizures, or a combination of both. He had intractable hiccups and episodes of vertigo, ataxia, slurred speech, and nystagmus. He was normotensive (blood pressure of 104/68 mmHg) and a febrile (temperature: 38.8°C).

Data

Full septic screen, including midstream urine, chest X-ray, echocardiogram, and blood cultures were negative formal for active infection. Serum antiepileptic drug levels were within normal limits and cANCA was negative. Cerebrospinal fluid (CSF) analysis showed normal protein and glucose parameters and was acellular.

Imaging Studies

Postictal Electroencephalogram (EEG) was normal. Initial noncontrast brain computed tomography (CT) was normal. Brain magnetic resonance imaging (MRI) with gadolinium showed small ill-defined, nonenhancing high signal areas measuring 5–20 mm in several locations (Fig. 14.1).

1. With the presented data, what is your working diagnosis?

    (a) Miller–Fisher syndrome
    (b) Riley–Day syndrome
    (c) Alice in Wonderland syndrome
    (d) Ganser syndrome

2. What are the differential diagnosis of the underlying pathologic etiology?

Discussion

The clinical picture at this stage was thought consistent with the Alice in Wonderland syndrome, which is complicated with Wegener's granulomatosis. The features of Alice in Wonderland syndrome were first reported by Coleman in 1932, but it was

14 Vasculitis

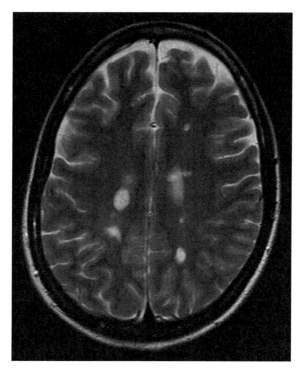

Fig. 14.1 Brain MRI with gadolinium showed small ill-defined, nonenhancing high signal areas measuring 5–20 mm in several locations

Todd who coined the term in 1955 to describe the phenomena of distorted space, time, and body image. Lewis Carroll made this phenomenon famous in "Alice's Adventures in Wonderland" (1865), and it has been suggested that Alice's transformations were based on Carroll's own migrainous symptomatology; however, this remains controversial.

Alice in Wonderland syndrome has been associated with migraine, epilepsy, drug intoxication, cerebral mass lesions (particularly involving the occipital and temporoparietal lobes), psychiatric disease, viral infections, pyrexia, and vasculitis. Perceptual errors of body schema and objects (kinesthetic illusions or metamorphopsia), people appearing smaller (micropsia) or bigger (macropsia) than normal visual hallucinations (*Lilliputian hallucinations*) and acceleration of deceleration of the passage of time have been attributed to Alice in Wonderland syndrome. It may also be associated with vertigo. The etiology and anatomic basis are not fully understood. Body image distortion, vertigo, and metamorphopsia have been described from posterior parietal stimulation. Positive visual phenomena of flashing lights and colored visual spectra equated to a kaleidoscope and negative visual phenomena (scotoma) are both established occipital lobe phenomena. In addition, headache and vomiting may have an occipital origin. These symptoms prompted more imaging. Brain MRI showed diffuse white matter high signal abnormalities demonstrating dramatic interval progression involving the occipital, parietal, and temporal lobes in addition to bilateral cerebellar legions with gadolinium.

Vasculitis is histologically defined by the presence of blood vessel inflammation, often with ischemia, necrosis, and occlusive changes. It can affect any blood vessel, arteries, arterioles, veins, venules, or capillaries. It can be observed in a wide variety of settings, either occurring secondarily to another process or as the pathologic foundation of a primary vasculitic disease (1) (Table 14.1). The primary systemic vasculitides comprise a broad group of disease entities that are uniquely identified by the nature of their clinical, histopathologic, or therapeutic characteristics. Individual diseases often predominantly affect blood vessels of a particular size, the pattern of which influences their clinical manifestations and has been used in their classification (2) (Table 14.2).

The pathophysiology of the vasculitides remains poorly understood and may vary between different diseases. For each disease, however, immunologic mechanisms appear to play an active role in mediating the necrotizing inflammation of blood vessels. Based on current understanding of the inflammatory response, it can be hypothesized that cytokine-mediated changes in the expression and function of adhesion molecules together with inappropriate activation of leukocytes and endothelial cells are key factors influencing vessel inflammation and damage. Although the primary events that initiate this process remain largely unknown, recent advances have begun to allow investigators to examine the effector mechanisms involved in disease pathogenesis.

Wegener's granulomatosis is a necrotizing, granulomatous vasculitis that affects small to medium-sized vessels. The disease can occur at any age and appears to affect men and women in equal proportions. Wegener's granulomatosis is a multisystem disease that has a predilection to involve the upper and lower respiratory tract and kidneys. More than 90% of patients first seek medical attention for symptoms related to the upper and/or lower airways. Nasal and sinus mucosal inflammation may result in cartilaginous ischemia with perforation of the nasal septum and/or saddle nose deformity. Pulmonary radiographic abnormalities can include single or multiple nodules or infiltrates, cavities, and ground glass infiltrates. Glomerulonephritis is present in 20% of patients at the time of diagnosis but develops in 80% at some point during the disease course. Renal involvement is detected by the presence of an active urine sediment with microscopic hematuria and red blood cell casts and has the potential to be rapidly progressive and asymptomatic. Before the development of treatment, patients with Wegener's granulomatosis had a mean survival time of 5 months, with death occurring from pulmonary or renal failure. Although effective therapy has brought the potential for long-term survival, relapse occurs in at least 50% of patients. The diagnosis of Wegener's granulomatosis is made by biopsy, with nonrenal tissues demonstrating the presence of granulomatous inflammation, necrosis, often with aggregates of neutrophils, and necrotizing or granulomatous vasculitis. Surgically obtained biopsy specimens of abnormal pulmonary parenchyma demonstrate diagnostic changes in 91% of cases. Biopsy of the upper airways is less invasive but demonstrates diagnostic features only 21% of the time. The characteristic renal histology is that of a focal, segmental, necrotizing, crescentic glomerulonephritis with few to no immune complexes.

Table 14.1 Names and definitions of vasculitides adopted by the Chapel Hill consensus conference on the nomenclature of systemic vasculitis

LARGE-VESSEL VASCULITIS	
Giant cell (temporal) arteritis	Granulomatous arteritis of the aorta and its major branches, with a predilection for the extracranial branches of the carotid artery. Often involves the temporal artery. Usually occurs in patients older than 50 and often is associated with poly myalgia rheumatica
Takayasu arteritis	Granulomatous inflammation of the aorta and its major branches. Usually occurs in patients younger than 50
MEDIUM-SIZED VESSEL VASCULITIS	
Polyarterities nodosa (classic poly arterities nodosa)	Necrotizing inflammation of medium-sized or small arteries without glomerulonephritis or vasculitis in arterioles, capillaries, or venules
Kawasaki disease	Arteritis involving large, medium-sized, and small arteries, and associated with mucocutaneous lymph mode syndrome. Coronary arteries are often involved. Aorta and veins may be involved. Usually occurs in children
SMALL-VESSEL VASCULITIS	
Wegener's granulomatosis	Granulomatous inflammation involving the respiratory tract, and necrotizing vasculitis affecting small to medium-sized vessels (e.g., capillaries, venules, arterioles, and arteries). Necrotizing glomerulonephritis is common
Churg–Strauss syndrome	Eosinophil-rich and granulomatous inflammation involving the respiratory tract, and necrotizing vasculitis affecting small to medium-sized vessels, and associated with asthma and eosinophilia
Microscopic polyangiitis (microscopic polyarteritis)	Necrotizing vasculitis, with few or no immune deposits, affecting small vessels (i.e., capillaries, venules, or arterioles)
	Necrotizing arteritis involving small and medium-sized arteries may be present. Necrotizing glomerulonephritis is very common. Pulmonary capillaritis often occurs
Henoch-Schönlein purpura	Vasculitis, with Ig-A dominant immune deposits, affecting small vessels (i.e., capillaries, venules, or arterioles). Typically involves skin, gut, and glomeruli, and is associated with anthralgias or arthritis
Essential cryoglobulinemic vasculitis	Vasculitis, with cryoglobulin immune deposits, affecting small vessels (i.e., capillaries, venules, or arterioles), and associated with cryoglobulins in serum. Skin and glomeruli are often involved
Cutaneous leukocytoclastic vasculitis	Isolated cutaneous leukocytoclastic angiitis without systemic vasculitis or glomerulonephritis

Glucocorticoids alone are ineffective in the setting of active Wegener's granulomatosis affecting a major organ, such as the lung, kidney, nerve, or eye, and must be combined with a cytotoxic agent. Patients who have active Wegener's granulomatosis immediately threatening to life should be treated with cyclophosphamide at 2 mg/kg per day in combination with prednisone at 1 mg/kg per day. With the use of such therapy, 91% of patients have had marked improvement, 75% achieved

Table 14.2 Potential mechanisms of vessel damage in selected primary vasculitis syndromes

Immune complex formation
Hepatitis B-associated polyarteritis nodosa
Henoch-Schönlein purpura
Essential mixed cryoglobulinemia
Production of antineutrophil cytoplasmic antibodies
Wegener's granulomatosis
Microscopic polyangiitis
Churg–Strauss syndrome
Pathogenic T-lymphocyte responses and granuloma formation
Giant cell (temporal) arteritis
Takayasu arteritis
Wegener granulomatosis
Churg–Strauss syndrome

a complete remission, and an 80% survival rate has been observed. In the setting of fulminant disease, 1 g/day solumedrol may be given in divided doses over a period of 3 days, in combination with 3–4 mg/kg per day cyclophosphamide for 3 days, after which time it is reduced to 2 mg/kg per day. After the first 4 weeks of treatment, if there is evidence of improvement, the prednisone is tapered on an alternate day schedule and discontinued by 6–12 months. In the first studied regimen, cyclophosphamide was given for 1 year past remission, after which time it was tapered and discontinued. Although cyclophosphamide is very effective, it is associated with substantial toxicity, including bone marrow suppression, bladder injury, infertility, myeloproliferative disease, and transitional cell carcinoma of the bladder. Recent studies have examined a staged approach, whereby cyclophosphamide is given until remission, which usually occurs at about 3–6 months, at which time it is switched to a less toxic medication for remission maintenance. The two maintenance agents with which there has been the greatest body of experience have been methotrexate at 20–25 mg/week 25 or azathioprine at 2 mg/kg per day. These are given for 1–2 years, after which time if patients remain in remission, they are tapered and discontinued. In patients who have active but nonlife-threatening disease or patients who are unable to tolerate cyclophosphamide, prednisone given together with 20–25 mg/week methotrexate has also been found to be efficacious at inducing remission. Methotrexate should not be given to patients with impaired renal function (creatinine clearance of <35 mL/min) or chronic liver disease.

Miller–Fisher syndrome is a variant of Guillain–Barre syndrome and manifests as a descending paralysis, proceeding in the reverse order of the more common form of Guillain–Barre syndrome. It usually affects the eye muscles first and presents with the triad of ophthalmoplegia, ataxia, and areflexia. Anti-GQ1b antibodies are present in 90% of cases.

Riley–Day syndrome is a disorder of the autonomic nervous system which affects the development and survival of sensory, sympathetic, and some parasympathetic neurons in the autonomic and sensory nervous system resulting in variable symptoms, including insensitivity to pain, inability to produce tears, poor growth, and labile blood pressure (episodic hypertension and postural hypotension).

Ganser syndrome is a rare dissociative disorder previously classified as a factitious disorder. It is characterized by nonsensical or wrong answers to questions or doing things incorrectly, other dissociative symptoms, such as fugue, amnesia, or conversion disorder, often with visual pseudohallucinations and a decreased state of consciousness.

Case 2

A 32-year-old woman was affected by a midline ulceration and a mucocele of the palatal mucosa without purulent discharge. No other symptoms were referred. A biopsy of the lesion that suggested Wegener's granulomatosis had already been performed. Chest radiograph and ANCA titers were normal. Past clinical history of the patient was unremarkable (Fig. 14.2).

Data

Evaluation of the biopsy sample demonstrated the foci of squamous metaplasia of the minor salivary gland ducts, thus confirming the diagnosis (Fig. 14.3).

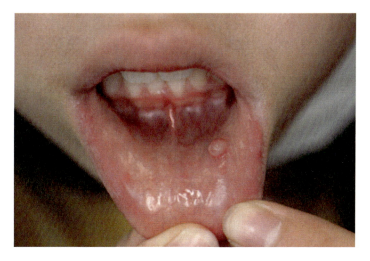

Fig. 14.2 Midline ulceration and a mucocele of the palatal mucosa without purulent discharge was observed

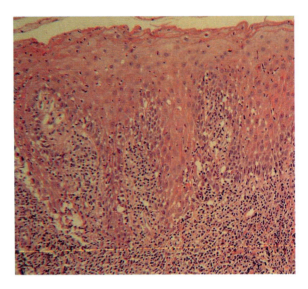

Fig. 14.3 The biopsy sample demonstrated foci of squamous metaplasia of the minor salivary gland ducts

Imaging Studies

An MRI scan demonstrated a lobulated submucosal lesion in the posterior third of the hard palate, which was hyperintense on T2 and hypointense on T1 weighted images; after contrast administration (Gd-DTPA), no abnormal finding has been detected. Bone was not eroded. The lesion abutted both of the major palatine nerve canals, with no signs of perineural spread.

1. Based on the imaging and clinical findings, what is the diagnosis of this case?

    (a) Sarcoidosis
    (b) Necrotizing sialometaplasia
    (c) Sjögren's syndrome
    (d) Lymphoma

2. How do you think about the absence of fever and purulent discharge?

    Based on the imaging and clinical findings, necrotizing sialometaplasia of minor salivary glands of the palate was suspected.

Discussion

Necrotizing sialometaplasia is a necrotizing inflammatory process that largely involved the minor salivary glands, which is potentially throughout the whole upper aerodigestive tract; although in up to 10% of cases it is also reported in major salivary glands (3).

The most common clinical manifestation of this condition is swelling and/or ulceration of the hard palate, which may be associated with pain. Infarct of salivary gland lobes with subsequent repair and metaplasia is commonly accepted basis of necrotizing sialometaplasia, although the pathophysiology is still unclear. Chemical injury, chronic or acute trauma, infection and atherosclerosis are some of the proposed causes. Necrotizing sialometaplasia is self-limiting, and spontaneous resolution is expected within 6–12 weeks. Treatment of symptoms is indicated for painful lesions.

An incisional biopsy is required to obtain diagnosis. At histology, lobular necrosis along with squamous metaplasia of ducts and acini are found. Necrosis areas, filled with mucus and debris, may be associated with an intensive inflammatory reaction.

MRI findings in the present case might reflect such a histological background. We hypothesize that T2 hyperintensity might be the hallmark of minor salivary gland necrosis, whereas the peripheral rim of enhancement might represent the inflammatory reaction. On MRI, a list of differential diagnosis should be considered when a submucosal palatal lesion is detected, including both inflammatory diseases and begnign and malignant neoplasm.

In this case, the mucosal ulceration and the fluid content of the lesion could suggest a palatal abscess. Conversely, the absence of fever and purulent discharge was inconsistent with this hypothesis. Wegener's granulomatosis was first suspected after pathological examination of biopsy sample. MRI findings of Wegener's granulomatosis of the oral cavity have not been described in the literature. Nonetheless, in the nose and paranasal cavities, MRI findings consist of submucosal lesions with hypothesis T2 signal and variable degrees of enhancement.

Minor salivary gland tumors include both benign (e.g., pleomorphic adenoma) and malignant (e.g., mucoepidermoid carcinoma and adenoid cystic carcinoma) histotypes, although the latter are much more frequent. A hyperintense T2 signal is quite common in pleomorphic adenoma (owing to its myxoid component) and can be observed in mucoepidermoid carcinoma (when intralesional hemorrhage occurs). Nevertheless, all of these lesions exhibit variable degrees of enhancement after contrast agent administration. The fluid-like appearance and absence of contrast enhancement (apart from the thin and regular peripheral rim) helped to exclude salivary gland neoplasm. The hard palate can be secondarily involved by sinonasal lymphoma. Bone involvement is frequent and may manifest as destruction (in up to 40% of non-Hodgkin's lymphoma cases) or permeative infiltration (tumor on both sides of a bone boundary without macroscopic erosion). Bone destruction is quite typical (78% of cases) in T/NK-cell lymphoma, a disease entity that has been described with several different names, including lethal midline granuloma, polymorphic reticulosis and nonhealing granuloma. The MRI signal pattern and lack of bone changes ruled out lymphoma in this case.

In conclusion, necrotizing sialometaplasia is a spontaneously resolving inflammatory condition that can mimic a neoplasm. Awareness of this disease entity is crucial for radiologists in order to avoid misinterpretation of imaging findings that may lead to undue surgical treatment.

Questions

Case 1

A 68-year-old woman had a history of allergic rhinitis, chronic sinusitis (documented by sinus radiography), and asthma for 20 years. She had been receiving inhaled corticosteroids and short prednisone bursts for 10 years. Since last month, the asthma became more severe and oral prednisone was started. The dose was gradually increased to 60 mg q.d. daily, and after control was achieved, it was quickly tapered to 5 mg q.d. in 1 month.

At that time, numbness and pain developed in the right hand at the thumb, index, middle finger, and thenar area, and 5 days later left foot drop developed that was consistent with mononeuritis multiplex of the right median and left peroneal nerves. There was also a recent 10 pound weight loss. Laboratory evaluation revealed a white blood cell (WBC) count of 20,200/μL with 55% eosinophils and an erythrocyte sedimentation rate (ESR) of 21 mm/h. The antineutrophil cytoplasmic antibody (ANCA) test was positive by fluorescence at a titer of 1:160 with a perinuclear pattern (pANCA). Blood urea nitrogen (BUN), creatinine, and urinalysis were normal. The antinuclear antibody (ANA) test was positive at a titer of 1:160 (homogeneous pattern) and serum protein electrophoresis (SPEP) showed no paraproteins. Chest radiography was normal. Stool examination for parasites and hemorrhage were both negative. Nerve conduction studies were consistent with left peroneal axonal neuropathy. The left sural nerve biopsy specimen demonstrated axonal degeneration as well as intramural eosinophilic, mononuclear, and lymphocytic infiltrate with thrombosis of adjacent vessels (Fig. 14.4).

1. What are the possible etiologies of numbness and pain developed in the right hand at the thumb?

    (a) Corticosteroid myopathy
    (b) Rhabdomyolysis
    (c) Fibromyalgia
    (d) Churg–Strauss syndrome

2. What medication do you administrate for this patient?

    (a) Antibiotics
    (b) Dantrolene
    (c) High dose of corticosteroids
    (d) Milnacipran

The etiology of Churg–Strauss syndrome is still unknown. Wechsler et al. described a syndrome resembling Churg–Strauss syndrome with pulmonary infiltrates, eosinophilia, and cardiomyopathy in association with the cysteinyl leukotriene receptor antagonist zafirlukast (4). After that, four cases of Churg–Strauss syndrome in patients receiving zafirlukast have been reported. In addition, a letter from Merk & Co, Inc.

14 Vasculitis

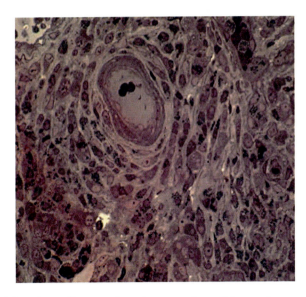

Fig. 14.4 The left sural nerve biopsy specimen demonstrated axonal degeneration as well as intramural eosinophilic, mononuclear, and lymphocytic infiltrate with thrombosis of adjacent vessels

to physicians in December 1998 indicated that signs and symptoms of Churg–Strauss syndrome have been reported with the use of another cysteinyl leukotriene receptor antagonist, montelukast. Pranlukast, a cysteinyl leukotriene receptor antagonist not available in the United States, was reported in association with Churg–Strauss syndrome in Japan (5). The significance of this association is not clear. A plausible explanation is that the introduction of the cysteinyl leukotriene receptor antagonist improved the asthmatic, leukotriene-mediated component of preexisting Churg–Strauss syndrome and allowed the reduction of the systemic corticosteroid dose, unmasking other manifestations of the syndrome. Churg et al. reported cases of formes frustes Churg–Strauss syndrome that followed the reduction of the systemic corticosteroid dose (6). This explanation is further supported by a letter from Glaxo Wellcome, Inc., to physicians in January 1999 stating that in rare cases, patients on inhaled fluticasone propionate may present with eosinophilic conditions and clinical symptoms consistent with Churg–Strauss syndrome, possibly due to the reduction of the systemic steroid dose. The reduction of the oral corticosteroid dose, however, did not precede the Churg–Strauss syndrome in all cysteinyl leukotriene receptor antagonist-associated reported cases. Four patients receiving zafirlukast were not on maintenance oral corticosteroids at the time of onset (5). Asthma and sinus disease were the unifying features in those cases. The duration of asthma before the onset of Churg–Strauss syndrome was variable from 1 to 20 years. The severity of asthma was also variable as assessed by history, spirometry, and oral corticosteroid requirements. The only medication that was common in most patients was inhaled corticosteroids.

This patient has allergic asthma and chronic sinusitis and pronounced eosinophilic vasculitis on the biopsy specimen, which is consistent with Churg–Strauss syndrome. Although peripheral eosinophilia is considered one of the primary diagnostic features of Churg–Strauss syndrome, there are reports of forms of the syndrome without it.

It is important to note that, in that report, all patients were receiving oral corticosteroids, which were thought to be masking some of the features of the syndrome. The practicing physician should be aware of the possibility that steroids may be masking a form of Churg–Strauss syndrome and that this syndrome can occur in patients, with mild to moderate asthma of short duration, who are using only inhaled steroids.

Case 2

A 55-year-old woman was referred for recurrent palpable purpura and cutaneous ulcers over her lower legs. Her disease started 3 years ago with erythematous papules and palpable purpuric lesions located over her lower legs, including the dorsa of her feet. The lesions were intensely pruritic. They usually evolved into shallow skin ulcers, some of them preceded with a short-lived bullous phase. Lesions used to crop in the late autumn and winter, and then subside in the spring leaving hyper- and hypopigmented atrophic scars. In the second year of her disease, she experienced similar lesions located on the upper back. The disease responded well to midpotency topical steroids only to recur shortly after stopping them. Otherwise, she feels healthy and denies any other health-related problems, including Raynaud's phenomenon. Family history was negative for autoimmune illness, including rheumatic and blistering diseases.

On her lower legs, we found several cutaneous ulcers covered with hemorrhagic crusts along with hyper- and hypopigmented atrophic scars and a few excoriated papules (Fig. 14.5). A multitude of hypopigmented oval atrophic scars were distributed over her upper back. The rest of physical examination, including accessible mucosal surfaces and peripheral pulses was normal.

Complete blood cell count with the differential, urinalysis, routine biochemical blood tests, liver and renal function tests, liver and muscle enzymes, autoantibody screen, immunoglobulins, complement, cryoglobulins, rheumatoid factor, syphilis serology, antiphospholipid antibodies, lupus anticoagulant, blood viscosity, (SPEP), throat swabs, antistreptolysin O (ASO) titers, chest X-rays, abdominal ultrasound, gynecologic exam, and stool examination for occult blood were all negative or within a normal range. Erythrocyte sedimentation rate was elevated at 45 mm/h. Her blood was checked up for pemphigus antibodies upon monkey esophagus, and they were found in a titer of 1: 320.

Endothelial cell swelling, fibrinoid necrosis, neutrophil infiltration, sparse karyorrhexis, erythrocyte extravasation, and some eosinophil infiltration around vessels (Fig. 14.6). Biopsy was taken from a periphery of the most recent, partially ulcerated,

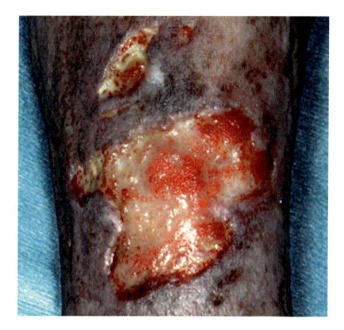

Fig. 14.5 On her lower legs showed several cutaneous ulcers covered with hemorrhagic crusts along with hyper- and hypopigmented atrophic scars and a few excoriated papules

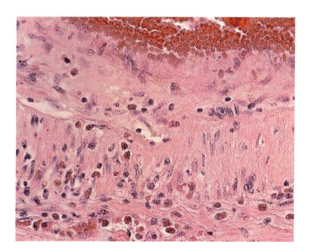

Fig. 14.6 Endothelial cell swelling, fibrinoid necrosis, neutrophil infiltration, sparse karyorrhexis, erythrocyte extravasation, and some eosinophil infiltration around vessels

lesion and processed for routine histopathology and direct immunofluorescence study. Histopathology showed partly ulcerated epidermis and foci of collagen necrosis with leukocytoclastic vasculitis of the dermal blood vessels. Direct immunofluorescence disclosed intercellular deposits of IgG in the epidermis along with IgG, IgM, C3, and

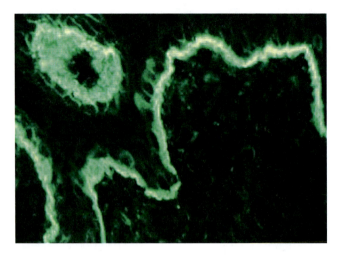

Fig. 14.7 Epidermal intercellular IgG deposits were found in the clinically uninvolved skin

fibrinogen deposits around dermal blood vessels in her lesional skin. Only epidermal intercellular IgG deposits were found in the clinically uninvolved skin (Fig. 14.7).

3. With the presented clinical course and data, what is your working diagnosis?

    (a) Varix of lower extremities
    (b) Cutaneous small-vessel vasculitis
    (c) Pemphigus vulgaris
    (d) Senear–Usher syndrome

4. How do you treat this patient?

    (a) Topical alprostadil alfadex ointment
    (b) Topical corticosteroid ointment
    (c) Pentoxiphylline
    (d) Cyclosporin

Cutaneous small-vessel vasculitis refers to a group of disorders usually characterized by palpable purpura and the result of necrotizing, mostly leukocytoclastic, vasculitis of dermal postcapillary venules (7). It is believed that the majority of cutaneous necrotizing vasculitides are a consequence of immune-complex deposition in the walls of the affected blood vessels. Yet, the etiology of the disorder remains elusive in up to 60–70% of patients. Pemphigus is a group of acquired autoimmune bullous dermatoses resulting from the production of autoantibodies directed to an array of epithelial adhesion molecules, which in turn result in the disruption of intercellular cohesion clinically manifesting as cutaneous or mucosal bullae and erosions (8). Pemphigus or pemphigus-related autoantibodies have been found in sera of healthy relatives of patients with this disease as well as in some other diseases, such as toxic epidermal necrolysis, thermal burns, and penicillin reactions. The case presented is unusual in several respects. The seasonal appearance of her vasculitic lesions was reminiscent of livedo vasculopathy, but her condition lacked some common features of the disease, i.e., livedo reticularis, atrophie blanche changes, and fibrin thrombi within the superficial blood vessels. Additionally, pain but not pruritus is a usual symptom in livedo vasculopathy. Several episodes of presumably vasculitic lesions over her upper back are quite unusual for livedo vasculopathy and even for cutaneous small-vessel vasculitis. The cause of her vasculitis could not be found despite a thorough examination. The incidental finding of intraepidermal intercellular deposits of IgG together with circulating pemphigus autoantibodies in a relatively high titer was surprising. Histologic examination of her lesional skin did not show any signs of acantholysis, and her history did not disclose any relatives with pemphigus. Occasional blisters she did notice surmounting some of her purpuric lesions might be a consequence of her pemphigus antibodies as well as of the vasculitic process. It may be argued that indirect immunofluorescence testing may give many false positives at some laboratories. However, a recent study comparing serodiagnosis of pemphigus vulgaris by standard immunofluorescence testing on monkey esophagus and a commercially available ELISA showed that, with immunofluorescence, none of 50 controls was positive. Cutaneous small-vessel vasculitis should be added to the list of skin conditions which might be accompanied by the appearance of pemphigus autoantibodies without overt clinical manifestations of pemphigus.

Case 3

A 47-year-old woman presented with a 2-month history of numerous, skin-colored, small papules that were distributed symmetrically on the proximal aspects of the extremities and upper trunk. They were not pruritic or painful. The nonremitting lesions began suddenly and preceded a flare in joint pain. Medical history included rheumatoid factor-negative arthritis that previously had been treated with nonsteroidal antiinflammatory medications and gold therapy, chronic obstructive pulmonary disease, and emphysema. Tobacco use had been discontinued for 5 years. No family history of skin disorders was reported. The patient denied recent travel or any new illness. Her medications included alprazolam and atorvastatin, which she has taken for 4 years. Metaxalone, which is a centrally acting skeletal muscle relaxant, had been started 5 months earlier. The patient also had been on vitamin B12, folate, and calcium carbonate supplements on a long-term basis.

Numerous, discrete, monomorphic, skin-colored papules were scattered in a symmetric pattern on the upper chest, posterior upper shoulders, posterior neck, and proximal extremities. On the extremities, the papules were arranged on the posterior upper arms, which included the axillary vaults, and superior medial thighs (Fig. 14.8).

A complete blood count, erythrocyte sedimentation rate, comprehensive metabolic panel, fasting lipid panel, and C-reactive protein were normal. Antinuclear and Sjögren single-stranded A and B antibodies and rheumatoid factor were negative.

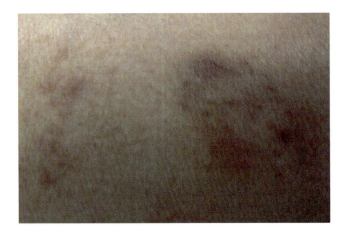

Fig. 14.8 The papules were arranged on the posterior upper arms, which included the axillary vaults, and superior medial thighs

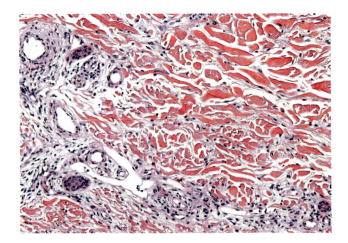

Fig. 14.9 There is a superficial and deep, perivascular and interstitial infiltrate of lymphocytes, eosinophils, and mononuclear histiocytes. Mononuclear histiocytes are scattered between collagen bundles and associated with mucin deposits, which are *highlighted* with a colloidal iron stain

Throughout the dermis, there is an interstitial infiltrate of histiocytes, lymphocytes, and eosinophils (Fig. 14.9).

5. With the presented clinical course and data, what is your working diagnosis?

   (a) Lyme borreliosis
   (b) Urticarial vasculitis
   (c) Necrobiosis lipoidica
   (d) Interstitial granulomatous dermatitis

14 Vasculitis 233

6. What is the appropriate staining for differential diagnosis?

   (a) Colloidal iron stain
   (b) Periodic acid-Schiff and diastase stain
   (c) Elastica van Gieson stain
   (d) Direct fast scarlet stain

Interstitial granulomatous dermatitis (IGD) is a histologic inflammatory reaction pattern with a large differential diagnosis that requires clinicopathologic correlation to identify the underlying cause (9). IGD is typically associated with autoimmune or connective-tissue disorders; such as rheumatoid arthritis, systemic lupus erythematosus, systemic vasculitis, and lymphoproliferative disorders. It may also be induced by systemic medication. First described in 1993, IGD with arthritis (IGDA) is an uncommon form of interstitial granulomatous dermatitis that often occurs in women with rheumatoid factor positive or seronegative arthritis. Other autoantibodies or an elevated erythrocyte sedimentation rate may or may not develop. The clinical presentation in IGDA was initially described as nontender, erythematous plaques that affected the trunk and extremities. In some cases, the plaques form palpable cord-like lesions, which are termed the rope sign, which is no longer considered pathognomonic for IGDA and may not be observed in all cases. The cutaneous clinical presentation is variable in spectrum and features papules to annular or linear plaques. Lesions are asymptomatic and often symmetrically distributed. Arthralgias and myalgias may occur before, after, or during the onset of the skin lesions. Histopathologic classification of IGDA is controversial. IGD is considered by some to be a unique diagnostic entity because it has never been reported to involve leukocytoclastic vasculitis, and histopathologic features have not been shown to vary greatly over time. Others, however, propose that IGDA represents a subgroup variant of palisaded neutrophilic and granulomatous dermatitis (PNGD), which is a spectrum of disorders that involve degeneration of collagen postulated to be immune complex-mediated. Rheumatoid arthritis and other collagen vascular or autoimmune diseases have been reported to occur concurrently with PNGD. In PNGD, early lesions involve a neutrophilic infiltrate with leukocytoclastic vasculitis. Older lesions tend to show a palisaded granulomatous infiltrate that surrounds centralized or scattered neutrophils and less commonly eosinophils nearby degenerated collagen. In IGDA, the dense dermal lymphohistiocytic infiltrate usually extends throughout the reticular dermis in contrast to granuloma annulare. Histiocytes can potentially form rosettes around degenerating collagen. In contrast to PNGD, the presence of neutrophils, mucin deposition, and signs of leukocytic vasculitis are not seen. Differential diagnosis of IGD with arthritis includes granuloma annulare, urticarial vasculitis, erythema chronicum migrans (*Lyme borreliosis*), rheumatoid neutrophilic dermatosis, mycosis fungoides (granulomatous slack skin), necrobiosis lipoidica, and granulomatous drug reactions. Implicated drugs include calcium channel blockers, angiotensin-converting enzyme inhibitors, beta-blockers, lipid lowering agents, antihistamines, anticonvulsants, antidepressants, sennosides, and tumor necrosis factor alpha inhibitors (lenalidomide, infliximab, etanercept, and adalimumab). Clinicopathologic correlation in this patient with arthritis is suggestive of IGDA. Interestingly, prior case reports of IGDA have not included a clinical description fully matching the patient's nonerythematous, skin-colored, papular, symmetric cutaneous eruption. However, the clinical presentation in IGDA is considered variable. An atypical granulomatous drug reaction was considered in the differential diagnosis, but the medication history did not support this diagnosis. Cutaneous manifestations of allergy to metaxalone have not been reported in the literature. Likewise, long-term medications alprazolam, atorvastatin, and dietary supplements have not been reported to invoke IGD.

The systemic vasculitides are rare disorders that can be presented to the allergist/immunologist as a range of different symptoms and signs. Recognizing the possibility of vasculitis is essential because many of these diseases can be potentially life/organ-threatening. Treatments are not well defined. It is important to remember that the treatment of vasculitis is fraught with considerable toxicity, and the risk/benefit ratio should always be factored into therapeutic decision making. In looking toward the future, studies of disease pathogenesis will increase our knowledge about the causes of vasculitis and generate hypotheses for the exploration of novel therapeutic approaches.

Answers

Case 1 (c)
Case 2 (b)

Questions

Case 1

1. (d)
2. (c)

Case 2

3. (b)
4. (c)

Case 3

5. (d)
6. (a)

References

1. Jennette JC, Falk RJ, Andrassy K, Bacon PA, Churg, J, Gross WL. Nomenclature of systemic vasculitides: proposal of an international consensus conference. Arthritis Rheum 1994;37:187–92.
2. Langford CA. Vasculitis. J Allergy Clin Immunol 2003;111:S602–12.

3. Carlson DL. Necrotizing sialometaplasia: a practical approach to the diagnosis. Arch Pathol Lab Med 2009;133(5):692–8.
4. Wechsler ME, Garpestad E, Flier SR, Kocher O, Weiland DA, Polito AJ, Klinek MM, Bigby TD, Wong GA, Helmers RA, Drazen JM. Pulmonary infiltrates, eosinophilia, and cardiomyopathy following corticosteroid withdrawal in patients with asthma receiving zafirlukast. JAMA 1998;279(6):455–7.
5. Wechsler ME. Pulmonary eosinophilic syndromes. Immunol Allergy Clin North Am 2007;27(3):477–92.
6. Churg A, Brallas M, Cronin SR, Churg J. Formes frustes of Churg-Strauss syndrome. Chest 1995;108(2):320–3.
7. Chen KR, Carlson JA. Clinical approach to cutaneous vasculitis. Am J Clin Dermatol 2008;9(2):71–92.
8. Murrell DF, Dick S, Ahmed AR, Amagai M, Barnadas MA, Borradori L, Bystryn JC, Cianchini G, Diaz L, Fivenson D, Hall R, Harman KE, Hashimoto T, Hertl M, Hunzelmann N, Iranzo P, Joly P, Jonkman MF, Kitajima Y, Korman NJ, Martin LK, Mimouni D, Pandya AG, Payne AS, Rubenstein D, Shimizu H, Sinha AA, Sirois D, Zillikens D, Werth VP. Consensus statement on definitions of disease, end points, and therapeutic response for pemphigus. J Am Acad Dermatol 2008;58(6):1043–6.
9. Jabbari A, Cheung W, Kamino H, Soter NA. Interstitial granulomatous dermatitis with arthritis. Dermatol Online J 2009;15(8):22.

Chapter 15
Cutaneous Mastocytosis

Jason R. Catanzaro and Haig Tcheurekdjian

Abstract Mastocytosis is a group of disorders characterized by an abnormal accumulation of mast cells in one or more organ systems. Cutaneous mastocytosis, by definition, is the restriction of mast cells to the skin although patients with this disease may have both cutaneous and systemic symptoms. Recognition of cutaneous mastocytosis is important, especially in children, as its prognosis is favorable in the majority of cases, and, while there is no cure, treatment options are available for symptomatic relief. Annual visits to monitor for signs of progression to systemic disease as well as patient education about potential triggers and consequences of mast cell degranulation are an important component of management.

Keywords Cutaneous mastocytosis • Urticaria pigmentosa • Mastocytoma • Tryptase • Telangiectasia macularis eruptiva perstans • Darier's sign

Case 1

The patient is a 3-year-old African-American female referred from her pediatrician for evaluation of dark spots on her extremities and trunk. These lesions are pruritic when rubbed, prominent during summer months, following warm baths, and occasionally interfere with sleep. The lesions appear on her chest, abdomen, and extremities, and were initially noted at 3–4 months of age. Her mother could not recall any flushing or blistering of lesions. The use of diphenhydramine and acetaminophen has only provided minimal relief.

H. Tcheurekdjian (✉)
Assistant Clinical Professor, Allergy/Immunology Associates, Inc, Cleveland, OH, USA
and
Department of Medicine and Pediatrics, Case Western Reserve University,
Cleveland, OH, USA
e-mail: haig.tcheurekdjian@gmail.com

The patient was the product of a full-term gestation and uncomplicated delivery. Past medical history is only remarkable for an episode of respiratory syncytial viral bronchiolitis at 1 year of age without residual respiratory symptoms. Her mother also notes that her daughter seems to develop hives during or following meals; however, she has been unable to determine which foods could be involved and wonders if a food allergy may be the underlying cause of both the hives and the lesions.

Review of the patient's environmental exposures demonstrates that she resides in a three bedroom home with new carpeting in the patient's bedroom, a single air conditioning unit in the living room and no pets or exposure to cigarette smoke. Family history is remarkable for atopic dermatitis in her 6-year-old brother. No one in the family is known to have any other skin disorders, asthma, or autoimmune disease.

Physical examination is notable for an active, well-nourished child with age-appropriate vital signs and normal growth and development. Her skin examination is remarkable for multiple reddish-brown, slightly elevated macules measuring between 0.5 and 6 cm noted on her extremities but mostly concentrated on her

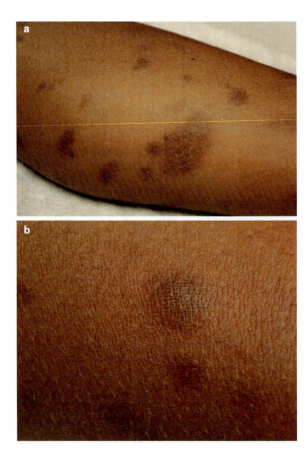

Fig. 15.1 (a) Skin lesions in a 3-year-old girl with (b) Darier's sign elicited with gentle rubbing of a typical lesion

chest, abdomen, and back (Fig. 15.1a, b). Darier's sign (macular lesion becomes a palpable wheal when rubbed) is present. There is no blistering.

Laboratory evaluation revealed a complete blood count of 9,000/mm^3 white blood cells ($N=6,000–16,000$/mm^3), 4,000/mm^3 neutrophils ($N=1,500–8,500$/mm^3), 4,500 lymphocytes ($N=2,000–8,000$/mm^3), 400/mm^3 monocytes ($N=200–600$/mm^3), and 100/mm^3 eosinophils ($N=100–300$/mm^3). Hemoglobin (g/dL) was 12.5 ($N=11.5–14.5$) with a hematocrit of 38% ($N=34–40\%$) and platelets of 200,000/mm^3 ($N=150,000–350,000$/mm^3). A complete chemistry panel including liver function tests was within normal limits.

With the Presented Data, What is Your Working Diagnosis?

The appearance of the lesions in association with pruritus and the presence of Darier's sign in an otherwise healthy young child are highly suggestive of cutaneous mastocytosis, namely, urticaria pigmentosa.

Differential Diagnosis

Given the appearance of the lesions, a broad differential diagnosis was considered including café-au lait spots, melanocytic nevi, guttate psoriasis, leukemia cutis, and non-Langerhans cell histiocytosis. The regularity of the borders and symmetry of the lesions made café-au-lait spots less likely, and the presence of significant pruritus made melanocytic lesions improbable as well. The possible diagnosis of guttate psoriasis, which presents as the acute eruption of multiple pruritic psoriatic lesions, was dismissed due to the presence of large lesions and lack of fine scales on the lesions. The more serious conditions of leukemia cutis (the infiltration of neoplastic leukocytes into the skin layers that may appear as brown macules) and non-Langerhans cell histiocytosis (brownish papules that are typically benign but may affect organs outside of the skin) are quite rare, and the normal laboratory evaluation argues against the former diagnosis, and the lack of papules or nodules argues against the latter.

Workup

Skin biopsy from a typical lesion, i.e., a symmetric lesion with regular borders in an area without direct sun exposure, was performed using lidocaine with epinephrine to minimize possible mast cell degranulation. Pathological examination demonstrated mast cell aggregates in the papillary dermis with >15 mast cells in a given aggregate. Serum tryptase was 3 ng/mL ($N=2–20$ ng/mL).

What is Your Diagnosis and Why?

The presence of mast cell aggregates in the absence of other abnormalities in the biopsy confirms mastocytosis. Furthermore, the normal physical examination outside of the skin and normal laboratory values (including tryptase), in the absence of any systemic signs or symptoms, confirms the diagnosis of cutaneous mastocytosis as opposed to systemic mastocytosis.

Case 2

The patient is a 10-year-old Caucasian female previously diagnosed with cutaneous mastocytosis who, following cashew ingestion, developed angioedema of the lips, periorbital edema, and dyspnea within 10 min of intake. Her father recalls that his daughter had a sudden orange complexion to her face. Upon arrival, emergency medical services found the girl unconscious. Prior to losing consciousness, she had one episode of non-bilious, non-bloody emesis. She received intramuscular epinephrine 1:1,000 dilution, 0.3 mL, supplemental oxygen, and 1 L of normal saline solution en route to the emergency department. Vital signs at that time revealed a blood pressure of 70/40 mmHg, heart rate of 130 beats/min, respiratory rate of 40 breaths/min, temperature of 98.8°F, and an oxygen saturation of 85% on a 100% non-rebreather mask. Prior to transfer to the pediatric intensive care unit, the patient received an additional intramuscular epinephrine injection along with intravenous methylprednisolone, diphenhydramine, and an additional 2 L of normal saline. A CT scan of her head for mental status changes was normal, and she was intubated for impending respiratory failure.

Past medical history was notable only for cutaneous mastocytosis diagnosed at 6 years of age based on skin biopsy. Her parents report that she has only occasional pruritus and on the rare occasion that she notices some tan discoloration of her skin she uses a topical corticosteroid cream. There was no history of anaphylaxis, cardiopulmonary disorders or atopic disorders in the past. The patient had last been seen by her dermatologist approximately 8 months prior and had her self-injectable epinephrine pen prescription refilled. She did later admit to not carrying this medication with her regularly. Her father noted no food allergies and believed that she had previously eaten cashews as well as other mixed nuts without incident.

Family history was notable for maternal asthma and a brother with eczema and possible food allergies. There was no family history of anaphylaxis.

Laboratory evaluation was notable for a complete blood count with 32,000/mm^3 white blood cells ($N=4,500-13,500$/mm^3), 23,640/mm^3 neutrophils ($N=1,200-7,700$/mm^3), 7,400/mm^3 lymphocytes ($N=1,200-4,800$/mm^3), 640/mm^3 monocytes ($N=100-1,000$/mm^3), and 320/mm^3 eosinophils ($N=0-700$/mm^3). Hemoglobin (g/dL) was 14 ($N=11.5-15.5$) with a hematocrit of 42% ($N=35-45\%$) and 364,000/mm^3 platelets ($N=150,000-400,000$/mm^3). A complete chemistry panel including liver function tests was within normal limits. Total serum tryptase measured approximately 2 h after inciting event was 85 ng/mL (*N*=0–20 ng/mL).

Upon admission to the pediatric intensive care unit, physical examination was remarkable for mild diffuse wheezing with good air exchange, abdominal distension, as well as multiple tan diffuse macules on her chest, abdomen, and thighs. Adjunctive therapies for the treatment of anaphylaxis included the continuation of corticosteroids and H1 antihistamines as well as the addition of H2 antihistamines and bronchodilators. Two days later, the patient was extubated following resolution of respiratory distress as well as normalization of hemodynamic status. The patient was discharged to the general pediatric inpatient service 4 days after the initial event.

With the Presented Data, What is Your Working Diagnosis?

The combination of angioedema, cardiovascular instability, and respiratory failure immediately after the ingestion of a food highly associated with allergic reactions is consistent with food-induced anaphylaxis. The presence of cutaneous mastocytosis may have contributed to more extensive mast cell mediator release leading to a more severe reaction than would have otherwise occurred.

Differential Diagnosis

Anaphylaxis is a life-threatening, IgE-mediated allergic reaction that frequently has a rapid onset and progression. There are a wide variety of etiologies of this severe reaction with the most common being medications, foods, stings from insects of the Hymenoptera order (i.e., bees, wasps, hornets, yellow jackets, and fire ants), latex, and blood products. Importantly, anaphylaxis may be idiopathic in greater than 50% of cases. Peanuts, tree nuts (walnuts, Brazil nuts, hazelnuts, etc.), shellfish, and fish are the most common causes of food-induced anaphylactic reactions.

Workup

During her inpatient stay, the patient had a serum tryptase of 3.1 ng/mL approximately 1 week after the inciting event. Two months later a repeat tryptase was 2.8 ng/mL. Biopsy slides were reviewed at that time demonstrating infiltration of the dermis with mast cells consistent with her previous diagnosis of urticaria pigmentosa (Fig. 15.2a, b). ImmunoCap (Phadia, Inc, Uppsala, Sweden) serum cashew IgE level was 10.3 kU/L, which is associated with an approximate 90% probability of being allergic to cashews. Upon discharge from the hospital, a personalized emergency action plan was provided to the patient and her family including the early

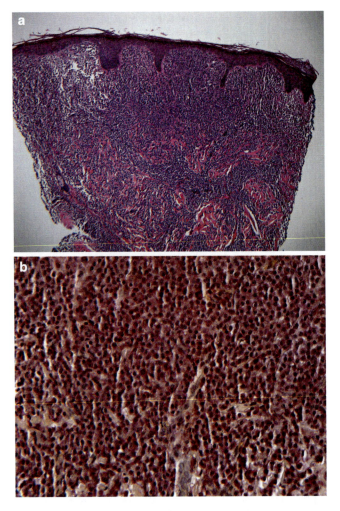

Fig. 15.2 (a) Skin biopsy (10× magnification) showing dense infiltration of mast cell aggregates in the papillary dermis consistent with urticaria pigmentosa. (b) Mast cells are confirmed with Leder stain (40× magnification)

administration of an epinephrine autoinjector with future events. The use of the epinephrine autoinjector was demonstrated to all family members.

What is Your Diagnosis and Why?

The patient experienced an IgE-mediated anaphylactic reaction to cashew amplified by increased baseline mast cell burden secondary to the presence of cutaneous mastocytosis. The rapid onset of systemic symptoms after the ingestion of cashews, plus the elevated serum cashew IgE level, supports the diagnosis of anaphylaxis. Furthermore, the return of tryptase values to normal levels after the episode of anaphylaxis and the absence of physical examination or laboratory evidence of mast cell infiltration affecting organs outside of the cutaneous system rule out systemic mastocytosis as contributing to this event.

Discussion

Mast cells are hematopoietic cells that reside close to blood vessels or nerve fibers with a life span of up to several months. The progenitor cells are detectable in the bone marrow and peripheral blood and undergo differentiation and maturation in vascularized tissues. Activation of the high-affinity IgE receptor (FceRI) on mast cell surfaces by specific antigens elicits the release of preformed mediators including histamine, heparin, tryptase, and chymase. Once activated, mast cells also produce various cytokines and arachidonic acid metabolites which include leukotrienes, prostaglandins, and platelet activating factor. Mast cells and their contents aid in the defense against bacterial, viral, and parasitic organisms and play a significant role in type I hypersensitivity reactions implicated in asthma, urticaria, and anaphylaxis.

Mastocytosis, a rare disease with a reported prevalence of 1 case in 1,000–8,000 patients seen in an outpatient dermatology clinic, is characterized by an abnormal accumulation of clonal mast cells in one or more organ systems. It can generally be classified into one of two types: systemic or cutaneous. Systemic mastocytosis is associated with infiltration of mast cells into multiple organs leading to a number of abnormalities including cytopenias, hepatomegaly, splenomegaly, pathological fractures, and gastrointestinal malabsorption. Cutaneous mastocytosis is limited to skin infiltration, although it may have both local and systemic symptoms caused by mast cell mediator release including flushing, pruritis, nausea, vomiting, diarrhea, dyspnea, and hypotension.

Mastopoiesis is regulated by the interaction between KIT, a transmembrane tyrosine kinase receptor, and various cytokines, including stem cell factor. The activation of KIT is critical for a number of mast cell functions such as induction of differentiation from hematopoietic progenitors, survival, chemotaxis, and the potentiation of IgE-mediated activation (1). Activating mutations, the most common being a point mutation in codon 816 of the *c-kit* gene, which encodes KIT, leads to the development of mastocytosis (1). The mutations, when found in any age group, are associated with lifelong persistent disease with or without systemic involvement. Children without this activating mutation generally have mild disease that is believed to result from transient dysregulation of local growth factors. Typically, their disease resolves by adulthood.

Cutaneous mastocytosis typically presents in four clinical variants: urticaria pigmentosa, solitary mastocytoma, diffuse cutaneous mastocytosis, and telangiectasia macularis eruptiva perstans. Urticaria pigmentosa, the most common presentation of cutaneous mastocytosis, presents with 0.5–1 cm tan to brown macules or papules with occasional nodules or plaques. Widespread distribution involves upper and lower extremities with general sparing of the face, scalp, palms, and soles. Half of the cases demonstrate Darier's sign when rubbed or scratched, and amplification of this sign may cause blistering at the dermal–epidermal junction through the action of chymase. In children, lesions typically lessen and symptoms improve over time, and those patients diagnosed at a younger age and with a smaller number of lesions have a higher probability of spontaneous remission. Adults who present with new-onset urticaria pigmentosa have an increased risk of systemic involvement.

Solitary mastocytomas of the skin are less common than urticaria pigmentosa and usually present within the first 3 months of life. Lesions typically present as single lesions and are similar in quality to those of urticaria pigmentosa but can be larger, measuring up to 3 cm in diameter. Bullae may be present, and flushing may occur after physical irritation of the tumor. Solitary mastocytomas generally have the highest concentration of mast cells of all types of cutaneous mastocytosis, showing as much as 150 times increase compared to normal skin. Spontaneous involution is frequently observed by adolescence.

Telangiectasia macularis eruptiva perstans is the least frequent form of cutaneous mastocytosis, accounting for less than 1% of cases. It occurs almost exclusively in adults and is characterized by tan to brown macules with telangiectasias. With telangiectasia macularis eruptiva perstans, there is an increase in the number of mast cells around capillaries and venules of the superficial vascular plexus (Fig. 15.3a, b). Typically, pruritis and blisters are not seen.

Diffuse cutaneous mastocytosis is a rare and severe variant predominantly seen in the first year of life. Discrete lesions are not described. Rather, there is a diffuse erythrodermic rash, and some individuals will exhibit skin with a thick, doughy appearance, accentuated in skin folds, due to extensive mast cell infiltration in the dermis. Bullous lesions may erupt spontaneously and can occur in the neonatal period. With the stabilization of the dermal–epidermal junction at 3–5 years of age, the blistering typically resolves. Diffuse cutaneous mastocytosis is more likely than other forms of cutaneous mastocytosis to be associated with severe systemic symptoms, because of the total volume of mast cells and, as such, these patients require close monitoring.

Symptoms of mediator release (i.e., recurrent flushing, pruritis, headache, palpitations, abdominal pain and diarrhea, dyspnea, and hypotension) are often observed in patients with systemic mastocytosis but can also be seen in cutaneous mastocytosis and are also typical of anaphylaxis due to an IgE-mediated allergic reaction. In fact, anaphylaxis in patients with mastocytosis is expected to be especially severe due to increased mediator release from those with high body mast cell number. Brockow et al. studied 120 patients with mastocytosis and found that the anaphylaxis risk in children with cutaneous mastocytosis increased in parallel to the extent and density of lesions and was nonexistent in children with limited skin disease or solitary mastocytomas (2). Severe blistering episodes on extensively infiltrated skin lesions appear to be the strongest intrinsic trigger for anaphylaxis in children with cutaneous mastocytosis (1). In this same study, among adults with mastocytosis, anaphylaxis

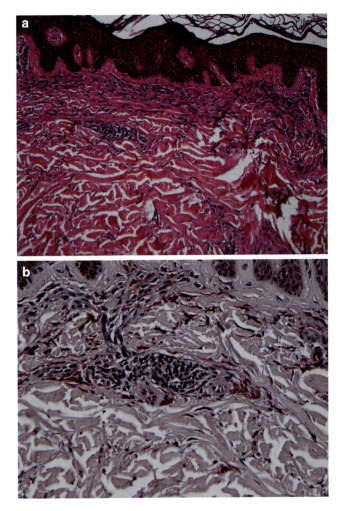

Fig. 15.3 (a) Skin biopsy (20× magnification) demonstrating diffuse infiltration of mast cells in the superficial dermis in telangiectasia macularis eruptiva perstans. (b) Mast cells are confirmed with Leder stain (40× magnification). Note the more spindled shape of the mast cells seen in telangiectasia macularis eruptiva perstans

occurred predominantly, but not exclusively, in those with systemic involvement (2). The major triggering factors for anaphylaxis in these patients did not differ from triggers in patients without mastocytosis. Thus, there is evidence that adults and children with extensive skin disease do have an increased risk of developing anaphylaxis.

The release of mast cell contents may be precipitated by a wide variety of IgE and non-IgE mediated mechanisms. Non-IgE-mediated mechanisms may include, but are not limited to, medications, physical stimuli (temperature change, pressure, rubbing, and exercise), alcohol ingestion, emotional stress, radiocontrast media, and infections. Medications that have been noted to induce release include opioid analgesics, aspirin/NSAIDs, anesthetic agents, and certain antibiotics, such as vancomycin. Of note, these patients typically tolerate acetaminophen, benzodiazepines, and local anesthetics without difficulty.

The diagnosis of cutaneous mastocytosis is based on clinical and histological findings together and can many times be established by an experienced physician after observation of a typical lesion. A focused history should include the duration of disease, factors provoking mediator release, an increase or decrease in activity of lesions over time, response of lesions to heat, stress, showers, certain foods or medications, and previous anaphylactic reactions. Review of symptoms should include attacks of flushing, syncope, heart palpitations, abdominal and/or bone pain, and pruritis as well as general symptoms of weight loss or fatigue which may be indicative of mast cell leukemia. A complete physical examination should include a meticulous skin examination with attention to findings that may indicate systemic involvement such as hepatomegaly, lymphadenopathy or splenomegaly. If lesions of urticaria pigmentosa are found, then the examiner may lightly rub a small area of the affected skin. The development of erythema or urticaria in this area (Darier's sign) is pathognomonic for the presence of mast cells within the lesion. Lesions consistent with mastocytomas, however, should not be disturbed as this may lead to generalized flushing and hives. In this case, the patient's history of symptoms noted upon disruption of these lesions should suffice. A biopsy of lesions may be performed to confirm the diagnosis.

Histopathological analysis of cutaneous mastocytosis reveals multi-focal or diffuse mast cell aggregates in the papillary dermis and extending into the reticular dermis (3). Mast cells can be identified on skin sections with hematoxylin and eosin stain but are better visualized by the use of special stains like Giemsa, Toluidine blue, or Astra blue that highlight mast cell granules. In addition, immunohistochemical staining for tryptase may be performed on skin sections.

Serum tryptase is a reliable diagnostic marker to estimate whole body mast cell burden. Typically, tryptase levels in healthy individuals range from 1 to 11.4 ng/mL and this normal range has been shown to be consistent between pediatric and adult populations as well as between atopic and nonatopic individuals (4). A tryptase level above 20 ng/mL is one of the diagnostic criteria for systemic mastocytosis and, additionally, these levels may be elevated in patients with myeloproliferative disorders, significant renal disease, and when measured within the first few hours of the inciting event of those experiencing an anaphylactic reaction.

The diagnostic evaluation must be expanded if there is a late presentation of skin lesions (>5 years of age), organomegaly, significant peripheral blood abnormalities, or significantly elevated serum tryptase levels (>20 ng/mL) as these suggest significant mast cell infiltration in the body and may be indicative of systemic mastocytosis (5). In this situation, a systemic workup including blood tests, imaging studies, and bone marrow biopsy should be performed for possible systemic mastocytosis diagnosis. Additionally, lesions that fail to resolve over time or annual increases of serum tryptase also warrant serious consideration for additional diagnostic workup. Unlike children who present with cutaneous mastocytosis, it is recommended that all adult patients who present with urticaria pigmentosa undergo bone marrow biopsy and aspiration. Furthermore, individuals with unexplained flushing or anaphylaxis, gastrointestinal abnormalities (e.g., peptic ulcer disease, malabsorption, or diarrhea), peripheral blood abnormalities, hepatomegaly, splenomegaly, lymphadenopathy, pathologic bone fractures or osteoporosis may be considered for workup for systemic mastocytosis regardless of the presence of skin lesions, particularly if there is an elevated baseline tryptase level (5).

Since no curative therapies are available, patients with cutaneous mastocytosis should be provided with education about avoidance of triggers that may induce mast cell release in addition to the treatment of symptoms. Practical measures for trigger avoidance include aggressive treatment of co-existent allergic disease, lukewarm baths for children, and careful selection of medications. In the authors' experience, a combination of guided skin testing and serum IgE testing based on history, and monitored, in-office challenges are required to fully evaluate food, drug, or hymenoptera allergy in these patients. Also, prior to surgical procedures, anesthesiologists must be informed about the mastocytosis to ensure avoidance of medications that may trigger mast cell degranulation.

Epinephrine is the primary treatment for life-threatening anaphylactic reactions. In addition to its direct actions of vasoconstriction, positive inotropy and bronchodilation, it acts to down regulate release of histamine and other mast cell mediators from mast cells, which may be especially important in patients with an increased mast cell burden. Intramuscular injection into the lateral thigh with 0.01 mg/kg of 1:1,000 epinephrine (maximum dose 0.3 mg) is recommended and may be repeated at 5–10 min intervals as needed. Epinephrine autoinjectors are available in 0.15 and 0.3 mg doses, and the manufacturers' recommend the use of the 0.3 mg dose only in individuals weighing 30 kg or more. Unfortunately, this would provide a sub-therapeutic dose to individuals weighing greater than 15 kg. Therefore, the authors use the 0.3 mg dose once an individual attains a weight of 20–25 kg.

All mastocytosis patients with definitive anaphylaxis, and those at heightened risk of anaphylaxis based on the criteria noted above, should receive an emergency kit that includes multiple doses of self-injectable epinephrine as well as H1 antihistamines. Oral and written instructions about using the kit, including training in using the self-injectable epinephrine, is mandatory.

Treatment options to relieve mediator related symptoms primarily include anti-histamines and topical glucocorticoids. First-generation H1-antihistamines are frequently used to prevent pruritus and urticaria, but second generation agents may be preferable due to their less sedating qualities. Additionally, psoralen ultraviolet A therapy or short-term use of topical glucocorticoids, applied under an occlusive dressing, may temporarily decrease the number of skin mast cells and reduce refractory symptoms of mediator release. It should be noted that the benefits of these therapies are only temporary, and caution should taken because of the side effects associated with chronic use of high potency glucocorticoids and the skin cancer risk associated with light therapy. Surgical intervention can provide definitive cure for solitary mastocytomas that are unresponsive to any of the above therapies.

The prognosis of cutaneous mastocytosis is related to the age at presentation and is excellent for children with onset of skin lesions within the first 2 years of life. Overall, more than 80% of children with cutaneous mastocytosis experience spontaneous resolution prior to the onset of puberty. Mastocytomas in children usually involute spontaneously after several years. Of the remaining children diagnosed in the first 2 years of life and whose disease persists into adulthood, 15–30% will develop systemic involvement. Those patients with cutaneous mastocytosis that develops after the age of 2 years tend to have persistent lesions, and approximately 90% of adult patients with skin lesions have evidence of systemic disease at the time of diagnosis. While patients with cutaneous mastocytosis have normal tryptase levels, it is recommended to follow levels annually, noting both the absolute level and trending of the level to address the possibility of progression to systemic disease which would necessitate a more exhaustive diagnostic search as noted above (6).

Questions

1. Which medication below should patients with cutaneous mastocytosis avoid?

   (a) Vancomycin
   (b) Ibuprofen
   (c) Codeine
   (d) Amphotericin B
   (e) All of the above

2. Which is not a mediator released from mast cells?

   (a) Histamine
   (b) Heparin
   (c) Catalase
   (d) Prostaglandin
   (e) Tryptase

3. Management of cutaneous mastocytosis involves which of the following?

   (a) Avoidance of triggers
   (b) Self-injectable epinephrine availability
   (c) Antihistamines
   (d) Treatment of co-existent allergic disease
   (e) All of the above

4. When is a bone marrow biopsy required in a child diagnosed with urticaria pigmentosa?

   (a) All children should have this
   (b) Hepatomegaly

(c) Tryptase 10ug/L
(d) Unresponsiveness to antihistamine therapy

5. What is the type of mutation most commonly noted in those with mastocytosis secondary to c-kit mutations?

   (a) Nonsense
   (b) Point
   (c) Missense
   (d) Deletion

6. Choose the correct statement.

   (a) Solitary mastocytoma is the most common form of cutaneous mastocytosis
   (b) Urticaria pigmentosa generally demonstrates a leather grain skin appearance
   (c) Urticaria pigmentosa generally spares the palms and soles
   (d) Urticaria pigmentosa lesions generally have the highest concentration of mast cells

7. The most common form of cutaneous mastocytosis is

   (a) Telangiectasia macularis eruptiva perstans
   (b) Diffuse cutaneous mastocytosis
   (c) Urticaria pigmentosa
   (d) Solitary mastocytoma

8. Approximately what percentage of adult patients with skin lesions have evidence of systemic mastocytosis at the time of diagnosis?

   (a) 10%
   (b) 30%
   (c) 60%
   (d) 90%

9. Which is not recommended for the treatment of skin lesions of urticaria pigmentosa?

   (a) Systemic corticosteroids
   (b) Topical corticosteroids
   (c) First generation anti-histamines
   (d) Second generation anti-histamines

10. Darier's sign is?

    (a) The presence of axillary freckling in a patient with neurofibromatosis type I
    (b) Elicited when slight rubbing of the skin results in exfoliation of the skin's outermost layer
    (c) Macular lesion becomes a palpable wheal when rubbed
    (d) Periumbilical bruising seen in acute dermatitis

Answers: 1(e), 2(c), 3(e), 4(b), 5(b), 6(c), 7(c), 8(d), 9(a), 10(c).

Acknowledgments We gratefully thank Kord Honda, MD, Assistant Professor of Dermatology and Director of Dermatopathology at Case Western Reserve University, for providing the images of mastocytosis histology.

References

1. Yanagihori H, Oyama N, Nakamura K, Kaneko F. c-kit mutations in patients with childhood-onset mastocytosis and genotype-phenotype correlation. J Mol Diagn. 2005; 7:252–257.
2. Brockow K, Jofer C, Behrendt H, Ring J. Anaphylaxis in patients with mastocytosis: a study on history, clinical features and risk factors in 120 patients. Allergy 2008; 63:226–232.
3. Akay B, Kittler H, Sanli H, Harmankaya K, Anadolu R. Dermatoscopic findings of cutaneous mastocytosis. Dermatology 2009; 226–230.
4. Komarow H, Hu Z, Brittain E, Uzzaman A, Gaskins D, Metcalfe DD. Serum tryptase levels in atopic and nonatopic children. J Allergy Clin Immunol. 2009; 124(4):845–848.
5. Heide R, Beishuizen A, De Groot H, Den Hollander JC, Van Doormaal JJ, De Monchy JGR, Pasmans S, Van Gysel D, Oranje AP. Mastocytosis in children: a protocol for management. Pediatr Dermatol. 2008; 25(4):493–500.
6. Valent P, Sperr W, Schwartz L, Horny H. Diagnosis and classification of mast cell proliferative disorders: delineation from immunologic diseases and non-mast cell hematopoietic neoplasms. J Allergy Clin Immunol. 2004; 114:3–11.

Chapter 16
Cutaneous Lupus

Lisa G. Criscione-Schreiber

Abstract Rashes are among the most common manifestations of systemic lupus erythematosus (SLE), affecting up to 85% of individuals with SLE. Cutaneous lupus without systemic features is even more common than SLE. In many patients, cutaneous involvement can be widespread and debilitating, requiring systemic treatment. Here, two challenging cases of cutaneous lupus are described.

Keywords Cutaneous lupus · Systemic lupus erythematosus · Acute cutaneous lupus erythematosus · Subacute cutaneous lupus erythematosus · Bullous lupus

Case 1

A 42-year-old woman with a 20-year history of systemic lupus erythematosus (SLE) was admitted to the hospital with 4 days of lip swelling, sore tongue, and peeling lips. In addition, she had an erythematosus eruption over her anterior chest, arms, and legs that she described as pruritic, burning, and painful. She denied new drug exposures, sick contacts, or recent fever. One month prior to this presentation, she developed periungual inflammation with subcutaneous nodules on the elbows and fingers. Two weeks prior to this presentation, she developed pleuritic chest pain. Thorough evaluation including a CT arteriogram ruled out pulmonary embolism, effusion or pneumonia. She was treated with oral prednisone 30 mg daily with resolution of the pleurisy and tapered rapidly off the steroids.

She came to the hospital at this time because the symptoms of the cutaneous eruption were identical to an episode that occurred 18 months earlier, which had been diagnosed as Stevens–Johnson syndrome and resulted in a 2-week-long hospitalization. The episode 18 months prior to admission started with a rash described as

L.G. Criscione-Schreiber (✉)
Division of Rheumatology and Immunology, Duke University, Box 3490 DUMC,
Room 4021 Duke South, Purple Zone, Durham, NC 27710, USA
e-mail: crisc001@mc.duke.edu

"pinpoint spots" on her arms, with a sensation of burning under the skin all over her body. The small lesions on the arm coalesced, turned red, developed blisters, and then peeled. She was hospitalized for the peeling rash, which eventually involved her entire body and oral mucosa, and was associated with a low-grade fever. She had not taken new medications before developing the rash but had been taking hydrochlorothiazide (HCTZ) and diclofenac. Skin biopsy during the hospitalization showed epidermal necrosis as well as periadnexal, perivascular, and interstitial lymphocytic infiltrate (Fig. 16.1). A diagnosis of Stevens–Johnson Syndrome was made and the patient received intravenous immunoglobulin for 3 days without improvement. The rash eventually

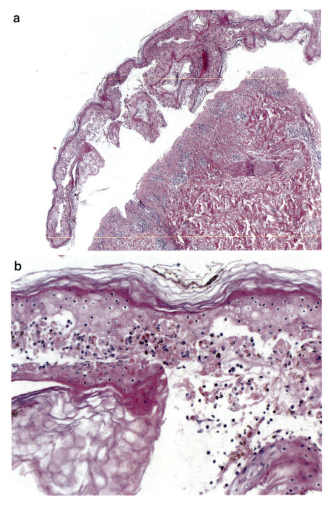

Fig. 16.1 TEN-like acute cutaneous lupus erythematosus, which had been originally diagnosed as Stevens–Johnson syndrome. (**a**) The epidermis is completely detached from the dermis. Extensive epidermal necrosis is evident with interstitial and periadnexal lymphocytic infiltrate (4×, hematoxylin and eosin). (**b**) At 20× magnification, ghost cells are seen throughout the epidermis (hematoxylin and eosin)

improved when she was treated with high doses of intravenous corticosteroids and wound care. Diclofenac, HCTZ, and hydroxychloroquine were discontinued.

In the 18 months since hospital discharge, she had experienced recalcitrant inflammatory arthritis related to SLE despite sequential treatment with weekly oral methotrexate, corticosteroid tapers, leflunomide, and a course of rituximab. During this interval, the patient also intermittently experienced macular and papular rashes including development of several annular lesions with evidence of scarring and hair loss on the scalp. These rashes were treated with topical corticosteroids and intermittent oral corticosteroids.

Serologic studies in the past revealed a high-titer positive antinuclear antibody, anti-Ro, and anti-double-stranded DNA antibodies with positive rheumatoid factor.

On admission, physical examination revealed T 37.0 C, HR 75 bpm, and BP 150/81 mmHg. Skin examination initially was notable only for swelling of both lips, lower more than upper, with superficial erosions. There was a single 3-mm oral ulcer on her inner lower lip without nasal mucosal ulcerations. There were numerous erythematous papules over her back and forearms. No lesions were noted on the palms or soles, no vesicles or bullae were present, and diffuse skin tenderness was absent. There was no conjunctivitis. White patches easily removed with a tongue blade covered the tongue. She had periungual inflammation with scattered periungual infarcts. The remainder of the general examination was unremarkable. There was no synovitis of any joints.

Over the first 48 h in the hospital, the patient developed multiple painful oral ulcerations involving the inner labial mucosa, buccal mucosa, and tongue as well as genital and peri-anal ulcerations. In addition, the areas of erythema on the skin evolved to scattered vesicles with increasing pain and tenderness of the skin of the trunk and extremities. Palpable purpura was absent. No palm or sole lesions or target type lesions were noted.

Data

Complete blood count revealed hemoglobin of 9.9 g/dL (normal range 12.0–15.5 g/dL), platelets of $215,000 \times 10^9$ (normal range 150–450), white blood cell count 4.9×10^9 (normal range 3.2–9.8); Westergren sedimentation rate was 70 mm/hr (normal less than 15 mm/hr) and serum creatinine 0.7 mg/dL.

Anti-dsDNA was markedly positive at 494 IU/mL (normal <100 IU/mL), complement C3 low at 55 (normal range 86–208), and complement C4 low at 7 (normal range 13–47). Serological studies at admission revealed positive antibodies against Ro, La, Sm, and RNP.

With the Presented Data, What Is Your Working Diagnosis?

This 42-year-old woman presented with severe oral ulcerations and a diffuse papular eruption that was rapidly progressive with increasing oral ulcerations, skin tenderness, and vesicles. The previous 18 months had been characterized by persistently active

SLE including inflammatory arthritis and serositis despite treatment. The clinical presentation, physical examination, and laboratory data led us to diagnose a lupus flare with severe mucous membrane and skin involvement.

Differential diagnosis. Diagnostic considerations of the cutaneous eruption included disseminated herpes simplex or varicella zoster infection, Stevens–Johnson syndrome secondary to a herpes simplex virus infection of the oral mucosa, Rowell's syndrome (SLE with erythema multiforme-like lesions), and SLE flare with mucosal and skin involvement.

Workup

Skin Biopsy

Punch biopsy from the left dorsal wrist showed hyperkeratosis and occasional dyskeratotic cells within the epidermis. Leukocytoclasis was present within the interstitium and around the vessels. The infiltrate consisted predominantly of neutrophils present in the superficial and deep dermis, and involving the superficial subcutis. The overall impression was of a neutrophilic dermatitis with prominent leukocytoclasis (Fig. 16.2).

What is Your Diagnosis and Why?

We made the diagnosis of bullous lupus for this admission. Clinically, this diagnosis was based on the rapid progression of the rash with vesicular transformation and worsening mucosal ulceration without conjunctivitis. Biopsy findings supported the diagnosis of bullous lupus. We re-reviewed the prior skin biopsies and clinical course, and surmised that the rash experienced 18 months earlier had also been a manifestation of SLE with epidermal necrosis.

Discussion

The classification of cutaneous lupus has traditionally been based on clinical findings and contains three groups: acute cutaneous lupus erythematosus (ACLE), subacute cutaneous lupus erythematosus (SCLE), and chronic cutaneous lupus erythematosus (CCLE). Recently, some authors have proposed a fourth class of cutaneous lupus, intermittent subtype of lupus erythematosus (ICLE), which includes the rash of tumid lupus (Table 16.1). Additional classification schemes for cutaneous lupus include histologic features. Histologic classification schemes differentiate between findings that are lupus-specific and findings that are not specific for SLE (and can be seen

16 Cutaneous Lupus

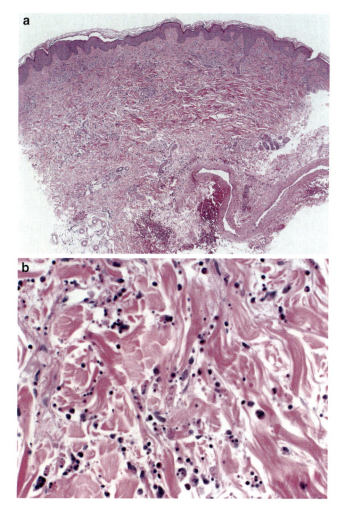

Fig. 16.2 Bullous lupus. (**a**) A neutrophilic infiltrate is present in the superficial and deep dermis. Lymphocyte infiltration is present within the interstitium and around vessels, and increased dermal mucin is seen (4×, hematoxylin and eosin). (**b**) Higher power view of the dermis shows several intact neutrophils with extensive nuclear dust (40×, hematoxylin and eosin)

in other diseases). Many of the histologic features of ACLE are not specific, namely interface dermatitis, which can be seen in other autoimmune disorders such as dermatomyositis. Clinically, ACLE includes the classic malar rash, which is characterized by erythema and cutaneous edema. ACLE also includes the category of bullous lupus, the name given to subepidermal blistering rashes sometimes observed in individuals with SLE (1).

SLE has an estimated incidence of up to 50/100,000 population per year. Isolated cutaneous lupus is more common than SLE and has been estimated to affect up to three times as many individuals as SLE (1). Among ACLE lesions,

Table 16.1 Classification of cutaneous lupus (adapted from Lin (1))

Subtype	Clinical manifestations
Acute cutaneous lupus erythematosus (ACLE)	Localized (malar rash)
	Generalized (includes bullous lupus)
	TEN-like
Subacute cutaneous lupus erythematosus (SCLE)	Annular
	Papulosquamous/psoriaform
	Other variants
Chronic cutaneous lupus erythematosus (CCLE)	Discoid lupus (localized or generalized)
	Lupus profundus/lupus panniculitis
	Chilblain lupus erythematosus
Intermittent cutaneous lupus erythematosus (ICLE)	Lupus tumidus

bullous lupus (BSLE) is distinctly rare, even among individuals with known SLE. In Vassileva's retrospective analysis, 1–3% of individuals with SLE developed bullous lupus (2).

Bullous lupus presents as an acute blistering eruption. As with all cutaneous lupus, sun-exposed areas are the most commonly affected, but the rash also has a predilection for the neck, upper trunk, and upper extremities. Bullous lupus frequently involves mucous membranes. Affected patients describe the rash as burning and painful, but not pruritic.

The diagnosis of bullous lupus can be missed when relying on pathologic diagnosis without a clinical correlation. Classically, the histologic diagnosis of cutaneous lupus is most associated with lymphocytic, not neutrophilic, infiltration with the near universal presence of interface changes. In contrast, bullous lupus is characterized by subepidermal vesicles and neutrophil microabscesses at papillary tips. The blisters contain neutrophils and fibrin. Dermal edema is present. The characteristic lymphocytic infiltrate of cutaneous lupus is generally seen in bullous lupus as well and is located in the superficial and middle dermis as a perivascular infiltrate. By histology, the features of bullous lupus are very similar to those of dermatitis herpetiformis (DH), with neutrophilic infiltrate at papillary tips. However, immunostaining in bullous lupus reveals diffuse staining in both lesional and non-lesional skin (the lupus band), while in DH, immune deposits occur only at the papillary tips. Clinically, bullous lupus can be differentiated by DH from the absence of pruritis and the presence of other clinical manifestations of SLE. Bullous lupus is often associated with lesional antibodies to type VII collagen, which is also targeted in epidermolysis bullosa acquisita (EBA). However, EBA is not associated with SLE and does not have the characteristic rapid response to dapsone seen in bullous lupus (3).

Thus, in this patient, the clinical presentation was consistent with bullous lupus, and the pathologic findings supported this diagnosis. We wondered how this presentation related to the episode 18 months earlier, when she had a clinically similar rash with a very different histologic appearance. The biopsy 18 months earlier had shown epidermal necrolysis. When reevaluating that biopsy in the context of the current pathology, in addition to the extensive epidermal necrosis, there was an interface process with perivascular and periadnexal lymphocytic infiltrate. Thus, there were characteristic changes of cutaneous lupus coincident with epidermal necrolysis. Even among cases of bullous lupus, findings of toxic epidermal necrolysis (TEN) are rare. Cases of TEN have been reported in patients with SLE over the years; although many described cases could have been precipitated by drugs or infections, many reported cases occurred independent of any toxic exposures (4, 5). "TEN-like ACLE" is a name suggested for the disorder of bullous skin lesions with epidermal sloughing accompanied by histologic features of epidermal necrolysis extending from interface dermatitis. In 2004, Ting and associates proposed definition of a spectrum of apoptotic pan-epidermolysis (ASAP) to describe vesiculobullous skin lesions in individuals with SLE (6). Their classification scheme focuses on separating histologic features of TEN associated with classical cutaneous lupus rashes from other autoimmune vesiculobullous skin diseases occasionally seen in individuals with SLE, including dermatitis herpetiformis-like lesions, EBA-like lesions, and bullous pemphigoid-like lesions.

TEN-like ACLE should be suspected in a patient with known SLE who develops a rapidly progressive blistering rash associated with burning pain. The lack of an inciting trigger such as a new medication does not eliminate this diagnosis as a possibility. In addition to serologic measures of SLE activity such as complete blood count, urinalysis, inflammatory markers, serum complement levels, and anti-dsDNA levels, a skin biopsy is essential to diagnose TEN-like ACLE. The biopsy will reveal subepidermal blistering with epidermal necrosis, neutrophils within blisters, and lymphocytic infiltrate at the dermal–epidermal junction and perivascular areas, as was seen in this patient. Direct immunofluorescence microscopy reveals the presence of a lupus band.

When TEN-like cutaneous lupus is suspected, treatment with intravenous immunoglobulin and systemic corticosteroids may be administered, although the use of intravenous immunoglobulin in isolated TEN has not been definitively proven effective (7). In patients with bullous lupus or TEN-like SCLE with significant neutrophilic infiltrate on biopsy, treatment with dapsone should be attempted.

In our patient, we started dapsone treatment when the skin biopsy revealed neutrophilic dermatitis with leukocytoclasis in the setting of a clinical course most consistent with bullous lupus. Within 24 h of starting dapsone therapy, new oral and cutaneous lesions were halted. By 48 h, the oral and genital ulcers had disappeared and the skin lesions improved rapidly. Four days after starting dapsone therapy, the patient was discharged from the hospital. Unfortunately, despite dapsone therapy, the patient developed a recurrent rash several weeks later that also involved the palms and soles. At that time, she was treated with high-dose intravenous steroids and we started treatment with mycophenolate mofetil, quickly advanced to 1,500 mg twice daily (this drug is not FDA approved for the treatment of SLE). In the 7 months since that hospitalization, she has not had recurrent cutaneous lupus.

Questions

1. All of the following are clinical classes of cutaneous lupus rashes except:
    (a) SCLE (subacute cutaneous lupus erythematosus)
    (b) BLE (bullous lupus erythematosus)
    (c) ACLE (acute cutaneous lupus erythematosus)
    (d) CCLE (chronic cutaneous lupus erythematosus)

2. Which of the following is NOT a classic histologic feature of cutaneous lupus?

   (a) Interface dermatitis
   (b) Lymphocytic perivascular and periadnexal infiltrate
   (c) Diffuse immunoglobulin in involved and uninvolved skin (lupus band)
   (d) Extensive dermal mucin
   (e) Neutrophilic infiltrate with nuclear dust

3. Which of the following is the treatment of choice for bullous lupus and other neutrophilic dermatoses?

   (a) Intravenous immunoglobulin
   (b) Hydroxychloroquine
   (c) Mycophenolate mofetil
   (d) Dapsone

4. Which of the following cannot help differentiate cutaneous lupus from other similar disorders?

   (a) Response to Dapsone therapy
   (b) The lupus band test
   (c) Neutrophilic infiltrate at papillary tips
   (d) The presence of interface dermatitis

5. Bullous lupus can be differentiated from TEN-like ACLE by which feature?

   (a) The presence of burning, painful skin
   (b) The presence of mucosal ulcers
   (c) The presence of an inciting medication
   (d) The presence of epidermal necrolysis starting at the dermal/epidermal interface

Answers: 1(b), 2(e), 3(d), 4(a), 5(d).

Case 2

A 54-year-old woman was seen in the rheumatology clinic to evaluate a pruritic rash. The rash started about 8 weeks prior to the visit, with small pruritic areas on her forearms and thighs which scabbed then healed, leaving hyperpigmented areas. The rash gradually spread to involve the entire surface of her arms, legs, trunk, and neck, and was spreading up to her face, palms, and soles, with associated diffuse alopecia. Over-the-counter 1% hydrocortisone cream helped neither the pruritis nor the spread of the rash. This intensely pruritic rash prevented the patient from sleeping.

The patient had been diagnosed with SLE only 3 months earlier, when she presented to her primary care physician with rapidly progressive dyspnea and lower extremity edema after a 1-year absence from medical follow-up. When the serum creatinine was found to be elevated at 5.4 mg/dL, the patient was admitted to the hospital for hemodialysis and further evaluation. Urinalysis revealed numerous red blood cell casts with 4 g of proteinuria measured over 24 h. Renal biopsy revealed chronic glomerulonephritis, "full house" immunofluorescence staining, extensive glomerular scarring as well as changes from hypertensive nephropathy. Serologic evaluation during the hospitalization supported the diagnosis of lupus nephritis with high-titer positive antinuclear antibodies, positive anti-double stranded DNA antibodies, and positive anti-Ro (SSA) antibody. Based on very low activity and high chronicity by renal biopsy, the renal dysfunction was considered irreversible, and the patient was not treated with immunosuppressive therapy for lupus nephritis.

At the time lupus nephritis was diagnosed, the patient was asymptomatic with the exception of volume overload. She had noted mild fatigue and the dyspnea that brought her to medical care but denied hair loss, rashes, photosensitivity, mucosal ulcerations, arthralgia, myalgia, Raynaud's phenomenon, or pleuritic or positional chest pain. During the hospitalization, she also had enzymatic evidence of a recent myocardial infarction confirmed by nuclear study. After initiating hemodialysis, cardiac catheterization was performed, and a stent was angiographically placed in the right coronary artery. Numerous new medications were begun, including aspirin, atorvastatin, calcium acetate, clopidogrel, metoprolol, ramipril, and erythropoietin injections.

At the outpatient rheumatology appointment, the patient was not acutely ill appearing and was hypertensive at 194/89 mmHg. She had no oral or nasal ulcerations and no palpable lymphadenopathy. Lungs were clear to auscultation, and cardiac examination revealed symmetric pulses, a regular rate, with a 2/6 systolic ejection murmur. She had no peripheral edema. There was no swelling, warmth, or tenderness of any joints. She had mild diffuse alopecia with no evidence of scale, scarring or erythema. Skin exam was notable for slightly raised markedly hyperpigmented plaques over the dorsal surfaces of the arms, back, chest, abdomen, and diffusely over

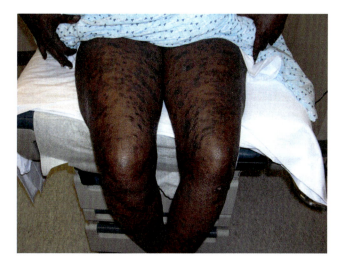

Fig. 16.3 Hyperpigmented plaques on the legs of the patient described in Case 2. Mild silvery scale is present over many lesions. Signs of cutaneous trauma are evident in several lesions

the legs (Fig. 16.3). Lesions were predominantly oval to round plaques with many that coalesced. There was mild overlying silvery scale. There were signs of cutaneous trauma with numerous crusted lesions. There was no periungual inflammation. The palms, soles, and lips had a hyperpigmented macular rash.

With the Presented Data, What Is Your Working Diagnosis?

In this individual, a drug-induced rash is a strong possibility, especially since it is intensely pruritic. Involvement of the palms and soles can occur with syphilis as well as a number of viral illnesses; however, macular hyperpigmentation is frequently seen in patients of color, and this patient had no evidence of active inflammation of the palms or soles and no symptoms of a viral illness. Cutaneous eruption secondary to the pruritis associated with renal failure was another possibility. The annular, scaly plaques had the appearance of psoriasis which raised the possibility of a new diagnosis of psoriasis. Given the patient's past medical history, however, the diagnosis of psoriaform ACLE was possible. The clinical appearance and distribution of the rash were not consistent with the discoid type of lesions that can sometimes be seen in patients with SLE. Most commonly, a skin eruption in an individual with known SLE is due to lupus.

Workup

Complete blood count revealed a white blood cell count of 3.1×10^9 (normal range 3.2–9.8) with a normal eosinophil percentage. Hemoglobin was slightly low at 11.8 g/dL (normal range 12.0–15.5 g/dL). Anti-dsDNA remained elevated. Complement C3, C4, and whole hemolytic complement were within the normal range.

Two punch biopsies were taken, one from the forearm (Fig. 16.4) and one from the upper arm. Both showed hyperorthokeratosis with focal vacuolization of the basal layer associated with a lymphocytic infiltrate. Follicular plugging was seen. There was a periadnexal lymphocytic infiltrate as well as lymphocytic infiltrate around superficial and deep vessels. By colloidal iron stain, dermal mucin was not significantly increased. Eosinophils were absent. These abnormalities were consistent with interface dermatitis with postinflammatory change.

What is Your Diagnosis and Why?

The biopsy findings considered with the clinical appearance and the patient's medical history were most consistent with SCLE. This rash may have been triggered by exposure to a new medication. There was significant postinflammatory hyperpigmentation.

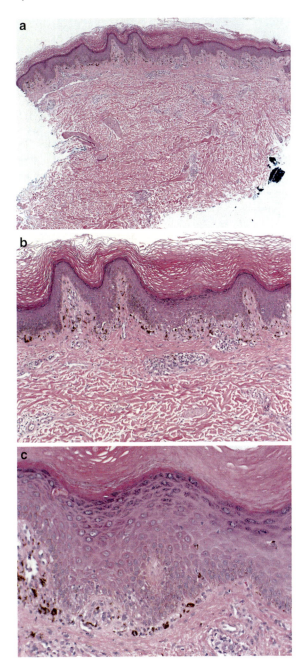

Fig. 16.4 Subacute cutaneous lupus erythematosus. (**a**) Interface dermatitis. Additional lymphocytic infiltrate around adnexal structures, superficial and deep vessels (4×, hematoxylin and eosin). (**b**) Higher power (10×) reveals melanin incontinence with dyskeratotic cells and lymphocytic infiltrate at the interface (hematoxylin and eosin). (**c**) Vacuolization of the basal layer with melanophages in the papillary dermis (20×, hematoxylin and eosin)

Discussion

SCLE is one of the four clinical subtypes of lupus-specific SLE rashes. SCLE is reportedly seen in up to one third of patients with SLE. SCLE is a nonscarring rash that is generally photosensitive and induced by exposure to ultraviolet light. However, SCLE can also be triggered by exposure to a variety of drugs and has been particularly associated with antihypertensives (thiazides, calcium channel blockers, ACE inhibitors, and beta blockers). Recently terbinafine has been associated with the development of SCLE. Of all the clinical subtypes, SCLE is most often associated with the presence of autoantibodies to Ro (SSA). The rash of SCLE is pruritic in some cases, especially when triggered by a drug reaction. In particular, the papulosquamous form of SCLE phenotypically resembles psoriasis and can be pruritic.

SCLE usually develops first as erythematous macules or papules. The lesions of SCLE start as small papules that can enlarge and coalesce into papulosquamous (psoriaform) plaques or into annular-polycyclic plaques. The papulosquamous variant, seen in our patient, is characterized by psoriasis-like lesions. The annular variant of SCLE features lesions with erythematous, slightly raised borders with mild central clearing. These papulosquamous and annular variants may overlap in the same patient. SCLE lesions heal without scarring but can leave behind changes in pigmentation.

The histologic features of SCLE are similar to the histologic features of discoid lupus. In both conditions, the epidermis can show atrophy and keratinocyte necrosis. In the dermis, there is generally a mild perivascular infiltrate and interface dermatitis. Basement membrane thickening is occasionally seen in SCLE but is more prominent in discoid lupus erythematosus (DLE). SCLE can include follicular plugging with keratin, though to a lesser extent than typically seen in DLE. As discussed above, at least half of skin biopsies in patients with SLCE show a granular lupus band at the dermal–epidermal junction (8).

As mentioned above, the autoantibody most associated with SCLE is anti-Ro (SSA). Although this particular autoantibody is not one of the American College of Rheumatology (ACR) criteria for SLE, it is associated with SCLE, photosensitivity, neonatal lupus, and sicca symptoms. Neonatal lupus skin lesions generally start several weeks after birth, and they may develop after exposure to ultraviolet light. Neonatal lupus rashes clinically and histologically resemble annular SCLE and generally involve the infants' face and scalp, especially the upper eyelids. Anti-Ro antibody positivity is also one of the ACR classification criteria for the diagnosis of Sjogren's syndrome, and individuals with Sjogren's syndrome frequently also develop a photosensitive, photodistributed rash.

Cutaneous lupus is generally photosensitive. Both UVA (long-wave UV light) and UVB (midrange UV light) contribute to the development of skin lesions. UVB, which penetrates only the epidermis, is absorbed by DNA causing direct damage. UVA penetrates to the dermis. UVA causes DNA damage and also leads to free radical production with eventual epidermal apoptosis. UV light also induces keratinocyte apoptosis (1, 9).

Apoptosis is important in the pathogenesis of both cutaneous lupus and SLE. In numerous studies, individuals with SLE demonstrate impaired ability to clear apoptotic cells. When cells undergo apoptosis, they form surface blebs. Proteins and other molecules that are usually sequestered inside cells and protected from the immune system are then displayed and available to the immune system for recognition. If apoptotic cells are not cleared and self-antigen binds autoantibodies, the resulting immune complexes can trigger immune responses implicated in the development of the clinical features of SLE (1, 10).

Prior to her presentation with SCLE, our patient started treatment with a number of medications for hypertension. One or more of the new drugs may have triggered the SCLE rash. The association of antihypertensives with the development of cutaneous lupus in individuals with anti-Ro positivity has been reported by a number of groups. In one detailed retrospective analysis, Srivastava and associates found that nearly 60% of individuals with anti-Ro antibodies developed cutaneous lupus. Of the individuals with cutaneous lupus and anti-Ro antibodies, 21% had been recently exposed to a new drug. Of these new drugs, several were antihypertensives, most commonly ACE inhibitors. The most commonly reported rash in this study was photodistributed erythema, followed by annular SCLE (11). It should be noted that these rashes are not allergic in nature and do not contain eosinophils, but rather the features are those of cutaneous lupus and occur after a pharmacologic trigger.

The treatment for SCLE depends on the extent of the rash. Topical therapies, most commonly corticosteroids, may be effective for treating mild and limited rashes. For more diffuse rashes, antimalarials are generally added to the topical treatment regimen. If the patient has a diagnosis of SLE, hydroxychloroquine therapy is nearly universally used. When treating with hydroxychloroquine, SCLE rashes may begin to improve within a few weeks' time. However, it is not uncommon for it to take 6–9 months to develop the full benefit of antimalarial therapy for cutaneous lupus. In refractory cases of cutaneous lupus, systemic corticosteroids or other immunosuppressive therapy may be used. When necessary, the choice of systemic immunosuppressive therapy is determined by considering the other manifestations of active SLE that require treatment. No systemic immunosuppressive therapies are currently approved for the treatment of SLE. In our experience, azathioprine is the most commonly used oral immunosuppressive used to treat refractory cutaneous lupus, though there are reports and we have clinical experience using a number of other agents including methotrexate, mycophenolate mofetil, and emerging biologic therapies. Thalidomide has been proven very effective for severe cutaneous lupus, especially in patients with severe CCLE (none of these drugs are FDA approved for the treatment of SLE).

This patient presented a challenging case because the rash of SCLE developed rapidly after the diagnosis of lupus nephritis, in association with positive anti-Ro antibodies and new use of numerous medications. The rash was clinically and histologically consistent with SCLE. Although we believed that new medications may have played a role in activating this patient's skin disease, it was necessary to maintain treatment with antihypertensive therapy. Thus, the patient's rash was treated with a combination of topical corticosteroids, a brief course of systemic corticosteroids (started at ½ mg/kg in a single daily dose), hydroxychloroquine, and oral antihistamines. None of the antihypertensive therapies were stopped. New skin lesions were arrested rapidly with treatment, and over the subsequent weeks many areas of active

SCLE gradually healed. The patient continued to experience generalized pruritis and continued to mechanically irritate lesions on the forearms, thighs, and upper back. Over the ensuing 5 years, the skin rash has completely cleared, with the exception of a few continued crusted lesions on the forearms and upper back due to continued cutaneous trauma. Areas not easily reached by the patient have all resolved without scarring, though the patient is left with hyperpigmentation in areas of previous rash.

Questions

1. Which autoantibody is most associated with SCLE?

    (a) Anti-RNP antibody
    (b) Anti- Ro antibody
    (c) Anti-double stranded DNA antibody
    (d) Antinuclear antibody

2. Which of the following is not an effect of UV light on the skin?

    (a) Causes melanocyte apoptosis
    (b) Induces keratinocyte apoptotis
    (c) Directly damages DNA in epidermal cells
    (d) Leads to free radical production in the dermis

3. Which of the following disorders feature rashes of SCLE?

    (a) Sjogren's syndrome
    (b) Scleroderma
    (c) Neonatal lupus
    (d) (a) and (b)
    (e) (a) and (c)
    (f) (b) and (c)

4. When topical agents fail to control SCLE, the following agent should be considered first-line treatment:

    (a) Dapsone
    (b) Prednisone
    (c) Azathioprine
    (d) Hydroxychloroquine

5. Which of the following is not a potential mechanism for cellular damage in cutaneous lupus?

    (a) Keratinocyte apoptosis from UV light
    (b) Impaired clearance of apoptotic skin cells
    (c) Necrosis of the lupus band
    (d) Direct DNA damage from UV light

Answers: 1(b), 2(a), 3(e), 4(d), 5(c).

References

1. Lin JH, Dutz JP, Sontheimer RD, Werth VP. Pathophysiology of cutaneous lupus erythematosus. Clin Rev Allergy Immunol. 2007;33(1–2):85–106.
2. Vassileva S. Bullous systemic lupus erythematosus. Clin Dermatol. 2004;22(2):129–38.
3. Patricio P, Ferreira C, Gomes MM, Filipe P. Autoimmune bullous dermatoses: a review. Ann N Y Acad Sci. 2009;1173:203–10.
4. Horne NS, Narayan AR, Young RM, Frieri M. Toxic epidermal necrolysis in systemic lupus erythematosus. Autoimmun Rev. 2006;5(2):160–4.
5. Paradela S, Martinez-Gomez W, Fernandez-Jorge B, Castineiras I, Yebra-Pimentel T, Llinares P, et al. Toxic epidermal necrolysis-like acute cutaneous lupus erythematosus. Lupus. 2007;16(9):741–5.
6. Ting W, Stone MS, Racila D, Scofield RH, Sontheimer RD. Toxic epidermal necrolysis-like acute cutaneous lupus erythematosus and the spectrum of the acute syndrome of apoptotic pan-epidermolysis (ASAP): a case report, concept review and proposal for new classification of lupus erythematosus vesiculobullous skin lesions. Lupus. 2004;13(12):941–50.
7. Faye O, Roujeau JC. Treatment of epidermal necrolysis with high-dose intravenous immunoglobulins (IV Ig): clinical experience to date. Drugs. 2005;65(15):2085–90.
8. Baltaci M, Fritsch P. Histologic features of cutaneous lupus erythematosus. Autoimmun Rev. 2009;8(6):467–73.
9. Kuhn A, Bijl M. Pathogenesis of cutaneous lupus erythematosus. Lupus. 2008;17(5):389–93.
10. Kuhn A, Krammer PH, Kolb-Bachofen V. Pathophysiology of cutaneous lupus erythematosus–novel aspects. Rheumatology (Oxford). 2006;45 Suppl 3:iii14–6.
11. Srivastava M, Rencic A, Diglio G, Santana H, Bonitz P, Watson R, et al. Drug-induced, Ro/SSA-positive cutaneous lupus erythematosus. Arch Dermatol. 2003;139(1):45–9.

Chapter 17
Psoriasis

Lloyd J. Cleaver, Nathan Cleaver, and Katherine Johnson

Abstract Psoriasis is a complex autoimmune-mediated disease typically characterized by erythematous papules and plaques with a silver scale. These lesions usually occur on the elbows, knees, scalp, legs, and sacrum, although other forms exist. Psoriasis is a disease whose mechanism is not fully understood, but results in an increased epithelium production by keratinocytes due to decreased cell cycle of 36 h as compared to the normal proliferative time of 311 h. Psoriasis follows an irregular course marked with exacerbations and remissions of unknown onset and duration. This condition ranges from a life-threatening erythrodermic form to a mild well-localized form. Topical steroids remain the primary therapeutic treatment in psoriasis, although systemic agents are available if necessary according to the severity. In general, treatment plans need to be individualized to meet the physician and the patient's long-term goals.

Keywords Silver micaceous scale • Auspitz's sign • Psoriatic arthritis • Epidermal hyperplasia with parakeratosis • Koebner phenomenon

Clinical Presentation

Case 1

A 76-year-old Caucasian male presents to the dermatology clinic due to intermittent irritating patches of thick skin. The patient states that these lesions usually appear on his elbows, knees, and scalp. He first developed these lesions at 31 years of age and

L.J. Cleaver (✉)
Department of Dermatology, Northeast Regional Medical Center,
A.T. Still University, Kirksville, MO, USA
e-mail: lcleaver@atsu.edu

has been dealing with them ever since. These lesions appear to improve during the summer months, and seem to flare up when stressed and with excessive alcohol consumption. The patient states that when he previously removed a lesion, pinpoint bleeding was noted at the site. The patient denies pruritus, tenderness, or joint pain.

The patient's past medical history includes hyperlipidemia. The patient denies smoking, but does admit to moderate alcohol use. The patient's family history is significant as his father had similar lesions.

Physical exam reveals an oval, violaceous 3.5×2.5 cm well-demarcated plaque with a silver scale on his right elbow. The patient also has similar lesions in his left axillae as well as the posterior scalp with flaking extending past his hairline. There is no tenderness, ulceration, or bleeding noted at these sites. Examination of the mucosal membranes reveals a geographic tongue, otherwise unremarkable.

What Is Your Working Diagnosis?

The patient's presentation is consistent with a chronic disease process. Due to the location of the recurrent lesions, the scaly appearance, and the erythematous plaques, a proliferative disorder is most likely the causative agent.

Differential Diagnosis

Plaque psoriasis, seborrheic dermatitis, squamous cell carcinoma in situ (Bowen's disease), cutaneous T-cell lymphoma, subacute cutaneous lupus erythematosus, hyperkeratotic eczema.

Workup

Obtaining a thorough history and physical exam provides an accurate clinical diagnosis. No skin biopsy is required.

What Is Your Diagnosis and Why?

In this case, the patient presented with plaque psoriasis. The complaint of "thick skin" is consistent with the disease process due to the increased activity of the keratinocytes. The fact that this patient's father had similar lesions suggests a hereditary component, which has been well documented in psoriatic patients. The patient's improvement with sunlight exposure, as well as his exacerbation secondary to alcohol use is consistent with psoriasis. The patient's past medical history also is significant for hyperlipidemia, which has been established as a comorbidity in psoriatic patients. On physical exam, plaque psoriasis is often described as being a well-demarcated plaque, erythematous or violaceous, demonstrating a positive Auspitz's sign. The patient's scalp lesion also extended beyond the hairline, differentiating psoriasis from seborrheic dermatitis.

Management and Treatment

The patient's psoriasis is considered mild-to-moderate. Due to the patient's scalp involvement, a tar preparation shampoo is to be used every other day. The initial therapy for the other psoriatic lesions will include a 1:1 mixture of a superpotent topical steroid and a vitamin D analog. This patient's individualized therapy will consist of mixing clobetasol 0.05% and calcipotriene for the elbow and axillae plaques. Once these plaques have responded to treatment, calcipotriene will be used as a maintenance therapy.

Case 2

A 37-year-old Caucasian female presents to the dermatology clinic with concerns over reddened, scaly patches of skin and a flaky scalp. She reports that she has been suffering from this skin condition for about 10 years, and she has only applied moisturizing lotion to the affected areas and used dandruff shampoo on her scalp. She denies any pruritus or bleeding in the affected areas. She does report, however, that her skin improved dramatically during her recent pregnancy and worsened shortly after childbirth. In addition, she complains of joint pain in both of her hands that has developed over the past 2 months. The joint pain has progressively worsened to include swelling and stiffness of the fingers.

Her past medical history is unremarkable. She does report a 30-pack-year smoking history but denies alcohol abuse. Family history is positive for skin cancer of unknown type in both her mother and father. There is no known history of other skin conditions.

The physical exam revealed extensive coalesced erythematous plaques on the bilateral extensor forearms and hands. Lichenification is noted on bilateral dorsal surfaces of hands, large areas on both knees, and bilateral helices with flakes and scales on the scalp. She also has nail pitting on both hands. On her left hand, her second finger's DIP joint is erythematous, swollen and tender to the touch. Similar findings are seen on the right hand's fourth digit.

What Is Your Working Diagnosis?

The patient's presentation of a chronic skin condition, the location of the lesions, and the characteristic scaling and lichenification of the plaques describe psoriasis.

In addition, the location of the swollen joints (DIP), swelling, and erythema are concerning for a psoriatic arthritis.

Differential Diagnosis

Psoriatic arthritis, gout, pseudogout, Reiter's syndrome.

Workup

1. Clinical picture and detailed history can diagnose psoriasis.
2. Obtain X-rays of hands to determine if there is bony damage present. If the patient complains of pain in any other joints or back, radiographs are necessary in those locations as well.

What Is Your Diagnosis and Why?

The patient presented with extensive psoriatic lesions on her scalp and limbs with lichenification, as well as swelling and erythema in her distal interphalangeal joints. Nail pitting is also common finding in psoriasis. The skin involvement, in combination with the arthritic joint findings, is indicative of psoriatic arthritis. It was imperative to obtain diagnostic studies to determine the extent of bony damage. Although the report of the study was unavailable, it most likely would have shown a "pencil-in-cup" deformity. Patient's smoking history may also be an exacerbating factor with respect to the psoriatic arthritis.

Management and Follow-Up

Psoriatic arthritis often requires consulting a rheumatologist to help manage the joint involvement. The rheumatologist and dermatologist will work together to help prevent further joint damage and improve the skin condition. In this case, the patient was initially treated with an NSAID and a topical preparation for the skin lesions. The NSAID provided relief initially, but her arthritis progressed to involve her wrists and more DIP joints and worsening erosions were seen on X-ray. The patient was then started on a TNF-α antagonist with eventual improvement of joint pain and swelling, improved skin condition, and improved overall quality of life.

Discussion

Background

Psoriasis affects up to 7.5 million, or 2.1% of the United States population. In the adult population, psoriasis occurs more frequently in Caucasians than in other ethnicities. 1.5 million of these affected individuals are considered to have moderate to severe forms (1) Psoriasis is classified into mild, moderate, and severe forms based on the affected body surface area (BSA). 0–3% of affected BSA is considered a mild form, 3–10% is considered moderate form, and >10% is the severe form. There have been two peaks of onset that have been reported. The first is at 20–30 years of age, with the second peak at 50–60 years of age. Approximately 75% of patients have the initial onset before the age of 40 (2) Psoriasis can also have extreme debilitating effects on individuals with regards to the physical, psychological, and social impacts.

Pathophysiology

Brief History

The science of psoriasis has been making progress in recent years with studies revealing that psoriasis is largely a T-cell mediated disorder. Initially, it was believed that psoriasis was a disease of keratinocytes, but recent evidence suggests an immunologically mediated mechanism. Clinically, this immunomodulatory model is consistent with the initial presentation of psoriasis and subsequent exacerbations, which are often due to inciting events that insult the immune system, such as infection, stress, or trauma.

Psoriasis can be classified into two main categories, Type I and Type II. Type I psoriasis is considered the familial form and is seen in the second or third decades of life. It is associated with certain HLA traits, particularly HLA-Cw6 (3). Type II psoriasis does not show familial clustering, nor does it have an HLA genotype association. Type II affects older individuals, manifesting in the fifth and sixth decades of life.

Molecular Pathogenesis

The initiation of psoriasis is dependent on predisposing factors, which include the combination of genotype and environmental stressors. When individuals with predisposing genotypes come into contact with factors such as microorganisms, drugs, smoking, skin trauma or physical stress, a cascade of events takes place. Keratinocytes in the epidermis become stressed and release cytokines and chemotactic peptides that began shaping an immune response. There is a formation of DNA-LL-37 complexes which function as autoantigens in the immunologic response, activation of plasmacytoid dendritic cells by the host's DNA, and production of key cytokines by innate immune cells (TNF-α, interferon-α, interferon-γ, interleukin-1β and interleukin-6). These cytokines activate the dendritic cells, which migrate to draining lymph nodes. There the dendritic cells present antigens and secrete mediators to differentiate naïve T-cells into Th1 or Th17 cells (3). These T-cells, considered "effector" cells, leave the lymph nodes, reenter the circulation and migrate into the dermis and epidermis.

A naïve T-cell can mature into a Th-1 cell via IL-12. Th1 cells release TNF-α and interferon γ, which contribute to psoriaform changes in the epidermis. In addition, the T-cell can mature into a Th-17 cell by the differentiation factors TGF-β or IL-6 (4). IL-23 is the growth and stabilization factor among other transcription factors that are involved in the development of Th17 cells (5). Once the cells become the Th17 subtype, they can become activated by IL-23 and causing the release of IL-17, IL 17-F, IL-21, I-6, and IL-22 (4, 6). These cytokine mediators affect the keratinocytes and promote proliferation, causing the vascular and epidermal changes seen in psoriasis.

Th-17 is a novel T-cell that has shown to serve an essential pathogenic role in psoriasis, as well as other autoimmune diseases. Prior to the discovery of the Th-17 cell, most of these diseases were believed to be due to Th-1 cells (4). In addition, one of the products of Th-17, IL-22, is emerging as the main cytokine involved in keratinocyte proliferation and it seems to be most specific for Th-17 cells. Transcripts for IL-17A and IL-22 have been documented in high levels in psoriasis lesions (4).

Psoriasis has unique findings when compared to unaffected skin. IL-23, which activates the Th17 cells, has shown to be overproduced by dendritic cells and keratinocytes in psoriatic individuals (4). In addition, there are greater numbers of Th-17 cells in the dermis when compared to Th-1 cells, although psoriatic lesions demonstrate a collective inflammatory environment populated by both Th1 and Th17 cells.

Research has shown that Th-1 cells' inflammatory product, IFN-γ and TNF-α, remains present throughout the treatment of psoriasis, and it is reduced late in psoriasis resolution. Therefore, it is believed that Th-17 cells drive keratinocyte proliferation, but Th-1 cells play a key role in maintaining the disease state and must also be eliminated for complete resolution.

Genetics

Genetics play a central role in the development of psoriasis. As mentioned earlier, Type I psoriasis (the familial type) is associated with HLA trait Cw6 (3). Genomic linkage analyzes have revealed nine chromosomal loci that are strongly associated with the development of psoriasis, and these are named PSORS1-PSORS9 (7). Genetic studies have revealed that single nucleotide polymorphisms (SNPs) have been found in the promoter region of TNF-α gene, as well as SNPs in the genes responsible for IL-12 and IL-23 (3). Polymorphisms have also been found in genes responsible for IL-13. IL-13 is important in the pathogenesis of psoriasis because it appears to halt the transformation of naïve cells into Th-17 cells. Therefore, the polymorphisms of IL-13 alter its function, allowing unrestricted transformation of T-cells into the Th-17 type (8).

Clinical Manifestations

Plaque Psoriasis

The plaque type is the most common form of psoriasis (Fig. 17.1). It accounts for 80–90% of patient with psoriasis. This form is characterized by well-demarcated, erythematosquamous plaques that are distributed somewhat symmetrically (9, 10).

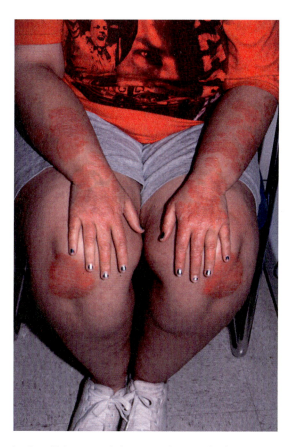

Fig. 17.1 The patient's well-demarcated plaques on the posterior forearms, hands, and knees are a common presentation of plaque psoriasis

These plaques are commonly seen on the scalp. The best way to differentiate scalp seborrheic dermatitis from plaque psoriasis is that psoriasis will have the scaling and plaques extend beyond the periphery of the hairline.

Erythrodermic Psoriasis

This type is sometimes referred to as exfoliative psoriasis. This form affects the majority of the skin surface and is characterized by inflammation of the skin with replacement of the skin surface with erythema, scaling, and exfoliation (Fig. 17.2). The appearance is often described as "fiery-red," with scaling of the skin in sheets rather than flakes. This is often associated with severe itching and pain, tachycardia, and hypo/hyperthermia. This is considered a dermatologic emergency due to secondary loss of protein and the possibility of opportunistic infections. Possible triggers include abrupt withdrawal of systemic steroids, allergic reaction to a medication, and severe sunburns. Repeated episodes of this type are uncommon, but can occur in up to 10% of psoriasis cases (9, 10).

Guttate Psoriasis

This type is characterized by small, erythematous papules of short duration (Fig. 17.3). These lesions usually affect children and young adults. These lesions

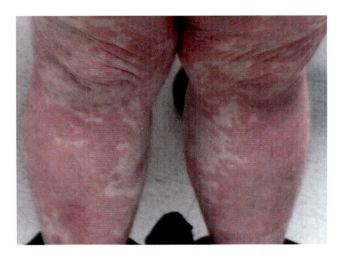

Fig. 17.2 This patient is in the resolving stage of erythrodermic psoriasis. Notice the diffuse erythema and coalescing plaques and pustules. In the acute form, prominent widespread scaling is a key diagnostic feature

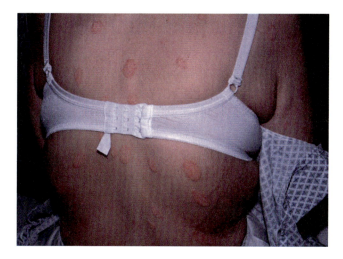

Fig. 17.3 Gutatte psoriasis has multiple lesions that are well-localized. As seen in this patient, a key feature of this form is the lack of coalescence

appear as "droplets" without coalescence, primarily on the trunk and limbs of the affected individuals, sparing palms and soles. This form has been associated with a recent infection, most commonly an upper respiratory tract, streptococcal sore throat, as well as reaction to antimalarials and beta-blockers (9, 10).

Pustular Psoriasis

This type is characterized by individual or multiple coalescing white pustules. These pustules are sterile, containing WBC's without any infectious implications. There are four variants within this category: Zumbusch pattern, annular pattern, exanthematic type, and the localized pattern. One localized variant involves only the palms and soles and occurs in less than 5% of patients. This pustular palmoplantar form of psoriasis appears as scaly erythematous plaques with pustules. These pustules can range in size, varying from 1 mm to 1 cm in size. 88% of patients presenting with this form are over the age of 60, with 70–90% of patients being female. Another type of pustular variant, the von Zumbusch psoriasis form, is characterized by widespread inflammation with diffuse generalized pustules located mainly in flexural areas. This condition has an acute onset of diffuse erythema with pain and tenderness. A few hours after the onset of erythema, pustules develop and last for 24–48 h until they dry out, giving a smooth appearance to the skin. This form has been related to the erythrodermic form of psoriasis due to its risks of secondary complications and known triggers (9, 10).

Inverse Psoriasis

This type of psoriasis is located in the armpits, groin, under the breasts, skin folds, and the buttocks. These lesions appear bright red, smooth and shiny. Due to its location, this form is often the most easily irritated due to excessive sweat. For this reason, scaling is rarely seen (9, 10).

Psoriatic Arthritis

This condition affects as many as 30% of patients with psoriasis. Skin lesions tend to occur before any joint symptoms begin. There are five clinical subtypes: symmetric arthritis, asymmetric arthritis, distal interphalangeal predominant, spondylitis, arthritis mutilans. Approximately 80% of individuals have asymmetric arthritis, usually affecting 1–3 joints. Any joint may be affected. Sausage digits are often seen with affected hand and feet joints. 15% of patients will have symmetric arthritis, with only 5% affecting distal interphalangeal joints exclusively (11).

Other Clinical Findings

During the active phase of the disease process, psoriatic lesions will often be pruritic. The edges of the plaques also appear to have an increased erythematous response. Nail changes are also extremely common, noted in approximately 50% in patients with psoriasis. The most common nail finding is pitting. The pits reflect an abnormal nail growth plate secondary to the psoriatic involvement. Nails can also have an "oil drop sign" which is a tan-brown color change that can be mistaken for onchomycosis (12). Many patients with psoriasis also present with mucosal abnormalities such as a geographic tongue. Auspitz's sign is when there is the presence of punctate bleeding when a hyperkeratotic plaque is physically removed. Koebner phenomenon is when skin lesions appear in sites of trauma. Psoriatic lesions typically occur at sites of trauma. They also commonly present with pruritus, inducing scratching which also results in a Koebner response.

Psoriasis and Other Comorbidities

Due to the systemic nature of psoriasis, comorbidities can play a large role in the disease process. A patient's social history is important to question because of the increased psoriasis risk associated with alcohol and nicotine abuse. Smoking has been specifically associated with an increased risk for pustular psoriasis. HIV positive and other immunocompromised individuals can often have severe forms and can further develop secondary complications from extensive skin involvement.

Psoriasis patients have been identified as having higher frequencies of hyperlipidemia, depression, hypertension, insulin resistance, diabetes mellitus, and homocysteinemia. These risk factors predispose patients to an increased risk of occlusive vascular disease, which results in an increased risk of myocardial infarctions. Some of the aforementioned comorbidities are criteria for metabolic syndrome, which has recently become a larger focus in the psoriasis population. It has been shown that metabolic syndrome has an increased prevalance in psoriasis patients, regardless of the severity of skin involvement (13). These comorbidities are thought to be a combination of the emotional afflictions of the skin condition and its effect on lifestyle. In addition, recent population based studies have indicated that psoriasis itself may be a risk factor for developing atherosclerosis and MI (14, 15).

Differential Diagnosis

If plaques are observed:

- Plaque psoriasis
- Lichen simplex chronicus
- Seborrheic dermatitis
- Squamous cell carcinoma in situ (Bowen's disease)
- Cutaneous T-cell lymphoma
- Tinea corporis (if raised)
- Lichen planus
- Subacute cutaneous lupus erythematosus
- Hyperkeratotic eczema
- Contact dermatitis
- Atopic dermatitis

If the guttate form is observed:

- Small plaque parapsoriasis
- Pityriasis lichenoides chronica
- Drug reaction
- Secondary syphilis
- Pityriasis rosea
- Candidiasis (if localized)

If erythrodermic presentation is observed:

- Pityriasis rubra pilaris
- Eczema
- Subacute cutaneous lupus erythematosus
- Sezary syndrome

If joint involvement is observed:

- Psoriatic arthritis
- Gout
- Pseudogout
- Reiter's syndrome

Management

History

A total body examination, including nails, scalp, and mucosal membranes should be the initial step in evaluation. Patients with suspected psoriasis should be questioned with regards to joint symptoms. History should also be obtained about whether similar lesions were seen in first-degree family members. According to recent studies, approximately 40% of patients with psoriasis or psoriatic arthritis have a family history of the disease in first-degree relatives (16). It is also important to identify potential triggers (i.e., alcohol, smoking), as well as ameliorating factors with respect to the cutaneous lesions. If psoriasis was previously diagnosed, were there any treatment regimens that have worked well in the past? Do these lesions itch, cause sleeplessness, or affect their daily activities? Has the patient started any new medications recently, including beta-blockers, antimalarials, or lithium? By obtaining a thorough history through these important points, a better understanding of the extent of the disease process as well as the psychological complications can be achieved.

Diagnostic Procedures

As mentioned before, a thorough physical exam is critical in appropriately diagnosing patients with psoriasis. Patients with a typical psoriasis presentation are easy to diagnose clinically, but sometimes lesions can pose difficulty when they resemble other disease manifestations. Lesions that require a more involved differential diagnosis include lesions that are asymmetric and solitary, evolving with pustular or erythematous components, and those lesions that are present on a patient with other diseases.

The most efficacious diagnostic tool for confirmation of psoriasis is a skin biopsy with histologic evaluation. In an initial psoriatic lesion, histopathology will often show a superficial perivascular infiltrate of lymphocytes and macrophages in the dermis, along with marked capillary dilation. The punctate bleeding seen in Auspitz's sign is due to the increased capillary response extending to the tip of the dermal papillae, which is only protected by a small number of epidermal cells; therefore, physical trauma exposes these capillaries within the dermis. Parakeratosis (stratum corneum retaining flattened nuclei), as well as epidermal acanthosis of the interpapillary ridges, presence of Munro microabscesses (presence of neutrophils in the epidermis), elongation and edema of the dermal papillae, and an increase in the number of mitoses are all seen in the active and stable lesions of psoriasis (16).

Other laboratory tools, including skin scrapings with KOH, complete blood count with differential, rheumatoid panels, and joint aspirates may be necessary in diagnosis. Radiographic plain films are part of the standard of diagnosis for psoriatic arthritis. These diagnostic studies and their indications is described below.

Single psoriatic lesions may resemble Bowen's disease, which is in situ squamous cell carcinoma. A biopsy of the lesion is required for definitive diagnosis. Other questionable lesions that can be confused with psoriasis include chronic eczematous changes, mycosis fungoides in the patch or plaque stage, and pityriasis rubra pilaris. All of these conditions require biopsies and histologic examination.

Psoriatic arthritis is considered a complication of psoriasis, and patients with psoriasis should be screened early to prevent joint damage. Laboratory tests for erythrocyte sedimentation rate (ESR) should be obtained, as well as rheumatoid factor. Patients with psoriatic arthritis often have an elevated ESR and are rheumatoid factor negative, as opposed to rheumatoid arthritis which is often rheumatoid factor positive. Radiographic imaging remains the "gold standard" for the assessment of bony changes in joints affected by psoriatic arthritis (17). Plain radiography can reveal the involvement of the interphalangeal joints of the digits, bony erosion, and new bone deposition resulting in the classic "pencil-in-cup" deformity, joint space narrowing, and bony spurs. The "pencil-in-cup" deformity occurs when the distal head of the interphalangeal joint becomes pointed and the adjacent surface becomes cup like due to erosive changes taking place in psoriatic arthritis. Preliminary studies indicate that MRI may be useful in determining severity of disease and outcomes with the treatment of biologics, but more detailed studies are required before MRI would become the standard of care (17).

It is important to properly identify psoriatic arthritis from Reiter's Syndrome because both can present with joint involvement and dermatologic manifestations. The two can often be distinguished by the clinical history because Reiter's Syndrome often has a history of infection 1–4 weeks before joint symptoms. An acute arthritis develops and is normally found in the knees and ankles, although finger involvement can be present and mimic psoriatic arthritis. These patients also can present with mucocutaneous lesions, genitourinary infectious diseases, and conjunctivitis. A CBC with differential can indicate leukocytosis and mild anemia. Acute phase reactants, ESR and CRP, can be abnormally elevated. There is also a strong association with the HLA-B27 haplotype, although this is neither diagnostic nor confirmatory (18). Microbiology of urine or stool may reveal Chlamydia or other bacterial pathogens if present. If a joint aspirate is performed, the synovial fluid will show elevated WBC's with cultures likely to be negative.

If there is clinical suspicion for syphilis, VDRL lab testing and skin biopsies should be ordered. Acute subcutaneous lupus erythematosus can be diagnosed through a rheumatologic panel of antibody testing. If a fungal infection is suspected, a scale scraping with KOH or a biopsy with fungal stains can appropriately identify any fungal elements present.

Treatment

Treatment for psoriasis has been changing as new research and medications have been developed. There are now a variety of medications and therapies that can be used depending on the patient's clinical picture. When choosing a therapy, it is important for the clinician to remember the goals of treating a patient with psoriasis. These goals include gaining rapid control of the disease, decreasing the amount and extent of involvement, maintaining the patient in remission and avoiding adverse effects of medications. Achieving these goals can hopefully improve the patient's quality of life.

There are four treatment strategies that are seen in the treatment of psoriasis: monotherapy, combination therapy, rotational therapy, and sequential therapy. Monotherapy is often used as an initial therapy. When it fails or toxicity develops, new agents can be added in a combination or rotational therapy. Combination therapy is often seen with a topical and a systemic or phototherapy and a systemic medication. The combination therapy allows for decreased chances of toxicity, and once a patient is in remission one drug may be removed for maintenance therapy. Rotation therapy involves periodically rotating therapies, usually at 1–2-year intervals. This mechanism can aid in long-term treatment, and it may help minimize chronic toxicity. Finally, sequential therapy involves a step-wise approach. Initially, a stronger agent is used to rapidly clear the psoriasis, followed by weaker, less toxic agents for maintenance therapy. In between the clearance and maintenance phases, treatments are used to minimize the risk of flares.

All of the available therapies have their unique benefits and side effects. Topical creams/ointments are the most safe and effective therapy available in the long-term management of psoriasis, although their use is limited to mild forms of the disease or as an adjunct in combination therapies. Corticosteroids are the most effective and can be continued as long as the patient has thick active lesions. Corticosteroids are thought to act by exerting an antiinflammatory, antiproliferative, and immunosuppressive action on gene transcription. If utilizing a superpotent Class I steroid, it is important to closely monitor the patient's progress as it can lead to skin atrophy with prolonged use. Alternative topical agents include tar, topical retinoids, and vitamin D analogs. Calcineurin inhibitors have also shown to be effective and can be used in corticosteroid sensitive areas such as facial or intertriginous areas. Using vitamin D analogs, such as calcipotriene, along with superpotent corticosteroids has shown increased efficacy and patient tolerance in clinical trials compared to using either agent alone (19).

For moderate to severe disease, the more aggressive modalities of phototherapy and systemic medications are necessary. However, these treatments have a nonselective mechanism of action and systemic therapy can cause vast multiorgan side effects. Phototherapy can be used for patients with moderate to severe disease as well as those with mild disease with complications. Patients with psoriatic arthritis are candidates for phototherapy but also require systemic medications. Systemic therapy is used if the psoriasis is moderate to severe, but there are additional factors that can determine its use in patients suffering from the disease. For example, if the psoriasis covers a "mild" surface area but is greatly impacting the patient's quality of life, a systemic therapy can be chosen. Two additional reasons for systemic therapy include the presence of psoriatic arthritis or disabilities related to the psoriasis. Traditionally, methotrexate, cyclosporine, and acetritin were the agents used for systemic therapy when the psoriasis was too extensive for topical therapy. Methotrexate is the most commonly prescribed traditional systemic therapy for psoriasis worldwide. It has been demonstrated to be effective even in the most severe forms of psoriasis, and has recently been studied as an adjunct to biologics to help prevent the development of autoantibodies to the medications (20). Cyclosporine is a highly effective treatment, although prolonged use of 3–5 years can cause glomerulosclerosis. Therefore, treatment is reserved for the length of 1 year, brief treatment for severe flares, and for rebound flares after discontinuation of biologics or steroids (21).

Biologics, such as efalizumab, alefacept, etanercept, infliximab, and adalimumab are medications that are derived from proteins of living organisms through recombinant technology and are extremely effective in targeting particular steps in the pathogenesis of psoriasis. Their mechanism of action is to either mimic or block the function of naturally occurring proteins (6); however, the high expense associated with these medications and the difficulty in obtaining insurance reimbursement make their use extremely limited. It is important to note that rotation therapy does not involve biologics because biologics tend to lose efficacy if they are discontinued and restarted (10).

Management of psoriasis is a battle against a chronic systemic immunologic process. Its treatment can become extremely frustrating for both patients and physicians. Fortunately, there are now several resources available to physicians when determining the proper treatment. Algorithms that take into account the variety of patient types, recommended therapies, side effects, and management options have been developed (10). When treating patients in practice, the patients should be fully educated about psoriasis, its predisposing factors, stressors to avoid, and the importance of health maintenance with the disease.

Conclusion

Psoriasis is a complex disease process that can have a variety of presentations. The underlying immunologic process is extremely complicated and continues to be an active topic in research with regards to mechanism of disease and development of appropriate therapies. A thorough history and physical exam is the most important aid in diagnosing psoriasis. Subtle physical findings can differentiate psoriasis from other diseases that present in a similar fashion. Depending on the severity and extent of the psoriatic lesions, mid to high potency topical steroids and various systemic therapies are available for treatment.

Questions

1. Which of the following physical findings is unique to psoriasis?

    (a) Koebner phenomenon
    (b) Nail Pitting
    (c) Auspitz's sign
    (d) Sausage digits

2. A 42-year-old Caucasian male presents with well-demarcated erythematous plaques with a silvery scale well localized to the hands bilaterally, but spares the remainder of his body. How would you describe the severity of the disease?

    (a) Mild
    (b) Moderate
    (c) Severe
    (d) Life-threatening

The severity of psoriasis is related to the amount of body surface area (BSA) affected. Mild is described as 0–3% BSA affected, moderate is 3–10% of BSA affected, with severe being >10% of BSA affected. In this case, the patient's hands were the only affected areas. Each hand, including the palms, dorsal surface, and digits, represent approximately 1% of the body's total surface area. The rule of 9's is used to assess the remainder of the body surface area affected. The rule of 9's state that the head accounts for 9%, each arm accounts for 9%, each leg accounts for 18%, the anterior trunk accounts for 18%, and the posterior trunk accounts for 18%.

3. What is the most common age of psoriasis onset?

    (a) 20–30
    (b) 30–40
    (c) 50–60
    (d) >60
    (e) A and C
    (f) B and D

4. Which of the following lab tests are often elevated in psoriatic arthritis patients?

    (a) Antinuclear Antibody test (ANA)
    (b) Rheumatoid Factor (RF)
    (c) Erythrocyte Sedimentation Rate (ESR)
    (d) Elevated WBC count

5. What is the most significant risk factor in the development of psoriasis?

   (a) Premature birth
   (b) Family history positive for father having psoriasis
   (c) Previous myocardial infarction
   (d) History of atopy (asthma, eczema, hay allergy)

6. What immunologic factor is NOT implicated in the pathogenesis of psoriasis?

   (a) Th-2 cells
   (b) Tumor Necrosis Factor – alpha
   (c) Th-1 cells
   (d) Th-17 cells

Research has shown that Th-1 and Th-17 cells are both involved in the pathogenic process of psoriasis. Until recently, Th-1 was thought to be the main cell involved in the immune response. However, Th-17 cells are now becoming more understandable and appear to be responsible for the epidermal changes seen in psoriasis. TNF-alpha is perhaps the most important inflammatory mediator, as it causes the psoriatic changes seen in the keratinocytes as well as the maturation of naïve immune cells. There is currently no clinical research to show that Th-2 cells are involved in the pathogenic process.

7. What is the most common location for psoriasis?

   (a) Elbows
   (b) Knees
   (c) Scalp
   (d) Trunk

The most common site for psoriatic manifestations is scalp seen in approximately 80% of patients. The next most common site is at the elbows, which 78% of patients have reported (9). The next most common sites in order of prevalence include the legs, knees, arms, trunk, lower part of the body, and the base of the back.

8. Which of the following is NOT seen on histology of psoriatic lesions?

   (a) Parakeratosis
   (b) Elongation and edema of the dermal papillae
   (c) Decrease in the number of cells undergoing mitoses
   (d) Munro's microabscess

9. A 56-year-old female with DMII and a history of numerous basal cell carcinomas presents with moderate psoriasis affecting the elbows, knees, and gluteal cleft. The patient has never had her psoriasis treated, but is now seeking treatment due to the increasing social distress it is causing her. She refused treatment previously because of her concerns regarding the side effects of "oral medications." What is the most appropriate initial therapeutic regimen for this patient?

   (a) Phototherapy
   (b) Calcipotriol cream twice daily for a period of 8 weeks

(c) Methotrexate
(d) Cyclosporine

Although psoriasis often requires aggressive treatment, it is critical to individualize therapy toward the patient. This patient requires a more conservative approach due to her concerns over medication toxicity as well as her comorbidities. Topical regimens are often the most appropriate first-line therapy, due to the lower toxicity profile when compared to systemic therapy. Another possible combination for this patient could be the use of a superpotent corticosteroid on weekends with the daily application of a strong retinoid. This patient would benefit from phototherapy; however, her history of skin cancer is a contraindication for this therapy. Methotrexate and Cyclosporine are both oral agents and have significant nephrotoxic profiles. For this reason, Cyclosporine is limited to 12-month use in the United States due to the risk of developing glomerulosclerosis.

10. What is a common trigger of psoriasis?

   (a) Alcohol
   (b) Severe sunburn
   (c) Stress
   (d) Smoking
   (e) All of the above

Answers: 1(c), 2(a), 3(e), 4(c), 5(b), 6(a), 7(c), 8(c), 9(b), 10(e).

References

1. Neimann, AL, Porter, SB. and Gelfand, JM. *The epidemiology of psoriasis*. 2006, Expert Rev Dermatol, 1(1):63–75.
2. Paller, A. and Anthony, M. Papulosquamous and Related Disorders. *Hurwitz Clinical Pediatric Dermatology*. 3rd edn. Philadelphia, PA: Elsevier Saunders; 2006:85–94.
3. Nestle, F, Kaplan, D. and Barker, J. *Psoriasis*. 2009, N Engl J Med, 361:496–509.
4. Blauvelt, A. *Pathophysiology of psoriasis: recent advances on IL-23 and Th17 cytokines*. 2007, Curr Rheumatol Rep, 9:461–467.
5. Korn, T. *IL-17 and Th17 Cells*. 2009, Annu Rev Immunol, 27:485–517.
6. Tzu, J. and Kerdel, F. *From conventional to cutting edge: the new era of biologics in treatment of psoriasis*. 2008, Dermat Ther, 21:131–141.
7. Bowcock, AM. and Krueger, JG. *Getting under the skin: the immunogenetics of psoriasis*. 2005, Nat Rev Immunol, 5:699–711.
8. Cargill, M. et al. A large-scale genetic association study confirms IL12B and leads to the identification of IL23R as psoriasis-risk genes. 2007, Am J Hum Genet, 80:273–290.
9. Van de Kerkhof, PCM. Clinical Features. *Textbook of Psoriasis*. Oxford, UK: Blackwell Science Ltd.; 2003:3–29.
10. VanVoorhees, A. Psoriasis and Psoriatic Arthritis Pocket Guide. www.psoriasis.org. [Online].
11. Sege-Peterson, K. and Winchester, R. Psoriatic Arthritis. *Fitzpatrick's Dermatology in General Medicine*. Vol 2, 5th edn. New York, NY: McGraw-Hill Inc; 1999:522–533.
12. Jiaravuthisan, MM, Sasseville, D. and Vender, RB. *Psoriasis of the nail: anatomy, pathology, clinical presentation, and a review of the literature on therapy*. 2007, J Am Acad Dermatol, 57:1.

13. Gisondi, P. *Prevalence of metabolic syndrome in patients with psoriasis: a hospital-based case-control study.* 2007, Br J Dermatol, 157:68–73.
14. Ludwig, RJ. *Psoriasis: a possible risk factor for development of coronary artery calcification.* 2007, Br J Dermatol, 156:271–276.
15. Gelfand, JM. *Risk of myocardial infarction in patients with psoriasis.* 2006, JAMA, 296:1735–1741.
16. Gladman, DD, Anhorn, KA, Schachter, RK. and Mervart, H. *HLA antigens in psoriatic arthritis.* 1986, J Rheumatol, 13:586.
17. Fitzgerald, O. *Firestein: Kelley's Textbook of Rheumatology: Psoriatic Arthritis.* [ed.] 8th edn. s.l., Saunders Elsevier; 2008.
18. Wu, I. and Schwartz, R. *Reiter's syndrome: the classic triad and more.* 2003, J Am Acad Dermatol, 59(1):113–121.
19. Papp, KA, Guenther, L, Boyden, B. and Larsen, FG. *Early onset of action and efficacy of a combination of calcipotriene and betamethasone dipropionate in the treatment of psoriasis.* 2003, J Am Acad Dermatol, 48:48–54.
20. Atzeni, F. and Sarzi-Puttini, P. *Autoantibody production in patients treated with anti-TNF.* 2008, Expert Rev Clin Immunol, 4:275–280.
21. Carey, W. *Relapse, rebound, and psorasis adverse events:an advisory group report.* 2006, J Am Acad Dermatol, 54(4 Suppl 1):S171–S181.

Chapter 18
Scleroderma

Elena Schiopu and James R. Seibold

Abstract Scleroderma is a descriptive construct that defines a large family of diseases characterized clinically by thickening of the skin. Systemic sclerosis (SSc) is a complex disease affecting multiple organ systems and is the most representative and prevalent of this spectrum of disorders. Generalized subcutaneous morphea (GSM, morphea profunda) is a form of localized scleroderma that tends to spare the internal organs. We are presenting two cases illustrating the aforementioned clinical entities.

Keywords Scleroderma • Fibrosing disorders • Morphea

Case 1

Our patient is a 33-year-old female who was referred to our clinic by her local rheumatologist for clarification of diagnosis. The patient had been healthy and had her first child 6 months prior to meeting with us. Toward the end of her pregnancy, she noted some acral edema and fatigue which she related to third trimester effects. Soon after she delivered, she noted the onset of triphasic Raynaud's phenomenon (RP), persistent hand swelling, and fatigue. Three months later, she noted skin tightness initially over her fingers and hands but then rapidly involving her upper and lower extremities, face and trunk, associated with hypo- and hyperpigmentation of the involved areas. There were no complaints of shortness of breath, heartburn, sicca symptoms, fevers, weight loss, joint swelling or stiffness, and rashes.

E. Schiopu (✉)
Division of Rheumatology, University of Michigan,
24 Frank Lloyd Wright Drive, Lobby M, Suite 2500, PO Box 481, Ann Arbor, MI 48106, USA
e-mail: eschiopu@umich.edu

Social and environmental history. She never smoked nor used alcohol or drugs. She had traveled only in the USA. She was a clerical worker in a physician's office with no relevant chemical exposures.

Physical examination. She appeared pleasant but anxious. Vitals: Ht: 48 in, Wt: 98.4 lbs, BP 131/70 mmHg, pulse 88 beats per minute. HEENT: mouth aperture was 65 mm (normal 46–54), the tongue was hypopapillated but the salivary glands were not enlarged. There was cyanosis of the hands and her feet at room temperature but no ulcerations or loss of digital pulp. Her nailfold capillaroscopic exam revealed dilated and distorted capillaries with frequent areas of drop out (Fig. 18.1). Her peripheral pulses were normal and symmetrical. There was skin thickening scored by palpation using the Modified Rodnan Skin Score (MRSS) scale wherein 0 is normal and 3 is the thickest as: fingers (2), hands (1), forearms (1), arms (0), face (1), chest (1), abdomen (1), thighs (0), legs (0), and feet (1); total was 13 (of a maximum of 51). There were palpable tendon friction rubs over her wrist extensors bilaterally. Flexion contractures were noted of the MCPs and PIPs of the fourth and fifth digits but no frank synovitis. Her cardiopulmonary examination was completely normal.

Diagnostic testing. Serum ANA was positive in a speckled pattern, with a titer of 1:2,560, while the rest of the serological testing, including the anti-Scl-70 antibody was negative. Her hemoglobin was decreased at 9.1 g/dl and her CK and aldolase levels were normal. Pulmonary function tests (PFT) revealed normal volumes, namely, a forced vital capacity (FVC) of 86% of predicted, a total lung capacity (TLC) of 94% of predicted, and a diffusion capacity (DLco) of 76% of predicted. The echocardiogram was completely normal; a high resolution CT (HRCT) scan of her lungs showed no evidence of parenchymal lung disease.

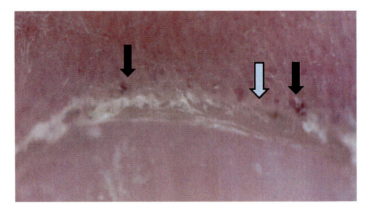

Fig. 18.1 Nailfold capillaroscopy showing capillary dilatation (black arrows) and areas of no capillaries (dropout) (blue arrow)

What Is Your Initial Impression About This Patient?

In summary, our patient is a 33-year-old female with postpartum progressive skin thickening, RP, anemia, and positive ANA.

Plan. The patient was advised to start a proton pump inhibitor. She was referred to occupational therapy for hand exercises, to gastroenterology for consideration of upper endoscopy and was also asked to monitor her blood pressure weekly. The plan was to follow her on an every 3 month basis with repeated PFTs and skin scores.

During the subsequent clinic visits, the patient noticed new onset pyrosis, progression of the skin thickening over the lower extremities and worsening bilateral hands flexion contractures (Fig. 18.2). Her fatigue and discomfort were markedly increased. Her MRSS worsened to a total score of 27. Her skin hypopigmentation progressed as well. She continued to have multiple painful tendon friction rubs. On examination, she was noted to now have end-inspiratory rales at the lung bases.

She received a blood transfusion when her hemoglobin dropped to 8 mg/dl and she underwent her first upper endoscopy. A diagnosis of gastric antral vascular ectasia (GAVE) was made, and the patient received argon photocoagulation (APC) treatment which was repeated two more times over the next 8 weeks, before complete resolution of her lesions. Pictures of her pre- and posttreatment gastric antrum are attached (Fig. 18.3). Her anemia resolved but she started noticing more shortness of breath and more effort intolerance.

Serial PFTs showed deterioration of the patient's ventilatory capacity (Table 18.1).

The 11% drop on the FVC (from June of 2007 to April of 2008) coupled with the patient's subjective functional worsening prompted us to obtain a repeated HRCT of the chest. There was interval development of very mild posterior basilar

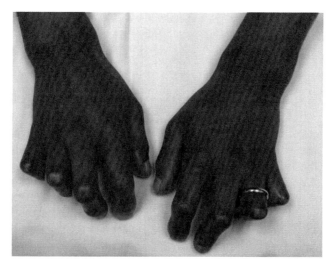

Fig. 18.2 Hands of our patient with scleroderma: sclerodactyly and flexure contractions

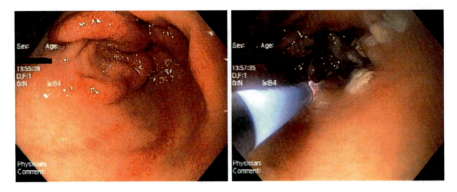

Fig. 18.3 Gastric antral vascular ectasia (GAVE) pre- and posttherapy with argon photocoagulation (APC)

Table 18.1 Serial PFTs showing deterioration of the ventilatory volumes

	FVC (%predicted)	TLC (%predicted)	DLco (%predicted)
06/2007	86	94	76
10/2007	81	91	73
01/2008	77	88	68
04/2008	75	91	91

FVC forced vital capacity, *TLC* total lung capacity, *DLco* diffusion capacity

interlobular septal thickening, best visualized on prone images, consistent with very early scleroderma-related nonspecific interstitial pneumonitis (NSIP) (Fig. 18.4). The patient was started on mycophenolate mofetil (MMT) at 2 g daily and prednisone 5 mg daily and continued for 18 months. At the end of the treatment, the patient's skin had softened, her FVC improved by 10%, and her pain level improved dramatically. She is currently trying to conceive a second child.

Differential Diagnosis

Systemic Lupus Erythematous. Although the positive ANA, arthralgias/myalgias, RP and skin changes could all be part of the classification criteria for lupus, the patient did not have the typical malar rash, lymphopenia/leucopenia, and autoantibodies.

Nephrogenic Systemic Fibrosis. NSF has been recently described in patients with severe renal insufficiency and multiple gadolinium exposures; aside from skin thickening, the clinical picture includes interstitial lung disease (ILD), yellow, raised plaques on the sclera and joint stiffness. Our patient had normal renal function and was never exposed to gadolinium.

Dermatomyositis. DM is a complex multisystem disease characterized by muscle inflammation and typical rashes. RP, nailfold capillary changes, and calcinosis

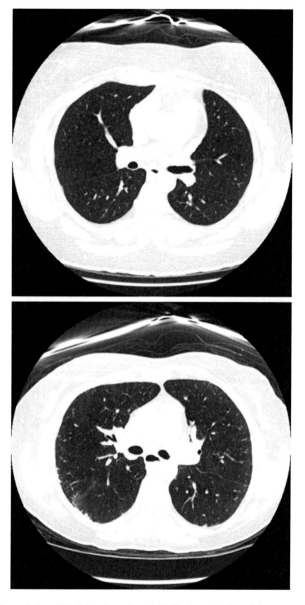

Fig. 18.4 High resolution CT of the chest done initially (top view) and the repeated HRCT done a year later (below) showing early NSIP changes

are present as well. Our patient did not complain of muscle weakness and her muscle enzymes were normal.

Scleredema Adultorum of Buschke. Most commonly associated with long standing Type 1 diabetes mellitus, this entity has been described to involve the skin of the upper back extending to the extremities and face. It is not associated with RP. Our patient did not fit this clinical picture.

Chronic Graft vs. Host Disease. This is a condition associated with hematopoetic cell transplantation; it is a T-cell mediated condition clinically characterized by sclerodermatous changes, bronchiolitis obliterans and GI involvement. Our patient did not undergo bone marrow transplant.

With the Presented Data, What Is Your Diagnosis and Why?

The review of the clinical presentation, the multitude of organ-systems involved and the distribution and extent of skin thickening led us to a diagnosis of *diffuse cutaneous systemic sclerosis (DcSSc).*

Our patient had an explosive onset of symptoms in the unique setting of the last trimester of her pregnancy. Over a few months duration, she developed RP, arthralgias and myalgias, weight loss, and rapidly progressive skin thickening. Within another few months, she became anemic due to the GI bleed caused by her GAVE – another common complication of the early stages of diffuse scleroderma. A year after her initial presentation, she developed ILD which was successfully stabilized with immunosuppressive therapy. Although pregnancy was initially thought to cause the initial symptoms, our patient continued to accrue various new organ involvements after the child birth. The natural history of diffuse scleroderma includes an acute inflammatory stage and the degree of internal organ involvement during the initial stage dictates the quality and length of survival. The rapid progression of the skin thickening from extremities to the trunk allowed us to classify our patient's scleroderma as having the diffuse form of SSc.

Discussion

SSc is a chronic connective tissue disease of unknown etiology with an estimated prevalence of 1 in 10,000, affecting women 5–6 times more frequently than men. Microchimerism (presence of circulating cells transferred from one individual to another during conditions like pregnancy) has been implicated in the pathogenesis of SSc (1, but no definite causality has been established. The clinical heterogeneity coupled with the unpredictable course makes diagnosis of SSc and prognosis assignment very difficult. The pathogenesis of SSc is complex and involves an interplay between endothelial injury leading to wide spread vasculopathy, autoimmune disturbance, and abnormalities in the components of the connective tissue (2). Vascular injury is probably the earliest event and might be triggered by endothelial-specific autoantibodies or reactive oxygen radicals generated during ischemia/reperfusion (3). Both the innate and the adaptive immune systems play a role in SSc: T-cell activation is present in the early inflammatory stages of the disease and highly specific autoantibodies are detected in the serum of SSc patients.

The activated fibroblasts are responsible for fibrosis and accumulation of extracellular matrix molecules in SSc, which explains its clinical manifestations.

SSc has been classified in two major subgroups based on the amount of skin involvement: diffuse and limited (formerly known as CREST) (4). In limited SSc, scleroderma ski change is limited to the hands and face, RP is present for years before fibrosis appears, and pulmonary hypertension is a late and frequent complication. The diffuse form is characterized by the explosive onset of symptoms, rapidly progressive skin thickening, and early internal organ involvement. Although useful, this classification does not comprise the full heterogeneity of the clinical manifestations of scleroderma. The degree of involvement of the internal organs is the major determinant of prognosis.

Raynaud's phenomenon and digital ulceration. RP is the most common initial manifestation of SSc (5); it is representative of the scleroderma-related vasculopathy and is characterized by excessive vasoconstriction in response to cold stimuli. Digital ulcers can be the result of digital vascular occlusion and constitute a major clinical burden because of increased pain, hand dysfunction, and risk of infection potentially leading to amputation. The current off-label therapies are focused on vasoactive agents, antiplatelet medications, and antibiotics if needed.

Renal involvement (scleroderma renal crisis, SRC). SRC occurs in 5–10% of the SSc patients and the clinical picture is one of the abrupt onset of hypertensions associated with microangiopathic hemolytic anemia and relatively bland urinary sediment. With the increased use of the ACE inhibitors and tighter BP control, the mortality due to this complication has decreased significantly (6), but SRC remains one of the few true rheumatological emergencies. The diffuse subtype of SSc, speckled pattern of the ANA, and the use of high dose corticosteroids (prednisolone or equivalent >15 mg/day) are associated with SRC.

Gastrointestinal involvement in SSc. GI involvement in SSc is the second most common clinical feature after Raynaud's and is present in as many as 90% of patients. It is thought that the GI impairment is due to initial microvascular damage, leading to neurogenic impairment and myogenic dysfunction with the end result being smooth muscle atrophy and subsequent fibrosis. Dysphagia, pyrosis (esophagus), early satiety (stomach), bloating and diarrhea (small bowel), and constipation (large bowel) are the clinical manifestations. The most common cause of iron-deficiency anemia in the early stages of SSc is hemorrhage from GAVE, also known as "watermelon stomach" due to its endoscopic appearance. The diagnosis is made by upper endoscopy which also allows for the prompt treatment of this condition with argon plasma coagulation (APC).

Pulmonary involvement in SSc. Pulmonary manifestations of SSc are the leading cause of morbidity and mortality in SSc and include parenchymal involvement (interstitial lung disease, ILD) and vascular involvement (pulmonary arterial hypertension, PAH). The key clinical issues are early detection of these complications and determination of the relative contribution of each process to the symptoms. The clinical signs of pulmonary involvement include shortness of breath on exertion and subsequently at rest, nonproductive cough, fatigue, and sometimes pleuritic chest pain. The physical exam could elicit fine end-inspiratory crackles (ILD), or signs of right heart failure such as jugular venous distention, right ventricular heave, and an accentuated P2 (PAH). PFTs play a key role in defining the nature of the pulmonary involvement: fibrotic disease is characterized by a restrictive pattern with decreased FVC and TLC, while the vascular involvement (PAH) can be suspected in the presence of impaired DLco (7). The introduction of HRCT scan of the chest increased the sensitivity of radiographic diagnosis: ground glass appearance denoting fine fibrosis (predominant or mixed with reticular abnormalities) and little or no honeycombing are the most common features (NSIP).

Doppler echocardiography is extensively used as a screening tool for PAH, but the diagnostic gold standard remains the right heart catheterization (RHC). The presence of PAH is indicated by a mean pulmonary artery pressure (mPAP) of ≥25 mmHg with a normal pulmonary wedge pressure. According to the WHO classification, patients with SSc can develop PAH as part of the connective tissue disease (Group I) or PH secondary to the ILD (Group III).

The treatment options for the ILD are perceived as either an attempt to modify the natural history of the disease (in the diffuse subset) or an acceptable organ directed intervention (in the limited subset). Numerous negative clinical trials (exploring methotrexate (MTX), D-penicillamine, azathioprine, relaxin) set the stage for the overall impression that the SSc-related ILD is a quintessentially untreatable complication. The effects of oral or intravenous cyclophosphamide on lung function and quality of life were modestly positive in randomized controlled trials and are subject of ongoing discussion about the subset of patients that improved (8). Encouraging observations have been reported with the use of MMT in terms of efficacy in SSc-ILD (9) and survival (10). Ongoing clinical trials are looking at autologous bone marrow transplant, comparisons between oral cyclophosphamide and MMT, and tyrosine kinase inhibitors as potential treatment options for SSc-ILD.

The treatment of SSc-PAH has made steady and unique progress with nine currently FDA approved therapies: four different synthetic prostacyclins (epoprostenol or treprostinil (parenteral) and iloprost or treprostinil (inhaled)), three endothelin receptor antagonists (bosentan, ambrisentan, and sitaxentan) and two phosphodiesterase inhibitors type 5 (sildenafil and tadalafil).

Summary and conclusion. SSc is a heterogenous group of diseases characterized by thickening of the skin and multiple organ involvement. The important subsets of this disease are limited and diffuse scleroderma. The main cause of mortality and morbidity is the lung involvement. Although a cure does not exist, numerous clinical trials are underway and organ directed therapy is currently able to significantly improve the quality of life.

Questions

1. Which one of the following is the cause of systemic sclerosis?

    (a) Slow virus infection
    (b) None, it is an idiopathic disease
    (c) Radiation therapy
    (d) Pregnancy with male fetuses
    (e) B and D

18 Scleroderma

2. Which one of the following statements concerning the distinction between diffuse and limited scleroderma is true?

   (a) The diffuse form involves internal organ involvement while the limited form affects the outside of the body
   (b) The limited form of scleroderma could be linear, circumscribed or affecting the face (en coup de sabre)
   (c) The skin in the diffuse form of scleroderma affects the trunk and proximal areas, whereas in the limited form the scleroderma is limited to the face and fingers
   (d) The antibody profile in the limited scleroderma includes a positive ANA in a speckled pattern while the diffuse scleroderma is characterized by a positive anticentromere antibody
   (e) Raynaud's phenomenon is present ONLY in the limited form of scleroderma

3. What is the first step in evaluating a patient with SSc who presents to clinic complaining of fatigue and you find her hemoglobin to be 7.2 mg/dl?

   (a) Iron studies
   (b) BUN/Cr levels and advise the patient to monitor her BP at home weekly
   (c) Peripheral smear and LDH levels
   (d) Promptly arrange a blood transfusion and an upper endoscopy
   (e) Start patient on Iron and advise leafy vegetables daily

4. What is the gold standard for diagnosing pulmonary hypertension?

   (a) Patient's subjective sense of dyspnea
   (b) Doppler echocardiogram
   (c) Decreased DLco on pulmonary function tests
   (d) Right heart catheterization
   (e) Referral to a center of excellence in pulmonary hypertension

5. Which one of the following statement is true regarding scleroderma renal crisis?

   (a) It seems to be more associated with a speckled pattern ANA
   (b) The only clinical signs are increased BP
   (c) It is present in both the limited and diffuse forms of SSc
   (d) It used to be the first cause of mortality in scleroderma before the introduction of ACE inhibitors
   (e) All of the above

Answer key: 1(b), 2(c), 3(d), 4(d), 5(e).

Case 2

We first met this delightful 67-year-old woman approximately 2 years ago. She was referred by her primary care doctor to our clinic with a presumptive diagnosis of scleroderma. More than 2 years earlier, she had noticed thickening of the skin on her forearms. Months later, she noticed that her shins were "shiny," and she noticed thickening of the skin on her calves as well. In the meantime, she started noticing small skin bumps on her forearms. Four months later, she developed her first ulceration in the lower extremities, in the medial malleolar region. She was referred to a dermatologist and a 5 mm deep biopsy of her forearm was done in an attempt to diagnose her condition. The report described a pattern of dermal sclerosis which was judged inconsistent with either scleroderma or morphea profunda.

When we further asked her about the changes affecting her skin, she mentioned that the initial skin tightness was accompanied by purple discoloration of the affected area, which over the course of a few months evolved into a mix of purple and ivory areas. She was initially given a prescription for prednisone (highest dose 40 mg daily), but after approximately 14 months it was stopped and she started MTX (20 mg/week orally). Six months later, she was also given a prescription for hydroxychloroquine (200 mg twice daily), in addition to the MTX.

This patient had never noticed RP, digital tip ulcers or other signs of vasulopathy. She had never had a malar rash or any other rashes. She never had photosensitivity, calcinosis, mouth or nose ulcers. She denied morning stiffness although she occasionally had joint pain and swelling affecting both of her knees. Her most important musculoskeletal complaint was her inability to stretch her knees and ankles because of the tightness of her skin which had progressively worsened over the last year. She has had reflux symptoms all her life but she denied aspiration events, abdominal pain, diarrhea, or constipation. She did not complain of dry eyes or mouth, and she did not have any systemic complaints, including fevers or weight loss.

She had a 50 pack year history of smoking, drank socially, and was never exposed to any chemicals. She mentioned that she is allergic to penicillin, demerol, and latex. She had not traveled outside the United States.

On physical exam, she was a slightly overweight female, weighing 261 lbs, 65.5 in tall, her pulse was 82, and the blood pressure was 155/65 mmHg. She seemed to be in no apparent distress. There were no malar or periorbital rashes, no telangiectasias, no RP, or nailfold capillary abnormalities. Her lungs revealed vesicular breath sounds bilaterally, and her heart examination was also within normal limits.

Her skin examination revealed morpheaform plaques of different colors, varying from purple-erythematous to ivory, involving the forearms up to her elbows and her legs up to the knees (Fig. 18.5). The overlying skin was indurated, with evident venous furrowing and lack of hair follicles. Her forearm skin has a coarse peau d'orange appearance. The range of motion (flexion/extension) in her wrists and ankles was markedly reduced. There were no signs of vascular instability, including Raynaud's, digital or lower extremity ulcers and livedo reticularis.

With the Presented Data, What Is Your Working Diagnosis?

This patient was 65-year-old at the time of presentation with a history of progressively worsening skin tightness that seems to have started in her forearms and legs, and

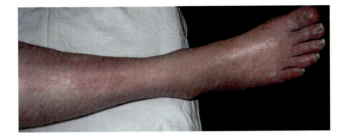

Fig. 18.5 Morpheaform plaques on lower extremities

impairing the movement of her wrists and ankles. There are two conditions that this type of presentation had been described: eosinophilic fasciitis and GSM, morphea profunda. The only way to differentiate the two entities is a deep tissue skin biopsy of the involved area to include the fascia.

Differential Diagnosis

Numerous conditions are characterized by thick skin and are generally referred to as being part of the scleroderma family of diseases. Aside from the systemic forms of scleroderma (e.g., systemic sclerosis), there are other forms of scleroderma in which the only organ involved is the skin: localized scleroderma or morphea. Linear scleroderma, morphea en plaque, progressive hemifacial atrophy (Parry-Romberg syndrome) should be considered in the differential diagnosis. The most important distinction that needs to be made is from SSc.

Workup

CBC with differential revealed normal white count and normal absolute eosinophil count. Her ANA was negative. We decided to obtain a wedge biopsy of her calf area which at the time seemed to be the most involved. The patient underwent a deep tissue biopsy successfully and without complications. The report outlined: scant lymphocytic inflammatory infiltrate in the dermoid and subdermoid area; there is inflammation present in the dermal subcutaneous junction and perivascular; presence of septal sclerosis was noted; no fascial inflammatory infiltrate (Fig. 18.6). The biopsy was descriptive of GSM, a form of localized scleroderma. Since there was still a significant degree of inflammation present on the biopsy and she seemed to have been progressively getting worse, we decided to switch the MTX to MMT, and we added corticosteroids to her regimen. We were able to wean the steroid within 6 months. By 18 months, her lesions had improved so substantially we stopped the MMT as well.

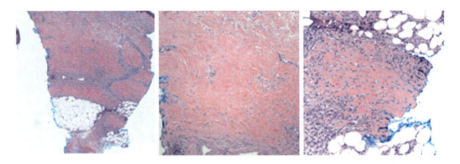

Fig. 18.6 Deep dermal and subcutaneous septal sclerosis with perivascular and perieccrine inflammation; deep dermal sclerosis with hyalinization of collagen bundles; subcutaneous septal sclerosis with hyalinzation of collagen and a lymphoplasmacellular infiltrate.

What Is Your Diagnosis and Why?

This patient has a medical history, physical examination, and histopathologic findings consistent with a rare form of localized scleroderma called morphea profunda or GSM. When patients present with symmetrical skin thickness involving forearms and legs, the only way to differentiate between eosinophilic fasciitis and GSM is a deep tissue biopsy, to include all the skin layers in "parfait-like" fashion from the epidermis to the fascia. The deep tissue biopsy could reveal the specific focus of the inflammation and fibrosis (fascia vs. the dermis) which in this case confirmed the diagnosis.

Discussion

Definition. Localized scleroderma, also named morphea, is a family of diseases characterized by skin thickening, increased collagen in the indurative lesions and minimal to no internal organ involvement.

Classification and Prevalence. There are numerous distinct forms of morphea based on the clinical picture and the levels of tissue involvement but the classification is still subject to interpretation. The most complete classification available to date has been described by Peterson and Su (Table 18.2) (11). An epidemiologic study from the same group showed that the incidence rate of morphea over the 33 years of age is as high as 3.6% per year (12), with a survival rate not different from the general population.

The term deep morphea describes a variant of morphea characterized by local inflammation and later sclerotic process that involves the deep dermis, fascia, or superficial muscle.

Clinical presentation. GSM is believed to originate in the panniculus or subcutaneous tissue. The lesions are deeper than the ones in the other forms of morphea. The natural history of the lesions involves a quick progression to sclerosis, often over a period of months. The plaques are mildly inflamed, hyperpigmented, symmetrical, and somewhat

Table 18.2 Classification of Morphea (11)

Plaque morphea
Morphea en plaque
Guttate morphea
Atrophoderma of Pasini and Pierini
Keloid morphea (nodular morphea)
[Lichen sclerosus et atrophicus]
Generalized morphea
Bullous morphea
Linear morphea
Linear morphea (linear scleroderma)
En coup de sabre
Progressive facial hemiatrophy
Deep morphea
Subcutaneous morphea
Eosinophilic fasciitis
Morphea profunda
Disabling pansclerotic morphea of children

ill-defined (12). On palpation, the sin feels thickened and bond down to the underlying fascia and muscles. Plaques are smooth and shiny, but there are also areas where bullae arise on the plaques.

Unlike systemic sclerosis, there is seldom involvement of the digits, and there are no vascular symptoms like RP, digital ulcers or distal phalangeal resorption. Flexion contractures of the joints are frequently present and patients often complain of arthralgias, myalgias, and muscle cramping. Internal involvement in GSM is not rare, but it is usually silent. The most commonly described are the impaired carbon monoxide diffusion in the lungs, and the peristaltic failure in the esophagus (13). Peripheral eosinophilia, anti single-stranded DNA (ssDNA) and antihistone antibodies (especially H1, H2A, and H2B) are distinct indicators of the disease.

Histological findings. The biopsy in GSM shows lymphocyte and plasma cell infiltration which is mainly perivascular and perieccrine. There is also collagenous tissue thickening and hyalinization of the subcutis. Eosinophils may be part of the cellular infiltrate. Deep dermis hyalinization at the junction between the dermis and the subcutaneous fat is common.

Pathogenesis. Localized scleroderma is a disease of unknown etiology. Although not fully elucidated, the proposed pathogenesis mechanism mimics the one described in SSc. The initial inflammatory stage is followed by fibrosis, caused by accumulation of extracellular matrix components, mainly type I and III fibrillary collagen. Transforming growth factor (TGF)-β and interleukin-4 are important cytokines in the activation of matrix production by dermal fibroblasts. Interleukin-4 is produced by T-cells and mast cells and exerts its effects on collagen and fibronectin synthesis by human dermal fibroblasts which makes it important in both normal wound healing and pathological fibrosis (14). Localized scleroderma fibroblasts present increased expression of TGF-β receptors which in turn induces skin fibroblasts to produce connective tissue growth factor (CTGF). CTGF mRNA expression was found to be elevated in fibroblasts present in the localized scleroderma lesions, while the adjacent nonaffected dermis was negative for CTGF mRNA (15). In response to an unknown initial injury, TGF-β, along with interleukin-4, in conjunction with CTGF produced by activated fibroblast, gives rise to a stimulatory loop with the end result being overproduction of the extracellular matrix.

Treatment. The treatment for localized scleroderma in general and GSM in particular is currently not satisfactory. The conditions is extremely rare, heterogeneous, difficult to diagnose and prone to remit spontaneously. The focus of the therapy so far has been to target various pathological phases of localized scleroderma. To date, most of the therapies have been reported as case series or open trials. Corticosteroids, UVA1, vitamin D analogs and MTX have all been used in the past. A combination of steroid and MTX has shown encouraging results (16). In fact, that is the preferred initial regimen for a patient with an established diagnosis of GSM. Due to its antiproliferative effect on the fibroblasts, 1, 25-dihydroxyvitamin D3 was tried with limited success. Reports of the effects of psoralens followed by UVA exposure (PUVA) are beneficial (17), and the level of dosing of the UVA therapy renders similar outcomes.

GSM has a longer, more protracted course and traditionally tends to be more resistant to therapy. Although the initial therapy with steroids and MTX is usually generally effective, there are cases where a next step is required. Successful use of MMT in cases of morphea that were resistant to MTX was reported (18). Patients who had failure of treatment after 4 months of MTX in combination with steroids showed clinical improvement and allowed reduction in the dose of cortiocosteroids and MTX. More sophisticated approach to this condition is being considered: one of the promising agents is imatinib mesylate, a tyrosine kinase inhibitor that interferes with the TGF-β signaling via c-Abl, blocking extracellular matrix synthesis both in vivo and in vitro.

Questions

1. What is the most important clue in the history of a patient presenting with skin tightness over his legs and forearms that the disease is NOT systemic?

    (a) Presence of heartburn
    (b) Joint pains
    (c) Car accident during his infancy
    (d) Lack of Raynaud's phenomenon

2. Which one of the following diagnoses would classify as "localized scleroderma"?

    (a) Generalized subcutaneous morphea
    (b) CREST syndrome
    (c) Scleroderma "en coup de sabre"
    (d) Mixed connective tissue disease
    (e) A and C only

3. GSM is microscopically similar to:

   (a) Cutaneous lupus
   (b) Linear scleroderma
   (c) The heliotropic rash in dermatomyositis
   (d) Eosinophilic fasciitis
   (e) Erythema nodosum

4. The most important element of the differential diagnosis between various forms of deep morphea is:

   (a) Clinical presentation
   (b) Presence of sclerodactyly
   (c) Deep tissue biopsy
   (d) Therapeutic response to steroids

5. The mortality in GSM is:

   (a) Extremely high since this is a paraneoplastic syndrome
   (b) Moderately high due to the joint and muscle involvement
   (c) Similar to that of the general population
   (d) None of the above

Answer key: 1(d), 2(e), 3(d), 4(c), 5(c).

References

1. Artlett, C., *Microchimerism and Scleroderma: An Update.* Current Rheumatology Reports, 2003. **5**: p. 154–9.
2. Varga, J. and D. Abraham, *Systemic sclerosis: A prototypic multisystem fibrotic disorder.* Journal of Clinical Investigation, 2007. **117**(3): p. 557–67.
3. Kahaleh, M., *Raynaud phenomenon and the vascular disease in scleroderma.* Current Opinion in Rheumatology, 2004. **16**: p. 718–22.
4. LeRoy, E., et al., *Scleroderma (systemic sclerosis): Classification, subsets and pathogenesis.* Journal of Rheumatology, 1988. **15**(2): p. 202–5.
5. Denton, C. and J. Korn, *Digital ulceration and critical digital ischaemia in scleroderma.* Scleroderma Care and Research Journal, 2003. **1**: p. 12–6.
6. Steen, V. and T. Medsger, *Changes in causes of death in systemic sclerosis, 1972–2002.* Annals of Rheumatic Diseases, 2007. **66**: p. 940–4.
7. Steen, V., et al., *Isolated diffusing capacity reduction in systemic sclerosis.* Arthritis and Rheumatism, 1992. **35**(7): p. 765–70.
8. Tashkin, D., et al., *Cyclophosphamide versus placebo in scleroderma lung disease.* New England Journal of Medicine, 2006. **25**(354): p. 2655–66.
9. Zamora, A., et al., *Use of mycophenolate mofetil to treat scleroderma-associated interstitial lung disease.* Respiratory Medicine, 2008. **1**(102): p. 150–5.
10. Nihtyanova, S., C. Black, and C. Denton, *Mycophenolate mofetil in diffuse cutaneous systemic sclerosis – A retrospective analysis.* Rheumatology, 2007. **3**(46): p. 442–5.
11. Peterson, L., A. Nelson, and W. Su, *Classification of morphea (localized scleroderma).* Mayo Clinic Proceedings, 1995. **70**: p. 1068–76.

12. Person, J. and W. Su, *Subcutaneous morphoea: A clinical study of sixteen cases.* British Journal of Dermatology, 1979. **100**: p. 371–80.
13. Dehen, L., et al., *Internal involvement in localized scleroderma.* Medicine (Baltimore), 1994. **73**(5): p. 241–5.
14. Postlethwaite, A., et al., *Human fibroblasts synthesize elevated levels of extracellular matrix proteins in response to interleukin 4.* Journal of Clinical Investigation, 1992. **90**(4): p. 1479–85.
15. Igarashi, A., et al., *Connective tissue growth factor gene expression in tissue sections from localized scleroderma, keloid, and other fibrotic skin disorders.* Journal of Investigational Dermatology, 1996. **106**(4): p. 729–33.
16. Uziel, Y., et al., *Methotrexate and corticosteroid therpay for pediatric localized scleroderma.* Journal of Pediatrics, 2000. **136**: p. 91–5.
17. Grundman-Kollmann, M., et al., *PUVA-cream photochemotherapy for the treatment of localized scleroderma.* Journal of the American Academy of Dermatology, 2000. **43**(4): p. 675–8.
18. Martini, G., et al., *Successful treatment of severe or methotrexate-resistant juvenile localized scleroderma with mycophenolate mofetil.* Rheumatology, 2009. **48**(11): p. 1410–3.

Chapter 19
Autoimmune Blistering Diseases of the Skin and Mucous Membranes

Timothy Patton and Neil J. Korman

Abstract Autoimmune blistering diseases of the skin and mucous membranes are characterized by the presence of tissue bound and circulating antibodies that are directed against specific proteins present in the skin. The different diseases that compose this category of conditions vary in their clinical presentation, prognosis, and response to therapy.

Keywords Pemphigus vulgaris • Mucous membrane pemphigoid • Paraneoplastic pemphigus • Desquamative gingivitis • Direct immunofluorescence

Case 1

Our patient is a 55-year-old male without significant past medical history who presented with complaints of painful oral erosions and widespread cutaneous blisters. The oral lesions began 2 months prior to presentation, and he began to develop skin lesions within the last few weeks. Prior to our examination, the patient had received multiple topical and systemic therapies for what was variably diagnosed as oral aphthous ulcers, herpes virus infection, cellulitis, and allergic contact dermatitis. There was no response to multiple therapies including systemic valacyclovir, cefadroxil, and fluconazole, but there was transient improvement primarily in the skin lesions when he was treated with a 3-week tapering course of oral prednisone.

Past medical history: The patient had no significant past medical history and was not on any medications at the time of his visit. He had not taken any new medications prior to the onset of the oral lesions.

Family history: Noncontributory, no history of autoimmune or other skin disease. There were no first degree relatives with a history of malignancy.

T. Patton (✉)
Assistant Professor, Department of Dermatology, University of Pittsburg,
Pittsburg, PA, USA
e-mail: pattontj@upmc.edu

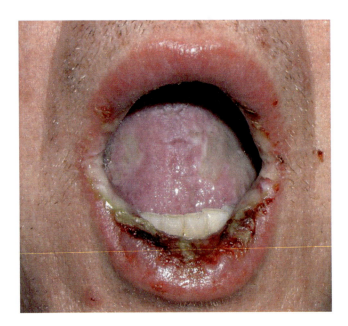

Fig. 19.1 Erosions of the tongue with hemorrhagic crusting and erosions of the lips

Social history: The patient worked as an engineer and he denied tobacco or ethanol use.

Review of systems: The patient reported pain from the oral and cutaneous erosions, but denied fevers or pruritus. He reported the recent onset of shortness of breath.

Exam: There were erosions and ulcerations on the tongue, the labial and buccal mucosa, and the palate. There was hemorrhagic crusting present on the lips (Fig. 19.1). The cutaneous examination revealed widespread erythematous plaques, flaccid bullae, and focal hemorrhagic crusting over the trunk and proximal extremities involving approximately 10% of the body surface (Fig. 19.2). The lungs were clear to auscultation and percussion, and the rest of the physical exam was unremarkable.

What Is the Differential Diagnosis?

The differential diagnosis includes widespread allergic contact dermatitis, erythema multiforme (EM), Stevens–Johnson syndrome (SJS), bullous pemphigoid (BP), and pemphigus vulgaris (PV).

Allergic contact dermatitis: While allergic contact dermatitis may present with widespread erythematous plaques and bullae, it is usually pruritic, which was not a symptom in this patient. Furthermore, intraoral ulcers and erosions are uncommon in patients with allergic contact dermatitis.

Erythema multiforme: EM is most frequently caused by the herpes simplex virus (HSV), which can cause widespread oral erosions and ulcerations. The skin lesions of EM commonly include erythematous plaques and vesicles. Classically, the skin

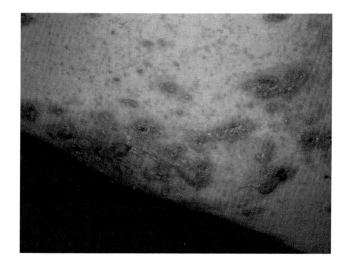

Fig. 19.2 Erythematous plaques, flaccid bullae, and hemorrhagic crusting on the lower abdomen

lesions present in EM are target lesions that are present on the acral surfaces of the skin. It would be somewhat unusual to have EM occur as an ongoing process for over 2 months, and at least a partial response to systemic valacyclovir would occur in most patients.

Stevens–Johnson syndrome: SJS is often caused by medications and less commonly by infections. It may also present with mucous membrane erosions along with cutaneous lesions. Patients with SJS are often quite ill and may develop constitutional symptoms along with internal organ involvement. As our patient was not on any medications at the time of presentation, SJS is a less likely diagnosis.

Bullous pemphigoid: BP can present with widespread erythematous plaques and bullae. The bullae of BP tend to be tense as opposed to flaccid, and most patients have significant pruritus. Oral lesions can occur in up to 30% of BP patients, and so the involvement of the mucous membranes in this case does not necessarily exclude BP.

Pemphigus vulgaris: PV commonly presents as oral erosions that may progress to involve the skin. Cutaneous lesions of PV present as flaccid bullae and erosions, and the most common sites of involvement include the scalp and the flexural surfaces. While pruritus is relatively uncommon in patients with PV, most patients do have pain from their eroded lesions.

What Is the Appropriate Workup in This Patient?

The patient underwent two skin biopsies, one which was sent for routine histology and another which was sent for direct immunofluorescence (DIF). When obtaining biopsies of the oral mucosa for histology, it is important to involve either oral surgeons or otolaryngologists as they are most skilled in oral cavity anatomy. The biopsy for standard histology should be obtained from involved mucosa, and it is critical that the biopsy for DIF be obtained from uninvolved tissue that has intact epithelium. A good place to biopsy for DIF that is often uninvolved is the lower inner lip. A culture for HSV was performed on the patient's oral erosions.

Test Results

Routine histology demonstrated suprabasilar acantholysis with minimal inflammation at the dermoepidermal junction (Fig. 19.3). DIF studies demonstrated cell surface deposits of IgG and C3 (Fig. 19.4). The HSV culture was negative.

Based on the Histology and Immunofluorescence Findings, What Is the Best Diagnosis in This Patient?

Based on the clinical, histological, and immunofluorescence findings, the best diagnosis is PV.

What Is the Appropriate Treatment for This Patient?

Due to the widespread nature of his disease and in order to prevent progression, the patient was admitted to the hospital and placed on high dose intravenous

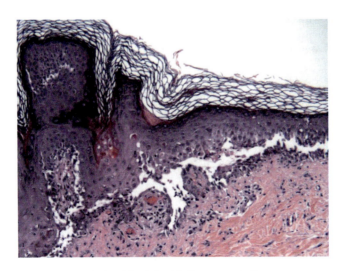

Fig. 19.3 Suprabasal acantholysis with minimal inflammatory infiltrate

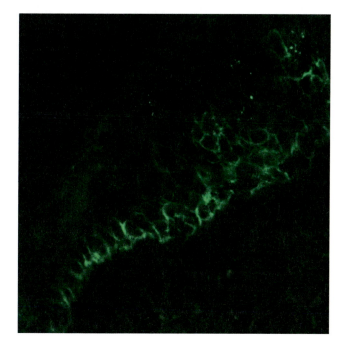

Fig. 19.4 Direct immunofluorescence demonstrating IgG deposition in a cell surface pattern

corticosteroids (60 mg methylprednisolone every 8 h). Baseline labs, including a thiopurine methyltransferase (TPMT) level, were ordered in anticipation of adding azathioprine as a steroid sparing agent. Within the next 3–4 days, the development of new bullae on the body ceased and the erosions began to reepithelialize. The TPMT level was 21 units/ml packed RBCs (which is a high level). The patient was discharged to home on oral prednisone (80 mg given every morning) and azathioprine 250 mg/day (based upon a dosage of 2.5 mg/kg given for patients with high TPMT levels and a patient weight of 100 kg). Over the next several months, the patient had significant improvement in his skin disease and the steroid dosage was slowly taperevd. The oral disease, however, was more recalcitrant to this therapy. When the prednisone dose reached 20 mg/day, the patient began to develop new red scaling lesions on his proximal upper arms, abdomen, and elbows (Figs. 19.5 and 19.6). A skin biopsy of these new lesions demonstrated a lichenoid dermatitis without acantholysis with several necrotic keratinocytes present in the epidermis (Fig. 19.7).

What Is the Significance of Lichenoid Dermatitis in a Patient With Pemphigus?

Typically, the histology of PV is that of a noninflammatory process which demonstrates suprabasilar acantholysis. When a lichenoid infiltrate is present in a patient with pemphigus, it should raise the possibility of paraneoplastic pemphigus.

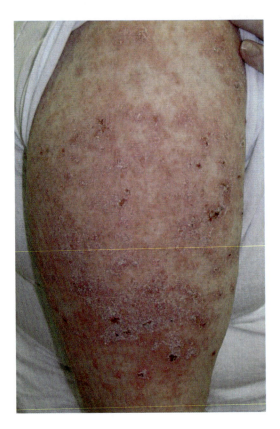

Fig. 19.5 *Red, scaling patches and plaques* with some hemorrhagic crusting on the right proximal upper extremity

With the Consideration of Paraneoplastic Pemphigus, What Should the Next Step Be in the Workup of the Patient?

The patient was sent for a computed tomography (CT) scan of the chest, abdomen, and pelvis to search for any underlying associated tumors. In addition, indirect immunofluorescence testing was performed using the patient's serum and rodent bladder as the substrate. The CT scan demonstrated a retroperitoneal mass encasing the aorta which closely involved the celiac trunk. Indirect immunofluorescence studies on murine bladder epithelium were positive for cell surface deposits of IgG (Fig. 19.8). A biopsy of the retroperitoneal mass was diagnostic for non-Hodgkins lymphoma.

Over a period of 2 months, the patient was treated with cyclophosphamide, adriamycin, vincristine, prednisone, and rituximab (CHOP-R) therapy resulting in a shrinking of his retroperitoneal mass and improvement of his skin and oral lesions. His lymphoma and pemphigus remain in remission 18 months following the treatment.

19 Autoimmune Blistering Diseases of the Skin and Mucous Membranes

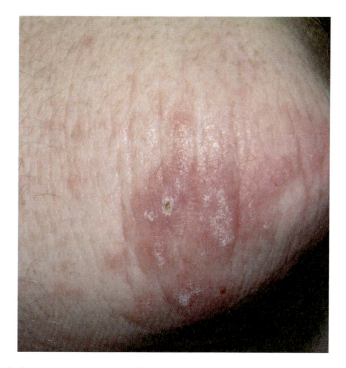

Fig. 19.6 *Red, scaling plaques* on the elbow

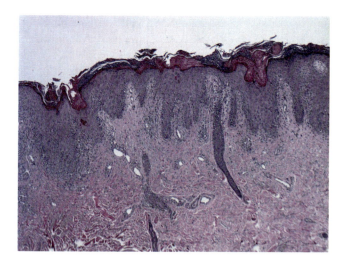

Fig. 19.7 Lichenoid dermatitis with necrotic keratinocytes

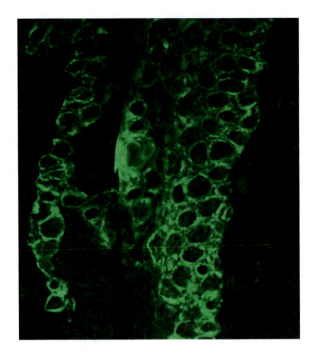

Fig. 19.8 Indirect immunofluorescence demonstrating patient IgG bound to murine bladder epithelia

Discussion

Pemphigus is an autoimmune blistering disease caused by antibodies directed against cell surface proteins called desmogleins, which are part of the transmembrane portion of desmosomes. Desmosomes are structures present at the cell membrane of keratinocytes which help provide epidermal integrity (1). With their disruption by pemphigus antibodies, epidermal integrity is lost and blistering and erosions develop which, if widespread, can predispose patients to sepsis and if untreated can lead to death. There are two main subtypes of pemphigus: PV, which is associated with antibodies directed against desmogleins 1 and/or 3, and pemphigus foliaceous, which is associated with antibodies against desmoglein 1 (2).

Patients with PV typically present with oral erosions and/or flaccid cutaneous bullae or erosions. Patients with pemphigus foliaceous present with superficial cutaneous erosions (it is quite uncommon to observe intact vesicles or bullae) without oral disease.

The diagnosis of pemphigus is made by clinical history and physical exam, histology demonstrating acantholysis in either the deep (PV) or superficial (pemphigus foliaceous) epidermis, and the demonstration of tissue bound or circulating antibodies by either direct or indirect immunofluorescence. Tissue bound antibodies are demonstrated by DIF, whereby antibodies are detected in the perilesional skin of the patient. Circulating antibodies can be demonstrated by several methods, including indirect immunofluorescence, enzyme-linked immunosorbent assay (ELISA), immunoblot, or immunoprecipitation. Indirect immunofluorescence is performed using monkey esophagus, guinea pig esophagus, or human skin as the substrate. Commercial ELISA kits that are able to detect antibodies to desmogleins 1 and 3 exist but are not widely available. Immunoblot and immunoprecipitation studies are only performed at specialty laboratories.

In the precorticosteroid era, if left untreated, PV had a mortality rate of 60–90%. Initially, all patients with PV should be treated with systemic corticosteroids (3). Most patients are started on 1 mg/kg of prednisone per day. The addition of steroid sparing medications such as azathioprine or mycophenolate mofetil may be necessary to allow tapering of the corticosteroids while still maintaining control of disease. While some patients with milder disease may have their steroids successfully tapered with the adjunctive use of milder therapies, including dapsone and hydroxychloroquine, many will require treatment with more potent adjunctive therapies such as mycophenolate mofetil, azathioprine, cyclophosphamide, intravenous immunoglobulin (IVIg), and rituximab.

In paraneoplastic pemphigus, in addition to antibodies against desmogleins, antibodies are produced against additional desmosomal proteins, including desmoplakin, plakoglobin, and envoplakin, among others (4). Because these proteins are present in the lung epithelia in addition to the skin, up to 30–40% of patients can present with lung disease in addition to their skin disease. In severe cases of paraneoplastic pemphigus, end stage bronchiolitis obliterans can occur. The most common malignancies associated with paraneoplastic pemphigus are non-Hodgkins lymphoma and chronic lymphocytic leukemia. Rarer associated tumors include Castleman's disease (especially in pediatric patients), thymomas, sarcomas, and Waldenström's macroglobulinemia. The diagnosis of paraneoplastic pemphigus can be suggested on histology by the presence of both an interface dermatitis and acantholysis (5). Indirect immunofluorescence using a substrate other than monkey or guinea pig esophagus (such as rat bladder) is important in helping to establish the diagnosis of paraneoplastic pemphigus. Immunoblot or immunoprecipitation can also be used to demonstrate the presence of circulating antibodies which bind to the plakin proteins. These studies are not routinely available in most laboratories and require the services of specialized research laboratories. Paraneoplastic pemphigus is more recalcitrant to therapy than is PV and is very commonly fatal in patients with associated malignancies while patients with associated benign tumors may improve substantially or even go into remission if the tumor is removed.

Case 2

The patient is an 83-year-old female who presented with a 4-month history of oral erosions. Her erosions began on the upper gingiva and gradually spread to involve the hard palate and buccal mucosa, causing significant difficulty while eating. She denied food getting stuck in her throat while swallowing, a foreign body sensation in the eyes, or stridor. She denied the presence of genital or anal lesions.

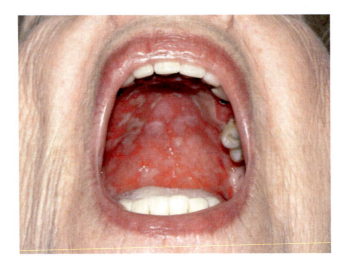

Fig. 19.9 Widespread erosions of the hard and soft palate

Past medical history: The patient had an extensive past medical history for which she was taking multiple medications. Her medical history and medication list at the time of the visit was as follows:

Medication (condition)
- Diltiazem (hypertension)
- Isosorbide (angina)
- Atorvastatin (hyperlipidemia)
- Esomeprazole (gastroesophageal reflux disease)
- Lisinopril (hypertension)
- Aspirin (coronary artery disease)
- Alprazolam (anxiety)

She was also taking multiple vitamins and supplements, including glucosamine, vitamin C, calcium, omega-3 fish oil, odorless garlic, and coenzyme Q10. None of her medications were started in close proximity to the time that she developed oral erosions.

Social history: The patient is a nonsmoker, nondrinker, retired housewife.

Exam: There were widespread erosions involving almost the entire hard palate (Fig. 19.9) and the bilateral buccal mucosal surfaces. There were a few small erosions on a background of bright red erythema on the upper and lower gingivae (Fig. 19.10). The conjunctival exam was normal without erythema or symblepharon formation. There were no cutaneous, vaginal or anal erosions.

What Is the Differential Diagnosis?

The clinical differential diagnosis includes oral erosive lichen planus, PV, Mucous membrane pemphigoid, and SJS.

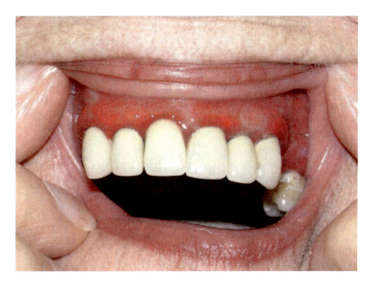

Fig. 19.10 *Bright red erythema and erosions* of the upper gingiva

This patient has desquamative gingivitis along with widespread oral erosions. In a patient with this type of presentation, it can be very difficult to distinguish between erosive lichen planus, PV, and MMP based on clinical findings alone (6). The majority of patients with PV present with oral lesions and more than 90% of patients will have oral lesions during the course of their disease. In lichen planus, Wickham's striae, which are reticular, lace-like plaques, may be present, but these are not usually seen in any of the other conditions. SJS patients usually have oral ulcers that extend onto the lips. Patients with SJS often have disease that involves more than one mucous membrane site. Since SJS is often caused by medications, and there were no medications that this patient had taken prior to the onset of oral mucosal disease, SJS is a less likely diagnosis.

What Is the Next Step in the Workup of the Patient?

Biopsies of both involved and uninvolved mucosal tissue are required to differentiate between these conditions. The tissue should be sent for both routine histology as well as DIF studies. When obtaining biopsies of the oral mucosa for histology, it is important to involve either oral surgeons or otolaryngologists as they are most skilled in oral cavity anatomy. The biopsy for standard histology should be obtained from involved mucosa, and it is critical that the biopsy for DIF be obtained from uninvolved tissue that has intact epithelium. A good place to biopsy for DIF that is often uninvolved is the lower inner lip.

Routine histology demonstrated submucosal blister formation with infiltration of neutrophils, lymphocytes, and eosinophils. DIF studies demonstrated linear deposits of both IgG and C3 at the epithelial–submucosal junction (Fig. 19.11).

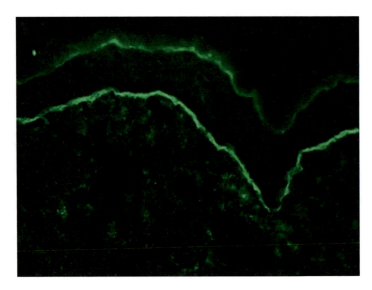

Fig. 19.11 Direct immunofluorescence of normal oral mucosa of the lower inner lip demonstrates linear IgG deposits at the epithelial/submucosal junction

With These Clinical and Pathologic Findings, What Is Your Best Diagnosis?

With the presence of a submucosal blister and linear deposits of IgG and C3 at the mucosal–submucosal junction, diseases within the pemphigoid spectrum should be considered. These include BP, epidermolysis bullosa acquisita (EBA), bullous lupus, and MMP.

BP classically presents with tense bullae which can be localized or widespread (Fig. 19.12). Involvement of the oral mucosa can occur in up to 30% of cases, but this oral disease is generally minor, and it would be extremely unusual for a patient with BP to exclusively develop oral lesions without any cutaneous disease.

EBA is an autoimmune blistering disease that can present with oral lesions and immunoreactants present at the mucosal/submucosal junction. There are different clinical presentations of EBA (7). The classic presentation of EBA is as a mechanobullous process, whereby bullae develop on sites of trauma or friction such as the knees, elbows, as well as the hands and feet (Fig. 19.13). EBA may also have an inflammatory presentation that makes it difficult to distinguish from BP. It also may present exclusively with oral lesions making it difficult to distinguish from MMP.

Bullous lupus erythematosus shares similar histologic and immunofluorescence findings, but is seen in patients with poorly controlled systemic lupus erythematosus and usually involves cutaneous sites – particularly the head, neck, and upper trunk. The inflammatory infiltrate is primarily composed of neutrophils instead of the mixed inflammatory infiltrate that was seen in this patient.

19 Autoimmune Blistering Diseases of the Skin and Mucous Membranes

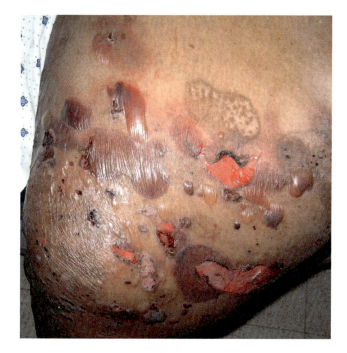

Fig. 19.12 Erosions, tense bullae, and hyperpigmented macules on the upper leg of a bullous pemphigoid patient

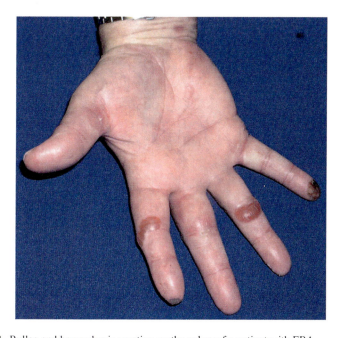

Fig. 19.13 Bullae and hemorrhagic crusting on the palms of a patient with EBA

Given the clinical, histologic, and DIF findings, the best diagnosis for this patient is MMP. Based upon the findings in this case, mucosal EBA cannot be completely excluded, but since MMP is more common than EBA, MMP remains the most likely diagnosis.

Is There Any Test That Can Be Performed to Differentiate Between MMP and EBA?

Indirect immunofluorescence performed utilizing salt split human skin is an excellent technique to differentiate between MMP and EBA. Patients with EBA will always demonstrate circulating IgG antibodies that bind to the dermal side of salt split skin, while patients with MMP will most often demonstrate circulating IgG antibodies which bind to both the dermal and epidermal sides of salt split skin or just the epidermal side. One less common form of MMP, in which patients have circulating IgG antibodies directed against epiligrin, will demonstrate circulating antibodies which only bind to the dermal side of salt split skin. This is clinically relevant because antiepiligrin MMP and internal malignancies have been associated (8).

Tests which can identify the specific antigen that is targeted by the patient's antibody, such as immunoblotting and immunoprecipitation, can differentiate between MMP and EBA, but these are not widely available and are generally performed only by research laboratories. Although an ELISA assay for the 180 kDa BP antigen has recently become commercially available, no such assay is yet available to assay for the EBA antigen.

Unfortunately, indirect immunofluorescence studies were negative in this patient and the salt split indirect immunofluorescence technique was unable to identify the presence of circulating antibodies.

With MMP as the Most Likely Diagnosis, How Should the Management of This Patient Proceed?

Therapy for MMP is determined based on the severity and location of disease (9). Patients with oral MMP generally have disease that tends not to scar and does not cause clinically significant problems. Patients with MMP involving the conjunctiva, esophagus, or larynx can develop severe sequelae, including blindness, esophageal stenosis, and total laryngeal scarring requiring a tracheostomy. Given the severity of these outcomes, aggressive therapy is warranted, most often involving a combination of prednisone and cyclophosphamide. Since our patient had no evidence of scarring present on her eye exam and she did not have any symptoms of esophageal or laryngeal involvement, we chose to pursue a more conservative, antiinflammatory therapy. This included topical clobetasol 0.05% gel along with oral dapsone at a dose of 50 mg daily initially with a gradual increase up to a dose of 150 mg daily.

After 3 months on dapsone, there was no improvement and dapsone was discontinued. At that time, doxycycline 100 mg twice daily, nicotinamide 500 mg three times daily and topical clobetasol 0.05% gel twice daily were given. After 3 months of this therapy, there was still no improvement in her oral ulcerations.

Given That Conservative Treatment Measures Have Failed, What Is the Next Step?

In patients with MMP who have purely oral disease that is much less dangerous than ocular, laryngeal, or esophageal disease, more aggressive therapy can be initiated as long as the patient is apprised of the possible risks of this treatment. Even though there was no scarring, the extent and severity of the patient's disease led us to consider more aggressive systemic therapy. A combination of prednisone (40 mg given once daily in the morning) along with mycophenolate mofetil (1,000 mg BID) for 3 months did not significantly improve her disease. A trial of azathioprine in place of mycophenolate mofetil was given starting at a dosage of 50 mg a day, but this was not tolerated due to the development of nausea and bloating. Based on the successful results of a small case series of patients (10), the antitumor necrosis factor alpha medication etanercept was given for 3 months but also did not improve her recalcitrant oral ulcerations. Throughout the entire period of therapy with both the conservative and more aggressive treatment, the patient did not develop any signs or symptoms that were concerning for a scarring process in her eyes, esophagus, or larynx. We discussed the possibility of pursuing the most aggressive therapy with either cyclophosphamide or rituximab, but the patient was reluctant to pursue these options, and we opted to treat with low doses of prednisone (between 10 and 20 mg per day) when the disease flared, with dexamethasone mouth elixir as topical therapy.

Eight months later, the patient presented with the complaint of a foreign body sensation in her right eye accompanied by redness and irritation. On exam, the conjunctiva of the right eye was injected, and there was symblepharon formation (Fig. 19.14), with entropion of the lower eyelid. She had forniceal shortening bilaterally, but there was no entropion of the left eyelid. She denied dysphagia or stridor.

With These New Ocular Findings, How Does This Change Therapy?

When ocular scarring develops in MMP patients, aggressive therapy is warranted. If left untreated, symblepheron formation can lead to such a degree of entropion that the eyelashes will continually traumatize the cornea, leading to corneal ulceration and ultimately to blindness. The prednisone dosage was increased to 40 mg given once daily in the morning and cyclophospamide was initiated at a dose of 25 mg a day and increased up to 75 mg daily. Within 4 weeks there was

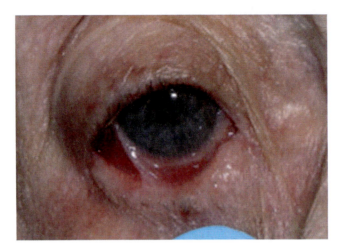

Fig. 19.14 Conjunctival erythema with symblepharon formation of the lower right eyelid

significant improvement in her ocular and oral disease. Regular careful monitoring of the complete blood count along with a urinalysis and a microscopic urine exam were performed to monitor for bone marrow suppression and the development of hemorrhagic cystitis. The prednisone dosage was slowly tapered over the next few months and was discontinued after 5 months. Cyclophosphamide was continued for 1 year, at which point her oral disease had improved significantly. There was no progression of her conjunctival scarring and her entropion improved. After 1 year, cyclophosphamide was successfully discontinued with no return in her disease as of 14 months following discontinuation.

Discussion

MMP is an autoimmune blistering disease in which antibodies are directed against proteins that are present at the dermoepidermal and/or mucosal/submucosal junction (11). Some of the proteins against which these antibodies are directed include epiligrin (also known as laminin 5 or laminin 332), BP antigen 2 (BPAg2 or collagen type XVII), alpha 6 integrin, and beta 4 integrin. Any mucous membrane surface can be involved and patients can present clinically with erosions or blisters on the gingiva, buccal and/or labial mucosa, palate, larynx, conjunctiva, esophagus, or anogenital mucosa. The major potential complication of this disease is scarring which can lead to significant morbidity, including blindness, and laryngeal, and esophageal stenosis requiring tracheostomy or gastrostomy, respectively. Scarring of the genital mucosa can lead to vaginal, anal, or urethral stenosis. Involvement of the skin may occur, most often manifested as bullae or erosions that heal with scarring on the upper body particularly on the head and neck.

The diagnosis of MMP can be made based on clinical history, physical exam, and histologic and immunofluorescence findings. Histology of the affected tissue will demonstrate a subepidermal (or submucosal) bulla with a mixed inflammatory infiltrate.

In patients who have milder disease, usually of the oral mucosa, scarring is minimal and conservative treatments, including topical therapy or systemic antiinflammatory medications, such as dapsone or tetracycline and nicotinamide, may be successful. If there is not an adequate response to these therapies in patients with milder disease, the decision to treat with more aggressive agents should be one that is made jointly with the patient after a thorough discussion of the potential side effects of the therapies as serious sequelae from the disease are unlikely to develop. In patients with more severe disease involving the eyes, larynx, or esophagus where the potential morbidity of scarring is significant combination therapy with systemic prednisone and cyclophosphamide is recommended (9). The enlistment of specialists such as ophthalmologists, gastroenterologists, and otolaryngologists to help monitor and manage the sequelae of scarring is essential. Once disease improves, the prednisone can be slowly tapered while the cyclophosphamide can be continued for another 6–12 months to achieve disease remission. IVIg and etanercept have been reported to be successful in some patients, but the responses do not seem to be as consistent as therapy with prednisone/cyclophosphamide combination therapy. Rituximab, an anti-CD20 chimeric antibody, holds promise as a therapy for MMP given its effectiveness in other immunobullous diseases, but reports of successful therapy at this time are limited (12, 13).

A specific subset of MMP patients, those with antibodies directed against epiligrin (laminin 5 or laminin 332), have been reported to be at risk for internal malignancy. In a study that examined 35 patients with antiepiligrin MMP, ten patients developed a solid organ malignancy (8). Unfortunately, tests which can identify the presence of antiepiligrin antibodies are not widely available.

Patients with MMP can present with a variety of clinical and immunologic findings. Therapy needs to be based on the severity of their disease and the willingness of the patient to accept risks associated with therapy. Aggressive therapy is indicated in patients with scarring of the eyes, larynx, or esophagus to prevent the development of long-term complications that may occur. Knowledge and experience with these aggressive therapies is essential for the best outcomes in these challenging cases.

Questions

1. All of the following tests are used to detect circulating antibodies EXCEPT:
    (a) Indirect immunofluorescence
    (b) Direct immunofluorescence
    (c) Immunoprecipitation
    (d) Western blot

2. Antibodies in patients with pemphigus vulgaris are directed against:

    (a) Desmogleins
    (b) Desmoplakin
    (c) Plakoglobin
    (d) Plakophilin

3. The first-line therapy in patients with pemphigus vulgaris is:

    (a) Topical corticosteroids
    (b) Systemic corticosteroids
    (c) Dapsone
    (d) Tetracycline

4. In pemphigus patients, the histologic finding that raises concern for paraneoplastic pemphigus is:

    (a) Subepidermal bullae
    (b) Vasculitis
    (c) Parakeratosis
    (d) Lichenoid infiltrate

5. In adults, the most common malignancy associated with paraneoplastic pemphigus is:

    (a) Castleman's tumor
    (b) Thymoma
    (c) Retroperitoneal sarcoma
    (d) Non-Hodgkins Lymphoma

6. The differential for desquamative gingivitis includes all of the following EXCEPT:

    (a) Eosinophilic granuloma
    (b) Pemphigus vulgaris
    (c) Mucous membrane pemphigoid
    (d) Lichen planus

7. In mucous membrane pemphigoid, antibodies to which of the following antigens is associated with a higher risk of internal malignancy?

    (a) Epiligrin
    (b) Type VII collagen
    (c) Plectin
    (d) Type XVII collagen

8. In scarring mucous membrane pemphigoid of the conjunctiva, which therapy is most appropriate?

    (a) Dapsone
    (b) Systemic corticosteroids plus cyclophosphamide

(c) Topical corticosteroids
(d) Tetracycline plus nicotinamide

9. Rituximab is a chimeric antibody that binds to which of the following proteins?

   (a) CD4
   (b) CD52
   (c) CD8
   (d) CD20

10. Serious sequelae that can develop in scarring mucous membrane pemphigoid include all of the following EXCEPT:

    (a) Corneal ulceration
    (b) Esophangeal stenosis
    (c) Intestinal stenosis
    (d) Laryngeal stenosis

Answer key: 1(b), 2(a), 3(b), 4(d), 5(d), 6(a), 7(a), 8(b), 9(d), 10(c).

References

1. Lin MS, Mascaró JM Jr, Liu Z, España A, Diaz LA. The desmosome and hemidesmosome in cutaneous autoimmunity. *Clin Exp Immunol.* 1997;107(Suppl 1):9–15.
2. Stanley J. "Pemphigus." Fitzpatrick's Dermatology in General Medicine. Ed. Wolff K et al. 7th ed. New York: McGraw-Hill, 2008.
3. Mimouni D, Anhalt G. Pemphigus. *Derm Ther.* 2002;15(4):362–8.
4. Anhalt GJ, Kim SC, Stanley JR, Korman NJ, Jabs DA, Kory M et al. Paraneoplastic pemphigus. An autoimmune mucocutaneous disease associated with neoplasia. *N Engl J Med.* 1990;323:1729–35.
5. Cummins DL, Mimouni D, Tzu J, Owens N, Anhalt GJ, Meyerle JH. Lichenoid paraneoplastic pemphigus in the absence of detectable antibodies. *J Am Acad Dermatol.* 2007;56(1):153–9.
6. Lo Russo L, Fierro G, Guiglia R, Compilato D, Testa NF, Lo Muzio L, Campisi G. Epidemiology of desquamative gingivitis: evaluation of 125 patients and review of the literature. *Int J Dermatol.* 2009;48(10):1049–52.
7. Woodley DT, Remington J, Chen M. Autoimmunity to type VII collagen: epidermolysis bullosa acquisita. *Clin Rev Allergy Immunol.* 2007;33(1–2):78–84.
8. Egan CA, Lazarova Z, Darling TN et al. Anti-epiligrin cicatricial pemphigoid and relative risk for cancer. *Lancet.* 2001;357(9271):1850–1.
9. Chan LS, Ahmed AR, Anhalt GJ et al. The first international consensus on mucous membrane pemphigoid: definition, diagnostic criteria, pathogenic factors, medical treatment, and prognostic indicators. *Arch Dermatol.* 2002;138(3):370–9.
10. Canizares MJ, Smith DI, Conners MS, Maverick KJ, Heffernan MP. Successful treatment of mucous membrane pemphigoid with etanercept in 3 patients. *Arch Dermatol.* 2006;142(11):1457–61.
11. Yancey K. "Cicatricial Pemphigoid." Fitzpatrick's Dermatology in General Medicine. Ed. Wolff K et al. 7th ed. New York: McGraw-Hill, 2008.
12. Schumann T, Schmidt E, Booken N, Goerdt S, Goebeler M. Successful treatment of mucous membrane pemphigoid with the anti-CD-20 antibody rituximab. *Acta Derm Venereol.* 2009;89(1):101–2.
13. Ross AH, Jaycock P, Cook SD, Dick AD, Tole DM. The use of rituximab in refractory mucous membrane pemphigoid with severe ocular involvement. *Br J Ophthalmol.* 2009;93(4):421–2, 548.

Chapter 20
Alopecia Areata*

Luciano J. Iorizzo III and Mary Gail Mercurio

Abstract Alopecia areata is a disease characterized by nonscarring alopecia, generally in circular patterns on the scalp. The disease appears to be caused by autoimmune attack on hair follicles mediated by T cells. Here, we present two cases of alopecia areata, one that responded quite well to treatment and another that was quite refractory.

Keywords Alopecia areata • Alopecia totalis • Alopecia universalis • Exclamation point hairs

Case 1

Case Presentation

A 65-year-old Caucasian female presented to the office with hair loss of approximately 4 months duration. She started noticing excessive hair fall when she brushed her hair and reported it was generalized to her entire scalp. She denied any pain or pruritus and denied pulling at her hair. Neither did the patient have a prior history of hair loss, nor did any members of her family.

The patient's past medical history was significant for anxiety and depression, type 2 diabetes, heart disease status post a stent placement 10 years earlier, hyperlipidemia, hypertension, and asthma. Her medications at presentation included glipizide, paroxetine, lisinopril, diltiazem, simvastatin, aspirin, gabapentin, and clonazepam. The patient otherwise felt well and was in her usual state of health. Her family and social histories were unremarkable.

---

* All treatments discussed in the chapter are off-label.

L.J. Iorizzo III (✉)
Department of Dermatology, University of Rochester, Rochester, NY, USA
e-mail: Luciano_Iorizzo@URMC.Rochester.edu

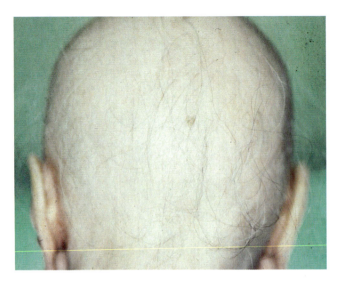

Fig. 20.1 The patient's presentation 1 month after initial presentation showing diffuse loss of scalp hair (alopecia totalis)

On initial physical exam, the patient had several 1–3 cm circular patches of nonscarring alopecia on the vertex of her scalp. Within 3 weeks, she lost all hair on her scalp with the exception of a few strands (Fig. 20.1). The remainder of the physical exam showed no hair loss of the eyebrows or eyelashes, and her nails were normal.

With the Presented Data What Is Your Working Diagnosis?

The patient is a 65-year-old woman who had no history of hair loss in the past. Given the clinical picture and history, the patient had alopecia areata, totalis type.

Differential Diagnosis

Alopecia areata is generally a relatively straightforward diagnosis to make based on history and physical exam. In this particular patient with a history of anxiety and depression, trichotillomania should be considered. However, in trichotillomania we usually see irregular-shaped patches of alopecia with hairs of different lengths from breaking, and our patient had quite regular, discrete patches of alopecia before total loss. Also included in the differential diagnosis is tinea capitis; however, our patient had no evidence of scale or crust on the scalp. Medications can cause a telogen effluvium, but this does not begin as discrete patches of hair loss or progress to the extent seen in this case.

Work-Up

TSH was within normal limits.

What Is Your Diagnosis and Why?

This patient had a history and physical exam consistent with alopecia areata as she had very discrete, circular patches of alopecia appearing suddenly. Anytime a clinician sees very discrete patches of alopecia, alopecia areata should be strongly considered as the diagnosis. At the patient's initial visit, triamcinolone 10 mg/mL was injected into patches of alopecia on the patient's scalp. The patient returned to our clinic 1 month later with progression of her disease with almost complete hair loss on the scalp (Fig. 20.1). She had a positive hair pull test for the few hairs that remained. Because of the extreme hair loss, the patient was started on systemic therapy with prednisone at 50 mg a day. During the course of the patient's treatment, she started to regrow hair (Fig. 20.2), and over the course of a 4-month prednisone taper, the patient had almost complete regrowth of hair (Fig. 20.3). As the next case demonstrates, some patients have little to no response to alopecia areata treatments.

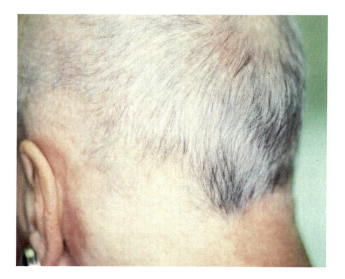

Fig. 20.2 The patient 2 months after beginning treatment with prednisone showing significant hair regrowth

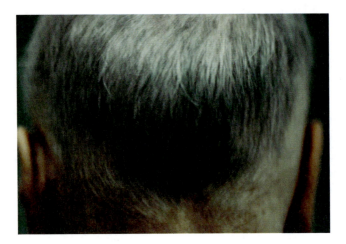

Fig. 20.3 The patient 4 months after beginning treatment with prednisone showing almost complete hair regrowth

Case 2

Case Presentation

A 37-year-old Caucasian female was referred to our office for management of hair loss. The patient had been diagnosed with alopecia areata 8 years ago when she had an approximately 3-cm patch of alopecia on her scalp. The area was injected with intralesional corticosteroids and grew back without any complications. She had no hair loss for several years until 5 months prior to presenting to our office. At that point in time, the hair loss was far more extensive on the crown of the patient's scalp. Prior to presentation to our clinic, she had treatment with intralesional corticosteroids; however, she had no regrowth. Upon presentation to our office, the patient noted additional hair loss on a daily basis. She had no changes in her medications and no new stressors in her life.

The patient's past medical history was significant for a previous case of alopecia areata, hypothyroidism, a basal cell carcinoma on her back, and a spinal fusion. Her medications included levothyroxine and a multivitamin. She took no herbal or other supplements. Her family history was significant for autoimmune diseases including systemic lupus erythematosus and pernicious anemia. On the review of systems, the patient was feeling more tired than usual. Her social history was noncontributory.

Physical examination revealed a circular patch of alopecia on the crown of the scalp measuring in its largest dimensions 16 × 12 cm (Fig. 20.4). A hair pull test was positive around the entire periphery of the patch. There was also a much smaller circular patch of alopecia on the midline frontal scalp measuring 1.5 cm. The rest of the exam was noncontributory with no hair loss of the eyebrows or eyelashes.

20 Alopecia Areata 327

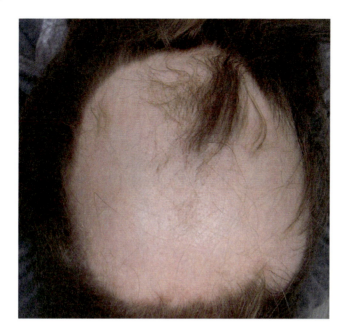

Fig. 20.4 The patient 3 months after initial presentation to our clinic after multiple ineffective therapies showing significant hair loss

Data

Thyroid stimulating hormone was 58.46 uIU/mL 3 months prior to presenting to our clinic and 1.45 uIU/mL 3 weeks after presenting to our clinic (reference range: 0.35–5.50).

With the Presented Data What Is Your Working Diagnosis?

The patient is a 37-year-old woman who had a prior history of alopecia areata and hypothyroidism and was manifesting symptoms and laboratory data suggestive of hypothyroidism at her initial presentation to us. Given the clinical picture and history, the patient had alopecia areata. She had been treated with intralesional corticosteroids prior to presenting to our clinic without any effect. Unfortunately, this is not an uncommon occurrence with alopecia areata.

Differential Diagnosis

As was previously noted, alopecia areata is usually a straightforward diagnosis based on history and physical exam. In this patient, who had alopecia areata previously, we were certain of the diagnosis. However, other things to consider again are trichotillomania, but our patient did not have any significant stress prior to her hair loss and she has no psychiatric history. Extensive hair loss like that seen in our patient could be androgenic; however, that would not usually happen so quickly and in this pattern in a female. Hair loss can also be seen in syphilis, but we had no history to lead us to this direction. Additional disease to consider could once again be tinea capitis or a telogen effluvium.

Work-Up

No additional work-up was needed in this case.

What Is Your Diagnosis and Why?

Given that the patient had a large, very well-circumscribed patch of alopecia on the scalp with a history of previous alopecia areata and hypothyroidism, she was diagnosed with alopecia areata. Although the diagnosis is relatively easy to make without confirming histologically with a biopsy, it can be quite difficult to treat, which is why this case is presented. Prior to presenting to our office, the patient had already been treated with intralesional corticosteroids without response. Because of this and her extensive involvement, we started her on prednisone 50 mg a day for 5 days followed by 40 mg a day until her follow-up appointment in 1 month. The patient returned to clinic 1 month later with additional hair loss.

As she was unresponsive to prednisone, we tapered her off the prednisone and started her on tretinoin 0.1% cream twice a day for an irritant effect, and oral methotrexate. The patient was on methotrexate orally starting at 10 mg once a week for 1 month, then 12.5 mg once a week for 1 month, and then 15 mg once a week for 2 months without an effect on her condition, so the medication was stopped. The tretinoin was stopped after about 1.5 months as the patient had no response.

One month after starting the methotrexate, the patient started narrow band ultraviolet light B (NBUVB) phototherapy. She received treatments twice a week for 8 weeks, stopped this treatment, and then started the Excimer laser (308 nm wavelength). The patient was treated with the Excimer laser about twice a week. One month into these treatments is when we stopped her methotrexate. She also started using topical minoxidil around that time. The patient had Excimer laser treatments for a total of 3 months while her hair continued to fall. At her last visit with us, the patient was considering stopping all therapies for her alopecia areata as nothing worked to help her condition. The patient was then lost to follow-up.

Discussion

Definition/Epidemiology

Alopecia areata is an autoimmune condition causing nonscarring hair loss, usually in circular areas on the scalp. It can progress to the complete loss of scalp hair (alopecia totalis) or loss of all body hair (alopecia universalis) (1). It occurs worldwide. Very few studies have been performed on the incidence and prevalence of the disease, but in the U.S. it has been reported to have a lifetime incidence of 1.7% (2), while in China the incidence was reported at 3.8% (3). The male-to-female ratio of the disease is about equal (2, 3). Alopecia areata is generally a condition of the young with one study reporting that 50.3% of patients had their first episode of the disease by age 20 and 83.8% of patients developed the condition before the fifth decade of life, with a mean age at diagnosis of 23.4 years (4). Another study found that 85.5% of patients developed alopecia areata before age 40 with the median age of diagnosis being 25.2 years (3). Safayi et al. observed no consistent trend in disease incidence with age; however, almost a third of the cases were observed at younger than 20 (2).

Presentation

Alopecia areata most frequently presents as the sudden loss of hair in one or more round or oval patches on the scalp (Fig. 20.5). The alopecia is nonscarring. At the margins of the patches, "exclamation point" hairs (hairs in which the distal end is broader than the proximal end) can be seen, but often normal hair is seen at the periphery of lesions. The disease can also present as alopecia totalis (loss of all scalp hair) and alopecia universalis (loss of all scalp and body hair) (1). Patients can lose their eyebrows and eyelashes as well (Fig. 20.6). Alopecia areata can present with only one discrete patch of hair loss and then progress to alopecia totalis (author's observation), and smaller patches can meet to form larger patches. The ophiasis pattern of hair loss presents as a band-like patch of alopecia along the posterior occipital and temporal scalp (1).

Hair pull tests (pulling the patient's hair to see if hairs can be extracted) at the periphery of lesions can positively correlate with disease activity. When and if hair regrows (see treatment), it often initially lacks pigment (1). Hair regrowth usually begins as fine white hairs within the lesion and at the periphery of patches of alopecia (author's observation).

Nail findings can be associated with alopecia areata. Nail pitting is the most common nail abnormality, which can occur in a transverse linear distribution on the nails (Fig. 20.7). Other nail findings include trachyonychia, Beau's lines, onychorrhexis, thinning or thickening, oncychomadesis, koilonychias, leukonychia, and a red, spotted lunula (1, 2).

As alopecia areata is an immune-mediated disease (see below), it has been associated with numerous autoimmune conditions. It has been associated with autoimmune

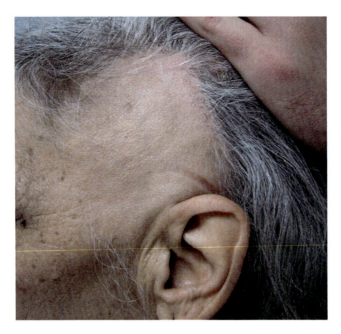

Fig. 20.5 Discrete patch of hair loss of the left temporal scalp in a patient with alopecia areata

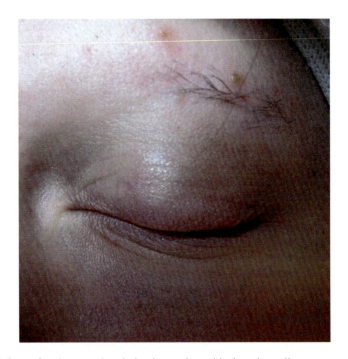

Fig. 20.6 Loss of eyebrows and eyelashes in a patient with alopecia totalis

20 Alopecia Areata

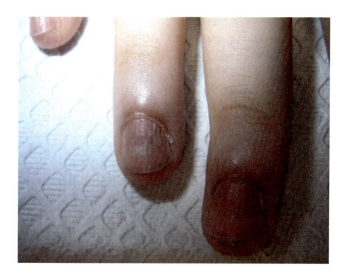

Fig. 20.7 Nail findings showing trachyonychia (longitudinal lines in the nail) in a patient with alopecia totalis

thyroid disease (a relatively common association) (Hashimoto's disease > Grave's disease), vitiligo, psoriasis, rheumatoid arthritis, ulcerative colitis, celiac disease, Sjogren's disease, autoimmune gastritis, lupus erythematosus, myasthenia gravis, and autoimmune blood diseases (1, 3, 5). Atopic dermatitis and allergic rhinitis have also been associated with alopecia areata (3, 5).

Pathophysiology/Genetics

Alopecia areata is mediated by T lymphocytes. In one study, investigators took scalp explants from patients with alopecia areata and implanted them onto SCID mice, and hair grew. Investigators were then able to induce alopecia areata in the human scalp explant on the mice by injecting activated lesional T cells from the humans. Both CD4+ and CD8+ T cells appear to be required for alopecia areata (6). There is likely a role for T cell-dependent melanocyte autoantigens in the pathogenesis of alopecia areata as well (7), and numerous cytokines have also been involved in the disease (1, 7). Although the exact pathophysiology of the disease is not known, it appears to be a TH1 autoimmune disease mediated by both CD4+ and CD8+ T cells with the autoantigen likely being associated with the melanocyte (6). (For a comprehensive review of the subject please, see references 6 and 7.)

There is certainly a genetic component to this immune response in alopecia areata. Blaumeiser et al. calculated the lifetime risk of developing the disease in an affected person's siblings, parents, and children to be 7.1, 7.8, and 5.7%, respectively. In the study, 28.1% of patients had a positive family history with a first-degree relative being affected, and 34.0% had a positive family history when second-degree relatives were included. There was no association between the severity of disease in relatives suffering from alopecia areata (4).

Also supporting the idea of a genetic component to alopecia areata is the fact that investigators have found HLA associations in the disease. A recent review article comprehensively looked at the genetics associated with alopecia areata. HLA-DQB1*03 has been seen in as many as 80% of U.S. patients with alopecia areata and it appears to be a general susceptibility gene. This link has also been seen in Turkish populations (7). Numerous additional HLA associations have also been reported (1, 6). Some HLA associations have also been proposed to be protective against alopecia areata including HLA-DRw52a and HLA-DRB1*03. MHC genes have also been implicated in alopecia areata and susceptibility loci have been found on chromosomes 6, 10, 16, and 18 (7). This evidence, along with the evidence showing family associations, shows there is a genetic component to alopecia areata.

Over the years, investigators have reported multiple disease triggers, with reports showing that biologic agents (which physicians initially thought would help in treating alopecia areata) can even trigger alopecia areata (1). However, in many cases a cause can never be identified. Psychological stress has long been considered to be a factor in the disease and patients can report stressful events before their hair loss started (3). Certainly, both genetic and environmental conditions are factors in disease development, and the disease is very likely polygenic.

Work-Up

Alopecia areata is relatively easy to diagnose based on history and physical exam. Other diagnoses to consider include trichotillomania, and if hair loss is diffuse, androgenic alopecia or telogen effluvium. However, it is usually quite easy to differentiate these conditions. One could also consider tinea capitis, secondary syphilis, or an autoimmune disease such as lupus. Occasionally, a skin biopsy is needed to diagnose the condition (Fig. 20.8). The classic histopathology findings include the presence of an inflammatory lymphocytic infiltrate in the peribulbar region ("swarm of bees"). Early on, there are an increased number of catagen and telogen follicles. In late stages there are "nanogen" hairs which represent an intermediate stage between vellus and terminal anagen hair follicles (1). If there is further doubt about the diagnosis, a fungal culture can be performed and serology for lupus and syphilis could be drawn.

As earlier noted, alopecia areata can be associated with many other autoimmune conditions. The authors think it is reasonable to order a thyroid-stimulating hormone level on newly diagnosed patients who do not already have autoimmune thyroid disease. Other diagnostic tests should be based on the patient's review of systems.

Management/Prognosis

It is unclear if any treatments for alopecia areata alter the long-term course of the disease, and evidence from randomized controlled trials shows that long-term prognosis is not affected by therapies (8). However, alopecia areata can eventually subside on its

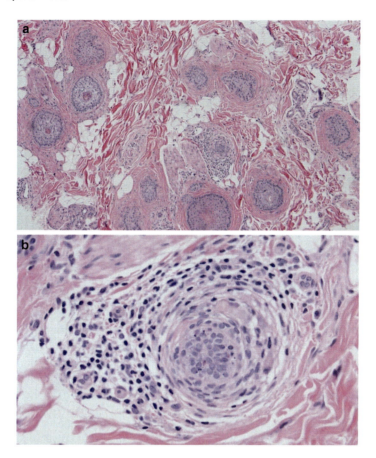

Fig. 20.8 (**a**, **b**) Histopathology of alopecia areata showing a lymphocytic inflammatory infiltrate in the peribulbar region ("swarm of bees"). Photo courtesy of Dr. Glynis Scott, University of Rochester

own and does not necessarily need to be treated. Data shows that in patients with small patches of hair loss, spontaneous remission can occur in up to 80% of patients. Additional data shows that as many as 34–50% recover hair within one year. However, in those with severe disease, <10% eventually recover and 14–25% of patients with alopecia areata can progress to alopecia totalis (9). Tosti et al. found that the more severe the initial presenting disease, the worse the prognosis, and this is the most important prognostic factor. However, in all disease severities in adults, some patients got worse and others got better (5). This gives all patients at least some hope of disease improvement, even in the most severe cases. In contrast to adults, when mild disease presented in childhood, there was a greater tendency for patients to progress toward severe disease, and the evolution of hair loss is even more difficult to predict than in adults (5).

As this disease can have a large psychological impact on patients, physicians have tried numerous treatments for alopecia areata, which shows that nothing works well all the time. There have been few randomized controlled trials that assess the efficacy of the different treatments. A Cochrane review article looked to identify randomized controlled studies on the subject (8). The article found 17 studies that met inclusion criteria. Treatments included topical corticosteroids, oral prednisolone, topical cyclosporine, psoralens with ultraviolet A light phototherapy (PUVA), intravenous thymopentin, photodynamic therapy, topical squaric acid dibutyl ester, topical minoxidil, oral inosiplex, oral imipramine, and topical latanoprost. (There are no randomized controlled studies on intralesional corticosteroids (which are one of the mainstays of treatment for alopecia areata), topical tacrolimus, systemic cyclosporine, dinitrochlorobenzene, diphencyprone, anthralin, cryotherapy, aromatherapy, antiviral agents, or other systemic immunosuppressive treatments.) None of these trials showed significant hair regrowth when compared to placebo. However, the authors were careful to point out that many of the included studies were small, and if there were an adequate number of subjects, statistically significant figures may have been obtained. Most of the studies included had a less than 6-month follow-up period, and when studies went beyond 6 months, the interventions had a poor affect on sustained hair growth. Additionally, most of the studies included heterogeneous groups of patients, so it may be possible that if there were subgroups in studies, certain patients may have responded differently.

Even though randomized controlled trials do not show that therapy has a significant effect on the disease, most patients still desire treatment. The main first-line treatment most commonly used by the authors is intralesional triamcinolone acetonide at a concentration of 10 mg/mL. Although there are no randomized controlled studies assessing the efficacy of this treatment (8), the authors have found this successful in many patients, and numerous uncontrolled trials have also found this to be successful (1, 3, 10). Initial results are usually seen in 1–2 months and injections are repeated every 4–6 weeks. This method of treatment is used for patchy hair loss, but is not generally administered for severe cases such as alopecia totalis or universalis, or rapidly progressing alopecia areata (1, 10). The most frequently encountered side effect of intralesional corticosteroid injection is atrophy of the skin and subcutaneous tissue.

Potent topical corticosteroids are one of the first-line therapies for patients with alopecia areata. Even though there is limited efficacy for their effectiveness, these remain a first-line treatment for widespread disease (1, 10). The authors start with clobetasol propionate 0.05% applied twice a day, sometimes under occlusion, when treating widespread disease. Topical tacrolimus, which is frequently used as a steroid sparing medication in atopic dermatitis, has not been shown to be beneficial in alopecia areata (1, 10), and the authors do not use this medication. Topical minoxidil, which is commonly added to topical corticosteroids, has failed to show significant regrowth in trials (10). The medication is quite safe for patients and the authors frequently encourage the use of topical minoxidil.

The authors have used systemic corticosteroids to treat severe alopecia areata as well, although it is used with caution. Systemic corticosteroids can have significant side effects, and although the authors find that many times patients do regrow hair, there is often a rebound hair loss when the corticosteroids are tapered. Data from studies agrees with the authors' findings (1, 10). In other autoimmune diseases that respond to systemic corticosteroids, steroid sparing agents are frequently added. This is the case with alopecia areata as well. Mycophenolate mofetil, methotrexate, or azathioprine could be added to a patient's prednisone and then the prednisone could be tapered, such as is done in many autoimmune diseases. This may help to decrease the relapse rate while taking someone off prednisone. The data for the efficacy of steroid sparing medications is not available, although some evidence suggests that mycophenolate mofetil is not effective (10). It is generally agreed upon that the negative side effects of cyclosporine do not usually outweigh the benefits of using the medication (1, 10).

Contact immunotherapy, which is the induction and periodic elicitation of an allergic contact dermatitis by topical application of a potent contact allergen, has been used to treat alopecia areata as well (1, 10). It is most frequently utilized when there is widespread disease and intralesional corticosteroids would not be practical. This therapy is believed to work via immunomodulation of the skin and hair at many different levels. Although there has only been a randomized controlled trial using squaric acid dibutyl ester (8), diphenylcyclopropenone (DPCP) has been frequently used for this purpose. Almost all patients have a contact allergic reaction to DPCP. Hair regrowth has ranged from 4 to 87% (1, 10). It is difficult to tell if this treatment has effective results, and the authors rarely use this treatment. Anthralin has also been used for an irritant effect, and in the largest trial of patients with alopecia areata, only 25% responded, which is not significantly higher than what would be expected from placebo (10).

Clinicians have tried PUVA as a therapy for alopecia areata. It did not show any benefits in a randomized controlled trial as noted above. Some studies show that PUVA has been up to 85% effective; however, additional studies suggest that it is no better than placebo (1, 10). We have used Excimer laser and NBUVB, but the effectiveness of these is not well tested, and in our limited experience with the Excimer laser and NBUVB for alopecia areata, we found limited efficacy.

Researchers initially thought that biologic medications would have an affect on alopecia areata. However, studies have failed to demonstrate any efficacy and they have even been shown to trigger the disease (1, 10). Given these results, biologic agents should not be used to treat alopecia areata.

Although there is not significant data to show that therapies for alopecia areata are effective in the long run, the authors believe that treatment is necessary for many patients because of the psychological impact of this disease. Treating patchy disease with intralesional corticosteroids seems to benefit many patients with resultant regrowth. For widespread disease where the use of intralesional corticosteroids is not practical, the use of topical high-potency corticosteroids with minoxidil is a reasonable alternative. After these medications, contact immunotherapy and topical irritants can be considered. Ultraviolet light treatments are then next-line treatment and in extreme cases we use systemic therapies, although their efficacy is not proven and they can have significant side effects. The choice of therapy for each patient should be evaluated on an individual basis.

Questions

1. Which of the following autoimmune diseases is most frequently associated with alopecia areata?

   (a) Systemic lupus erythematosus
   (b) Autoimmune thyroid disease
   (c) Sjogren's disease
   (d) Vitiligo
   (e) Rheumatoid arthritis

2. Which of the following is a poor prognostic factor for hair regrowth in alopecia areata?

   (a) Female sex
   (b) Smoker
   (c) Caucasian ancestry
   (d) More severe initial presenting disease
   (e) Obesity

3. Which treatment is a common first-line therapy for limited disease?

   (a) Topical tacrolimus
   (b) PUVA
   (c) Systemic corticosteroids
   (d) Contact immunotherapy with diphenylcyclopropenone
   (e) Intralesional corticosteroids

4. Which of the following is characteristic of alopecia areata?

   (a) Patients frequently pull their hair out
   (b) Patients have thinning of the hair
   (c) Patients have discrete, circular patches of hair loss
   (d) There is usually a thick scale on the scalp
   (e) It affects hairs in the telogen growth phase

5. Classic histopathology findings in alopecia areata include?

   (a) Follicular plugging
   (b) Scarring and obliteration of hair follicles
   (c) Early on, a decreased number of catagen and telogen hair follicles
   (d) The presence of an inflammatory, lymphocytic infiltrate in the peribulbar region, "swarm of bees"
   (e) Positive findings on bacterial stains

6. What is the most common nail abnormality in alopecia areata?

   (a) Thinning of the nails
   (b) A red, spotted lunula

(c) Trachyonychia
(d) Onychorrhexis
(e) Nail pitting

7. Which of the following is a commonly prescribed irritant that can induce regrowth in alopecia areata?

    (a) Anthralin
    (b) Paraben
    (c) Benzoyl peroxide
    (d) Azelaic acid
    (e) Tretinoin

8. Which of the following is a topical sensitizer used to treat alopecia areata?

    (a) Toluene blue
    (b) Paraphenylenediamine
    (c) Diphenylcyclopropenone
    (d) Octocrylene
    (e) Diethyltoluamide

9. Which of the following is the most common complication of intralesional corticosteroid injection?

    (a) Ecchymosis
    (b) Atrophy of the skin
    (c) Hypertrichosis
    (d) Acne
    (e) Infection

10. What is the most likely etiology of alopecia areata?

    (a) Autoimmune
    (b) Infection
    (c) Traumatic
    (d) Neoplastic
    (e) Metabolic

Answers: 1. (b), 2. (c), 3. (e), 4. (c), 5. (d), 6. (e), 7. (a), 8. (c), 9. (b), 10. (a).

References

1. Wasserman D, Guzman-Sanchez DA, Scott K, McMichael A. Alopecia areata. *Int. J. Dermatol.* 2007;46(2):121-131.
2. Safavi KH, Muller SA, Suman VJ, Moshell AN, Melton LJ,3rd. Incidence of alopecia areata in Olmsted County, Minnesota, 1975 through 1989. *Mayo Clin. Proc.* 1995;70(7):628-633.

3. Tan E, Tay YK, Goh CL, Chin Giam Y. The pattern and profile of alopecia areata in Singapore – a study of 219 Asians. *Int. J. Dermatol.* 2002;41(11):748-753.
4. Blaumeiser B, van der Goot I, Fimmers R, et al. Familial aggregation of alopecia areata. *J. Am. Acad. Dermatol.* 2006;54(4):627-632.
5. Tosti A, Bellavista S, Iorizzo M. Alopecia areata: a long term follow-up study of 191 patients. *J. Am. Acad. Dermatol.* 2006;55(3):438-441.
6. Hordinsky M, Ericson M. Autoimmunity: alopecia areata. *J. Investig. Dermatol. Symp. Proc.* 2004;9(1):73-78.
7. Gilhar A, Paus R, Kalish RS. Lymphocytes, neuropeptides, and genes involved in alopecia areata. *J. Clin. Invest.* 2007;117(8):2019-2027.
8. Delamere FM, Sladden MM, Dobbins HM, Leonardi-Bee J. Interventions for alopecia areata. *Cochrane Database Syst. Rev.* 2008;(2):CD004413.
9. MacDonald Hull SP, Wood ML, Hutchinson PE, Sladden M, Messenger AG, British Association of Dermatologists. Guidelines for the management of alopecia areata. *Br. J. Dermatol.* 2003;149(4):692-699.
10. Garg S, Messenger AG. Alopecia areata: evidence-based treatments. *Semin. Cutan. Med. Surg.* 2009;28(1):15-18.

Index

A
Acquired and idiopathic angioedema, 79
Acute cutaneous lupus erythematosus (ACLE), 254, 255
Allergic contact dermatitis (ACD). *See also* Rubber allergies
  armpit rash, 169–171
  chronic rash, 172–173
  definition, 173
  diagnostic patch testing, 174, 175
  fragrance allergen series, 176–177
  fragrance mix I and II, 175, 176
  ICDRG scale, 175
  pathophysiology, 174
  preservative
    2, 5-diazolidinylurea, 134–135
    formaldehyde, 131–133
    imidazolidinyl urea, 134
    MCI/MI, 135
    MDNG/phenoxyethanol, 135
    parabens, 135–136
    quaternium-15, 133–134
    standard series patch test, 131
  prevalence, 173–174
  red and splotchy rash, 171–172
Alopecia areata
  definition, 329
  epidemiology, 329
  hair loss
    differential diagnosis, 324–328
    hypothyroidism, 327
    medical history and medications, 323, 326
    physical examination, 324, 326, 327
  hair pull tests, 329
  histopathology, 332, 333
  immune-mediated disease, 329, 331
  management/prognosis, 332–335
  nail findings, 329, 330
  pathophysiology/genetics, 331–332
Alopecia totalis, 329, 330
Alopecia universalis, 329
American Contact Dermatitis Society, 156
Amoxicillin, 27
Angioedema
  ACE, 68
  acute and chronic angioedema, 67
  definition, 12
  differential diagnosis, 67
  Hageman factor (XIIa), 68
  idiopathic angioedema (*see* Idiopathic angioedema)
  INH deficiency, 68
  laboratory findings, 68–69
  management, 69–70
  mechanisms, 67
  vasoactive substance, 68
  without wheals, 18
Angiotensin converting enzyme (ACE)
  angioedema, 68
  HAE, 81
  laryngeal edema, 79
Antigen presenting cells (APCs), 158, 174
Antihistamines, 21–22
Aquagenic urticaria, 17
Asthma
  clinical presentation, 25
  diagnosis, 27
  differential diagnosis, 26
  follow up, 27–28
  physical examination, 26
  treatment, 25–26
  urticaria and angioedema, 26
  work-up, 27

Atopic dermatitis
    in adult, 193
    in childhood, 192
    diagnosis, 195
    eczema
        differential diagnosis, 187–188
        impetiginized lesions, 188–189
        management and follow-up, 190–191
        medical and social history, 187
        physical examination, 187–191
        review of systems, 187
        seborrheic dermatitis, 190
        subacute spongiotic dermatitis, 189
    genetics, 193–194
    histology, 193
    immunology, 194–195
    prevalence, 192
    rash
        autoimmune disease elimination, 186
        differential diagnosis, 185
        impetiginized lesions, 186
        management and follow-up, 186–187
        medical and surgical history, 183
        physical examination, 184, 185
        review of systems, 183
    risk factors, 192
    treatment
        antibiotics, 197
        calcineurin inhibitors, 197–198
        corticosteroids and antihistamines, 197
        HEPA filter, 196
        immunosuppressants, 198
        phototherapy, 197
        Staphylococcus aureus, 196
        topical corticosteroids, 196–197
Autoimmune blistering diseases, skin and mucous membranes
    desquamative gingivitis
        BP, 314, 315
        bullous lupus erythematosus, 314
        differential diagnosis, 312–313
        direct immunofluorescence, 313–314
        EBA, 314–316
        medical history and medications, 312
        MMP, 314, 316–317
        ocular findings, 317–318
        physical examination, 312
        treatment measures, 317
    lichenoid dermatitis (*see* Lichenoid dermatitis)
Autoimmune progesterone dermatitis, 19
Azathioprine, 198

B
Blue jean (nickel) ACD, 154
Bullous lupus, 256, 314
Bullous pemphigoid, 314, 315

C
Calcineurin inhibitors, 165
Candida albicans. See Recurrent vaginal candidiasis
C1 esterase inhibitor
    facial and throat swelling, 62, 63
    HAE, 14, 19
    recurrent angioedema, 66
Chronic cutaneous lupus erythematosus (CCLE), 254, 263
Chronic dorsal foot eczema, 142–143
Chronic idiopathic angioedema, 69
Churg–Strauss syndrome, 226–228
C1-INH. *See* Complement 1 inhibitor
Clavulanic acid, 27
Cobalt allergy, 13–14
Cold stimulation time test (CSTT), 39
Cold urticaria
    asthma, 25–28
    primary acquired (*see* Primary acquired cold urticaria)
    syncopal and near-syncopal, 28–31
Complement 1 inhibitor (C1-INH), 76
Complement 4 (C4) level, 76
Complete blood count (CBC)
    femoral medial condyle, nail gun, 116
    rashes, 186
    urticaria treatment, 22
Comprehensive metabolic panel (CMP), 186
Contact urticaria syndrome (CUS)
    atopic dermatitis, 47–48
    causative agent, 55–56
    chamber and chamber prick test, 54
    ICU, 51
    IgE–allergen interaction, 17
    medical history, 48–49
    NICU
        epoxy (epoxid) resins, 51, 52
        vs. ICU, 52, 53
        prostaglandin metabolism inhibition, 52
        substances, 51
    nonallergic IgE–independent group, 17
    open test, 54
    prevalence, 49–51
    radioallergosorbent test (RAST), 55
    staging, 53, 54
    tachyphylaxis, 55
    treatment-resistant hand eczema, 45–47
    use test, 54–55

Index

Corticosteroids
  ACD treatment, 149, 165
  chronic dorsal foot eczema, 142
Crohn's disease, 76
Cryopyrin, 33
CUS. *See* Contact urticaria syndrome
Cutaneous lupus
  bullous lupus, 256
  classification, 254, 256
  clinical presentation, 256–257
  DH, 256
  histologic features, 255
  pruritic rash
    complete blood count and punch biopsies, 260, 261
    diagnosis, 258–260
    skin examination, 259–260
  SCLE, 262–264
  SLE (*see* Systemic lupus erythematosus)
  TEN-like ACLE, 257
Cutaneous lymphocyte-associated antigen (CLA), 194
Cutaneous mastocytosis
  anaphylaxis, 247
  Darier's sign
    differential diagnosis, 239
    mast cell aggregation, 240
    physical examination, 238–239
    pruritic lesions, 237
    skin biopsy, 239
  diagnostic evaluation, 246–247
  histopathological analysis, 246
  intramuscular epinephrine
    allergic reactions, 241
    IgE-mediated anaphylactic reaction, 242–243
    medical and family history, 240
    physical examination, 241
    skin biopsy, 241–242
  mediator release, symptoms, 244
  medical treatment, 247
  non-IgE-mediated mechanisms, 245–246
  physical examination, 246
  prognosis, 248
  serum tryptase, 246
  telangiectasia macularis eruptiva perstans, 244, 245
  transmembrane tyrosine kinase receptor, KIT, 243
Cutaneous small-vessel vasculitis, 230–231
Cyclo-oxygenase 1(COX 1), 68
Cyclooxygenase-2 inhibitor valdecoxib, 95
Cyclosporin, 191, 198
Cyproheptadine, 40
Cytomegalovirus (CMV), 202

D
Darier's sign
  differential diagnosis, 239
  mast cell aggregation, 240
  physical examination, 238–239
  pruritic lesions, 237
  skin biopsy, 239
Delayed pressure urticaria, 16
Dermatitis herpetiformis (DH), 256
Dermatomyositis (DM), 290–291
Diffuse cutaneous systemic sclerosis (DcSSc), 292
Dimethyglyoxime (DMG)
  nickel-containing metal alloys, 164–165
  peri-umbilical dermatitis, 154, 155
Diphenylcyclopropenone (DPCP), 335
Doxepin, 21, 40
Duodenal ischemia, 76
Duodenal lymphoma/adenocarcinoma, 76

E
EACA. *See* Epsilon-aminocaproic acid
Eczema. *See* Atopic dermatitis
Edematous and erythematous lesions
  autoimmune progesterone dermatitis, 11
  chronic urticaria and angioedema, 9
  clinical presentation, 7
  differential diagnosis, 10
  management and follow-up, 11
  patient history, 10
  physical examination, 8–10
EIA. *See* Exercise-induced anaphylaxis
Enzyme-linked immunosorbent assays (ELISA), 218, 231
Epidermolysis bullosa acquisita, 314, 315
Epidermolysis bullosa acquisita (EBA), 256
Epigastric pain
  allergy service assessment, 76
  bowel syndrome, 73
  C4 level and C1-INH, 76
  diagnosis, 77
  medical and family history, 74
  pancreatitis, 76
  physical examination, 74–75
  PUD, 75–76
Epsilon-aminocaproic acid (EACA), 85
Erythema. *See* Toxic epidermal necrolysis
Erythema multiforme, 106–108, 115, 117
Erythrodermic psoriasis, 274

Excited skin syndrome (ESS), 173, 175
Exercise-induced anaphylaxis (EIA), 17

F
Familial atypical cold urticaria (FACU), 32–33
Familial cold auto-inflammatory syndrome (FCAS), 32–33
Familial delayed cold urticaria, 32–33
Filaggrin (FLG) gene, 194

G
Ganser syndrome, 223
Gastric antral vascular ectasia (GAVE), 289–290
Gold allergy, 160
Guillain-Barre syndrome, 222
Guttate psoriasis, 274–275

H
HAE. *See* Hereditary angioedema
Hair loss. *See* Alopecia areata
Heat urticaria, 16
Henoch-Schonlein purpura, 114
Hereditary angioedema (HAE)
   abdominal exacerbations, 83
   C1 esterase inhibitor, 14, 19
   epigastric pain (*see* Epigastric pain)
   erythema marginatum, 83
   facial and throat swelling, 63
   gastrointestinal tract, 81–82
   laryngeal edema, 77–80
   management and treatment
      danazol androgen and EACA, 85
      ecallantide (DX-88), 86
      fresh frozen plasma, 85
      Rhucin, 85
      short-and long-term prophylaxis, 84–85
   pathophysiology, 83
   recurrent cramping/colicky abdominal pain, 83
   subcutaneous/submucosal swelling, 80
   type I, II & III, 80
Hereditary C1 inhibitor (INH), 68
Herpes simplex virus (HSV), 202
Hevea brasiliensis, 143
High efficiency particulate air (HEPA) filter, 196
Histocompatibility Complex Type II Receptor (MHC II), 136
Human papilloma virus (HPV), 202
Human seminal plasma (HSP), 205–207
Hypothyroidism, 326–328

I
ICDRG. *See* International Contact Dermatitis Research Group
ICU. *See* Immunologic contact urticaria
Idiopathic angioedema
   facial and throat swelling
      acquired angioedema, 63–64
      C1 esterase inhibitor, 62, 63
      diagnostic testing, 60–62
      differential diagnosis, 62
      food allergy, 63
      HAE, 63
      IM epinephrine, 59–60
      medical history, 60
      medication induced angioedema, 63
      physical examination and medications, 60
      review of system, 60
      treatment planning, 61
   recurrent angioedema
      acquired angioedema, 66
      comprehensive laboratory evaluation, 66
      differential diagnosis and testing, 65
      doxepin, 64
      drug allergy, 64
      HAE type III, 66
      medical history, 64
      medication induced angioedema, 66–67
      physical examination, 65
      review of system, 64
      treatment planning, 65
      TSH, 66
IGDA. *See* Interstitial granulomatous dermatitis with arthritis
IgE receptors, 14, 68
IgE-specific enzyme-linked immunosorbent assay, 204
IL-17 cytokine, 159
Immediate pressure urticaria, 15
Immunologic contact urticaria (ICU), 51, 148
Interferon-gamma (IFN-γ? cytokine, 160, 194
International Contact Dermatitis Research Group (ICDRG)
   armpit rash, 170
   atopic dermatitis, 48
   chronic rash, 172
   dermatitis, 155
   patch test scoring, 175
   red and splotchy rash, 171
   treatment-resistant hand eczema, 46
Interstitial granulomatous dermatitis with arthritis (IGDA), 233–234
Intracellular adhesion molecule 1 (ICAM-1), 100
Inverse psoriasis, 276

K
Ketotifen, 40

L
Langerhan cells (LCs), 158–159, 174
Laryngeal edema
  ACE inhibitors, 79
  differential diagnosis, 78–80
  food allergy, 79
  hypothyroidism, 79
  ibuprofen, 77
  penicillin allergy, 77
  physical examination, 77–78
Leukocytoclasis, 254
Lichenoid dermatitis
  allergic contact dermatitis, 304
  bullous pemphigoid, 305
  erythema multiforme, 304–305
  IgG deposition, 306, 307
  medical and family history, 303
  medical treatment, 306–309
  paraneoplastic pemphigus (see Pemphigus)
  pemphigus vulgaris, 305
  physical examination, 304
  review of systems, 304
  skin biopsies, 305–306
  Stevens–Johnson syndrome, 305
  suprabasilar acantholysis, 306
Lymphocytes and eosinophils, 105

M
Methylchloroisothiazolinone/methylisothiazolinone (MCI/MI), 135
Methyldibromoglutaronitrile (MDNG)/phenoxyethanol, 135
MMP. See Mucous membrane pemphigoid
Muckle–Wells syndrome (MWS), 18
Mucosal surface allergy
  HSP hypersensitivity
    clinical evaluation, 203
    definition, 205
    differential diagnosis, 202
    ELISA inhibition, 204
    gel filtration chromatography, 203–204
    HPV DNA probe, 202
    IgE-mediated response, 206
    immunotherapy, 207
    SDS-PAGE, 205
    skin prick and serologic test, 206
    symptoms, 201–202, 205
  recurrent vaginal candidiasis (see Recurrent vaginal candidiasis)

Mucous membrane pemphigoid (MMP)
  diagnosis, 319
  vs. EBA, 316
  epiligrin, 318, 319
  mucosal–submucosal junction, 314
  ocular findings, 317
  patient management, 316
  treatment measures, 317
MWS. See Muckle–Wells syndrome

N
NACDRG. See North American Contact Dermatitis Research Group
Necrotizing sialometaplasia, 224–225
Nephrogenic systemic fibrosis (NSF), 290
Nickel and metal-based allergic contact dermatitis
  clinical presentation, 161–162
  cobalt, 160–161
  dermatitis, 154–155
  diagnosis and treatment
    calcineurin inhibitors, 165
    DMG test, 164
    NACDRG standard patch series, 162–164
    non-chelating barrier creams, 165
  European Union (EU), 157
  gold, 160
  immunology and pathophysiology, 158–159
  palladium, 161
  patient factors impact, 157
  peri-umbilical dermatitis (eczema), 153–154
  positive patch test, 156
  transitional metals, 156
Nifedipine, 22
Nonimmunologic contact urticaria (NICU)
  epoxy (epoxid) resins, 51, 52
  vs. ICU, 52, 53
  prostaglandin metabolism inhibition, 52
  substances, 51
Non-steroidal anti-inflammatory drugs (NSAIDs), 79
North American Contact Dermatitis Research Group (NACDRG), 142, 143
  armpit rash, 170
  atomic dermatitis, 48
  chronic rash, 171
  dermatitis, 155
  formaldehyde, 131
  MCI/MI and MDNG/phenoxyethanol, 135
  parabens, 136
  patch test, 162–164
  quaternium-17, 133

North American Contact Dermatitis Research Group (NACDRG) (*cont.*)
  red and splotchy rash, 171
  treatment-resistant hand eczema, 46

O
Oral antihistamines, 46, 149
Oral contraceptive pills (OCP), 11
Ordinary urticaria, 14–15

P
Palisaded neutrophilic and granulomatous dermatitis (PNGD), 233
Papulo-vesiculation, 161
Paraben paradox, 136
Parakeratosis, 193
Pemphigus
  desmogleins, 310
  diagnosis, 310
  paraneoplastic pemphigus
    chronic lymphocytic leukemia, 311
    computed tomography scan, 308
    murine bladder epithelium, 308, 310
    non-Hodgkins lymphoma, 311
    suprabasilar acantholysis, 307
    tissue bound antibodies, 310
Peptic ulcer disease (PUD), 75–76
Phenytoin (dilantin), 187
Physical urticaria. *See also* Cold urticaria
  challenge test, 20
  cholinergic urticaria, 15
  delayed pressure urticaria, 16
  dermographism, 15
  heat urticaria, 16
Pimecrolimus, 183, 187
Preservatives
  chronic recurrent dermatitis, 127–128
  cosmetic ingredient review, 130
  definition, 130
  diagnostic procedures, 136–137
  intermittent hand eczema, 129–130
  pathophysiology, 136
  types
    2, 5-diazolidinylurea, 134–135
    formaldehyde, 131–133
    imidazolidinyl urea, 134
    MCI/MI, 135
    MDNG/phenoxyethanol, 135
    parabens, 135–136
    quaternium-15, 133–134
  United States Food and Drug Administration (FDA), 130

Primary acquired cold urticaria (ACU)
  clinical manifestations, 34
  definition, 31
  differential diagnosis, 32–33
  history and physical examination
    cold stimulation time test (CSTT), 39
    signs and symptoms, 38–39
  pathophysiology, 34
  treatment
    aquatic activities, 40–41
    cyproheptadine and doxepin, 40
    steroid, 41
Prostate specific antigen (PSA), 203, 205
Provocative use testing (PUT), 171
Pruritic urticarial papules and plaques of pregnancy (PUPPP), 18–19
Pseudoephedrine, 105
Psoriasis
  Auspitz's sign, 276
  Bowen's disease, 279
  classification, 271
  comorbidities, 276–277
  differential diagnosis, 277–278
  erythrocyte sedimentation rate, 279
  erythrodermic psoriasis, 274
  guttate psoriasis, 274–275
  intermittent irritating skin patch, 267–269
  inverse psoriasis, 276
  medical treatment, 280–281
  pathophysiology
    genetics, 272–273
    molecular pathogenesis, 271–272
    type I and II, 271
  plaque psoriasis, 273–274
  psoriatic arthritis, 276
  pustular psoriasis, 275
  Reiter's syndrome, 279
  scaly and flaky skin patch, 269–270
  skin biopsy, 278
  total body examination, 278
  VDRL lab test, 280
Psoriatic arthritis, 276
Pustular psoriasis, 275

R
Rash
  allergic contact dermatitis (ACD)
    armpit, 169–171
    chronic, 172–173
    red and splotchy, 171–172
  atopic dermatitis
    autoimmune disease elimination, 186
    differential diagnosis, 185

Index 345

impetiginized lesions, 186
management and follow-up, 186–187
medical and surgical history, 183
physical examination, 184, 185
review of systems, 183
bullous and erythematous
   clobazam, 99
   cutaneous eruption, 97
   cytotoxic T lymphocytes, 100
   epidermal necrosis, 98–99
   immunological mechanism, 100
   photo-Koebner phenomenon, 99
   physical examination, 97
complete blood count (CBC), 186
pruritic
   complete blood count and punch biopsies, 260, 261
   diagnosis, 258–260
   skin examination, 259–260
Raynaud's phenomenon (RP)
DcSSc, 292
diagnostic testing, 288
differential diagnosis
   chronic graft *vs.* host disease, 292
   DM, 290–291
   NSF, 290
   scleredema adultorum, 291–292
   systemic lupus erythematous, 290
GAVE, 289–290
physical examination, 288
social and environmental history, 288
SSc
   CREST, 293
   digital ulceration and renal involvement, 293
   Doppler echocardiography, 294
   gastrointestinal involvement, 293
   medical treatment, 294
   microchimerism, 292
   pathogenesis, 292
   pulmonary involvement, 293–294
Recurrent vaginal candidiasis
   allergen immunotherapy, 210
   antifungal agents, 208
   chronic vulvovaginal hypersensitivity, 210–212
   differential diagnosis, 209
   IgE measurement, 209
   positive KOH preps, 208
   prostaglandin E2 (PGE$_2$) inhibition, 210
   risk factors, 209
   skin prick testing, 209
   treatment response, 212
Rheumatic juvenile arthritis, 114

Riley-Day syndrome, 11
Rubber allergies
   chronic dorsal foot eczema, 142–143
   clinical manifestations, 147–148
   diagnosis and treatment, 149
   Hevea brasiliensis, 143
   IgE-mediated allergy, 144
   immunology and pathophysiology, 145–146
   latex-accelerator complex and exposure, 144
   phospholipoprotein matrix, 144
   prevalence, 144–145
   recalcitrant hand eczema, 141–142

S
Schnitzler syndrome, 19
Scleroderma
   classification and prevalence, 298, 299
   clinical presentation, 298–299
   deep tissue skin biopsy, 296–298
   definition, 298
   dermal and subcutaneous septal sclerosis, 297, 298
   differential diagnosis, 297
   histological findings, 299
   medical treatment, 300
   pathogenesis, 299–300
   physical and skin examination, 296, 297
   RP
      DcSSc, 292
      diagnostic testing, 288
      differential diagnosis, 290–292
      GAVE, 289–290
      physical examination, 288
      social and environmental history, 288
      SSc, 292–294
   symptoms, 296
Scleroderma renal crisis (SRC), 293
Seminal plasma sensitizing proteins
   ELISA inhibition, 204
   gel filtration chromatography, 203–204
   IgE-specific enzyme-linked immunosorbent assay, 204
   SDS-PAGE and western immunoblotting, 205
Serum sickness
   femoral medial condyle, nail gun characteristics, 118–119
   complete blood counts, 116, 117
   differential diagnosis, 117
   drug allergies, 116
   intravenous solu-medrol, 117
   intravenous vancomycin, 115
   medical history, 116

Serum sickness (*cont.*)
  necrotic keratinocyte, 117, 118
  physical examination, 116
  Rocephin, 115
  vasculitis, 117
 immune complex detection, 120
 management/treatment, 120, 121
 pathophysiology, 119–120
 vs. serum sickness like-reactions, 121
 symptoms, 119
 type III hypersensitivity reaction, 119
 upper respiratory infections
  augmentin (amoxicillin/clavulanate) antibiotic therapy, 111, 115
  bilateral knee joint effusion, 114
  differential diagnosis and testing, 113–114
  keflex (cephalexin), 112
  medical history and physical examination, 112
  work-up, 114
Sodium dodecyl sulphate–polyacrylamide gel electrophoresis (SDS-PAGE), 205
Solar urticaria, 17
Spina bifida/spinal dysraphism, 144, 148–149
Stevens–Johnson syndrome, 117, 252–253. *See also* Toxic epidermal necrolysis
Subacute cutaneous lupus erythematosus (SCLE), 262–264
Sulfasalazine, 22
Sweet's syndrome, 6
Syncopal and near-syncopal
 cold environment exposure, 29
 diagnosis, 31
 differential diagnosis, 30
 physical stimuli, 28–29
 symptoms, 28
 treatment, 29
 work-up, 30–31
Systemic lupus erythematosus (SLE)
 clinical data, 253
 diagnosis, 253–254
 physical examination, 253
 skin biopsy, 254, 255
 Stevens–Johnson Syndrome, 252–253
 symptoms, 251

T
Tacrolimus, 165
Targetoid lesion
 biochemical analysis, 6
 clinical presentation, 3–4
 differential diagnosis, 5
 drug dosage, 5
 management and follow-up, 6
 physical examination, 4–5
 punch biopsy, 5
Telangiectasia macularis eruptiva perstans, 244, 245
Toxic epidermal necrolysis
 bullous and erythematous rash
  clobazam, 99
  cutaneous eruption, 97
  cytotoxic T lymphocytes, 100
  epidermal necrosis, 98–99
  immunological mechanism, 100
  photo-Koebner phenomenon, 99
  physical examination, 97
 erythema
  causative agent and corticosteroids, 96
  diagnosis, 93–94
  etiologic categories, 95
  herpes virus, 96
  mucosal pseudomembrane formation, 94
  multiple keratinocyte, 95
  prognosis, 96
  satellite cell necrosis, 92
  SCORTEN, 95
  targetoid lesions, 94
  viral diseases, 95
 erythema multiforme
  diagnosis, 106–108
  varicella vaccine, 106
 maculopapular eruption, 104–105
 upper respiratory infection
  ampicillin-sulbactam, 100
  epidermolytic exotoxin, 102
  intravenous immunoglobulin therapy, 103
  keratinocyte apoptosis, 103
  laboratory evaluations, 100–102
  Nikolsky sign, 100
  SCORTEN, 102, 103
Toxic epidermal necrolysis (TEN), 256–257
Triamcinolone acetonide, 142
Type IV delayed-type hypersensitivity reaction, 174

U
Urticaria
 angioedema without wheals, 18
 autoimmune progesterone dermatitis, 19
 clinical manifestation, 14
 contact urticaria, 17
 definition, 12
 diagnostics, 19–20

Index 347

history, 12
mechanical stimuli
  aquagenic urticaria, 17
  cold urticaria, 16
  delayed pressure urticaria, 16
  dermographism, 15
  exercise-induced anaphylaxis (EIA), 17
  heat urticaria, 16
  immediate pressure urticaria, 15
  solar urticaria, 17
  vibratory angioedema, 16
Muckle–Wells syndrome, 18
ordinary urticaria, 14–15
pathophysiology, 13–14
physical urticaria, 15
PUPP, 18–19
Schnitzler syndrome, 19
treatment, 21–22
vasculitis, 18
US Food and Drug Administration, 85

V

Vasculitis
allergic rhinitis, chronic sinusitis and asthma, 226–228
arthralgias and joint swelling
  Alice in Wonderland syndrome, 219
  brain MRI, 219–220
  imaging studies, 218
  migraine, 218
cyclophosphamide, 221–222
Ganser syndrome, 223
glucocorticoids, 221
granulomatous vasculitis, 220
Guillain–Barre syndrome, 222
midline ulceration and palatal mucosa mucocele
  biopsy, 223, 224
  clinical manifestation, 225
  imaging studies, 224
  minor salivary gland tumors, 225
  necrotizing inflammatory process, 224
primary systemic vasculitides, 220, 221
pulmonary radiographic abnormalities, 220
recurrent palpable purpura and cutaneous ulcers
  biopsy, 228–229
  complete blood cell count, 228
  hemorrhagic crusts, 228
  histopathology, 229
  IgG deposits, 229–230
  immune-complex deposition, 230
  pemphigus, 230–231
renal histology characteristics, 220
Riley–Day syndrome, 222–223
skin-colored papules
  diagnosis, 232–233
  IGD, 233–234
  medical history, 231
  perivascular and interstitial infiltrate lymphocytes, 232
vessel damage mechanisms, 220, 222
Vibratory angioedema, 16

W

Wegener's granulomatosis
Alice in Wonderland syndrome, 218–219
arthralgias and joint swelling, 218
cyclophosphamide, 221–222
diagnosis, 220
glucocorticoids, 221
midline ulceration, 223
necrotizing sialometaplasia, 225
Whole seminal plasma (WSP) proteins, 204

Z

Zollinger–Ellison syndrome, 75–76